Surgery: A Case-Based Approach

Surgery: A Case-Based Approach

Editor: Amy Walker

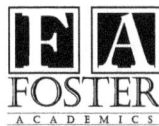

FA FOSTER
ACADEMICS

www.fosteracademics.com

www.fosteracademics.com

F A
FOSTER
ACADEMICS

Cataloging-in-Publication Data

Surgery : a case-based approach / edited by Amy Walker.
    p. cm.
Includes bibliographical references and index.
ISBN 978-1-63242-935-3
1. Surgery. 2. Surgery--Case studies. 3. Medicine. I. Walker, Amy.
RD31.5 .S87 2020
617--dc23

Foster Academics,
118-35 Queens Blvd., Suite 400,
Forest Hills, NY 11375, USA

ISBN 978-1-63242-935-3 (Hardback)

Contents

Preface

This book aims to highlight the current researches and provides a platform to further the scope of innovations in this area. This book is a product of the combined efforts of many researchers and scientists, after going through thorough studies and analysis from different parts of the world. The objective of this book is to provide the readers with the latest information of the field.

Surgery is a medical specialty which uses manual and instrumental techniques for investigating or treating a pathological condition such as disease or injury. This is done to improve bodily function and appearance, or repair unwanted ruptured areas. A surgical procedure is characterized by the use of anesthesia and surgical instruments, the maintenance of a highly sterile environment, and the act of suturing and stapling. Surgeries can be invasive or noninvasive. Laparoscopic surgery or angioplasty is a minimally-invasive surgery, while laparotomy is an open surgical procedure. Surgeries can also be classified based on their purpose, timing, body part that is excised, the type of procedure and the equipment used. Orthopedic surgery is performed on bones or muscles, while cardiac surgery is performed on the heart. Anesthesia can be local or provided as general anesthesia based on the procedure. Spinal anesthesia is administered when the surgical site is too deep or large for a local block. This book is compiled in such a manner, that it will provide in-depth knowledge about the techniques of surgery. The various studies that are constantly contributing towards advancing technologies and evolution of surgical practices are examined in detail. With state-of-the-art inputs by acclaimed experts of this field, this book targets students and professionals.

I would like to express my sincere thanks to the authors for their dedicated efforts in the completion of this book. I acknowledge the efforts of the publisher for providing constant support. Lastly, I would like to thank my family for their support in all academic endeavors.

Editor

Resolution of Uncontrolled Type 2 Diabetes after Laparoscopic Truncal Vagotomy, Subtotal Gastrectomy, and Roux-en-Y Gastrojejunostomy for a Patient with Intractable Gastric Ulcers

Laura F. Tait,[1] Gezzer Ortega,[2] Daniel D. Tran,[2] and Terrence M. Fullum[2]

[1] *Howard University College of Medicine, Washington, DC 20059, USA*
[2] *Division of Bariatric and Minimally Invasive Surgery, Howard University Hospital, Washington, DC 20060, USA*

Correspondence should be addressed to Laura F. Tait, laura.tait@bison.howard.edu

Academic Editors: D. J. Bentrem, J. M. Strzelczyk, and Y. Takami

Background. Laparoscopic Roux-en-Y gastric bypass (LRYGB) has been shown to be an effective treatment for type 2 diabetes mellitus (T2DM) in patients with morbid obesity. However, it is unclear just how effective the LRYGB procedure is on T2DM for patients with BMI less than $35 \, kg/m^2$. We report one obese patient with T2DM who did not meet the current NIH criteria for morbid obesity surgery. This patient underwent a laparoscopic truncal vagotomy, subtotal gastrectomy, and Roux-en-Y gastrojejunostomy for intractable gastric ulcers and subsequently had full resolution of her T2DM. *Methods*. A 48-year-old patient with a BMI of $34.6 \, kg/m^2$ underwent a laparoscopic truncal vagotomy, subtotal gastrectomy, and Roux-en-Y gastrojejunostomy for intractable gastric ulcers. The patient was seen 3 months preoperatively, followed for 24 months postoperatively, and evaluated for postoperative complications, weight loss, and improvement in comorbidities. *Results*. The patient had no postoperative surgical complications. Her BMI decreased from $34.6 \, kg/m^2$ to $22.3 \, kg/m^2$ by 24 months postoperatively. Significant improvements in her fasting blood glucose levels were seen 10 days postoperatively from a preoperative level of 147 mg/dl to 97 mg/dl. *Conclusion*. Patients with a BMI less than $35 \, kg/m^2$ and uncontrolled T2DM may benefit from a laparoscopic Roux-en-Y gastric bypass.

1. Introduction

Obesity is a growing epidemic and is strongly associated with an increase in the prevalence of comorbid conditions, including type 2 diabetes mellitus (T2DM), cardiovascular disease, and cancer. In the United States, the development of T2DM has been strongly linked to obesity, with 50% of T2DM patients having a BMI $>30 \, kg/m^2$ [1]. T2DM is now an epidemic, accounting for 90–95% of all cases of diabetes mellitus and affecting more than 246 million people worldwide. This number is expected to increase to 380 million people by the year 2025 [2, 3]. In the United States, the most common complications to long-standing, uncontrolled T2DM include heart disease, myocardial infarction, stroke, vision loss, renal failure, and peripheral artery disease often times resulting in amputations. While current medical therapies for T2DM can reduce the incidence of complications, they have not been effective in providing a

definitive cure [4]. Bariatric surgery has been shown to be the most effective therapy in the resolution of comorbid conditions including T2DM in obese patients [5].

The role of surgical therapy as the primary management of T2DM is promising but controversial. The mechanism of action has been studied, but there remains an unclear explanation as to what postsurgical effects are the most important in alleviating the disease [6]. Resolution of T2DM can be explained by changes in adipose tissue, leptin levels, and decreased stress on the intracellular endoplasmic reticulum by weight loss. Yet, significant improvement in glycemic control after bariatric surgery in patients with diabetes often precedes major weight loss through a weight-independent mechanism [2]. The malabsorptive surgical weight loss procedures have been proven to be the most effective in restoring euglycemia in obese patients. Roux-en-Y gastric bypass (RYGB), a common surgical weight loss procedure that is both restrictive and malabsorptive, has shown particular promise in the management of T2DM [2] by offering a potential cure.

The role of RYGB as a long-lasting and effective procedure for controlling T2DM in the morbidly obese is well defined. Currently, under the NIH guidelines, bariatric surgery is indicated when a patient's body mass index (BMI) is greater than $40 \, kg/m^2$ or greater than $35 \, kg/m^2$ with life-threatening comorbidities such as T2DM [6]. Only a few studies have investigated RYGB as being useful in the control of T2DM in the obese patient whose BMI is less than 35. Shah et al. 2009 reported the benefit of using Roux-en-Y gastric bypass (RYGB) in a prospective study involving 15 Asian Indian patients whose BMIs were less than $35 \, kg/m^2$. They achieved 80% remission of T2DM 1 month postoperatively and 100% euglycemia at 3-month followup [7]. We investigated one T2DM patient with a BMI lower than 35 who underwent a procedure very similar to a laparoscopic RYGB.

2. Case Report

The patient is a 48-year-old Caucasian female who underwent laparoscopic truncal vagotomy, subtotal gastrectomy, and Roux-en-y gastrojejunostomy for gastric and duodenal ulcers unresponsive to medication. Past medical history was significant for intractable gastric and peptic ulcer disease for 3 years, type 2 diabetes mellitus (T2DM), hypertension, hypercholesterolemia, gastritis, esophagitis, gastroparesis, and obesity. Her BMI was $34.6 \, kg/m^2$. She had a Zollinger-Ellison syndrome workup, which was negative. Her T2DM medications included Lantus 30 U once a day, Januvia 100 mg once a day, and Metformin 1000 mg twice daily. Three months prior to surgery, her HbA1c was 7.9% and fasting glucose was 147 mg/dL.

The patient underwent an uncomplicated laparoscopic truncal vagotomy, subtotal gastrectomy, and Roux-en-Y gastrojejunostomy. A subtotal gastrectomy was performed instead of an antrectomy because of her history of gastroparesis and multiple gastric ulcers. She had a small duodenal ulcer as well. Within 10 days of her bariatric procedure, rapid improvements in her fasting blood glucose levels, HbA1c, as well as her weight were noted. Her blood glucose, HbA1c, and BMI on day 10 postoperatively were 97 mg/dL, 7.2%, and $34.6 \, kg/m^2$, respectively. At her 2-month evaluation, her HbA1c had markedly improved to 6.5% and her BMI was $29.2 \, kg/m^2$. She remained off all insulin and hypoglycemic agents after her 10-day postoperative visit. Within 6 months, the patient's BMI had improved to $26.9 \, kg/m^2$ and she had a HbA1c of 6.1% (Figure 2). The only medication currently prescribed at that time was Metoprolol for her blood pressure. At one-year followup, the patient had blood glucose levels within the normal range (below 100 mg/dL) and was discharged from her endocrinologist due to resolution of her T2DM. The patient has had no further need of insulin or oral medications for blood sugar control since 10 days postoperatively, and her serum glucose values remained normal at her 18- and 24-month postoperative assessment (Figure 1).

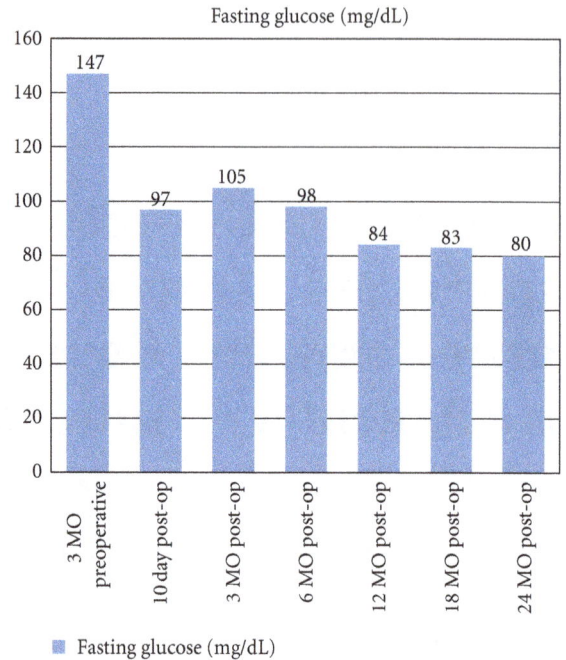

FIGURE 1: Patient's fasting glucose 3 months preoperatively through 24 months postoperatively.

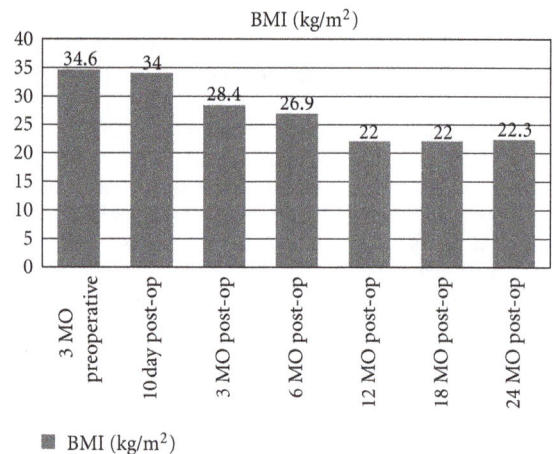

FIGURE 2: Patient's BMI 3 months preoperatively through 24 months postoperatively.

3. Discussion

Type II diabetes mellitus, a chronic and potentially fatal illness, may be improved with strict diet adherence, weight loss, and drug regimen, but optimal control or resolution of the disease is rarely achieved using these methods. Bariatric surgery has been successful in the treatment of type II diabetes mellitus. Recent studies have shown that bariatric surgery has antidiabetic effects with the normalization of serum glucose levels following bariatric surgery being measured long before any significant weight loss is observed. There is evidence that shows that greater than 80% of patients who undergo RYGB have a complete sustained

HbA1c (%)

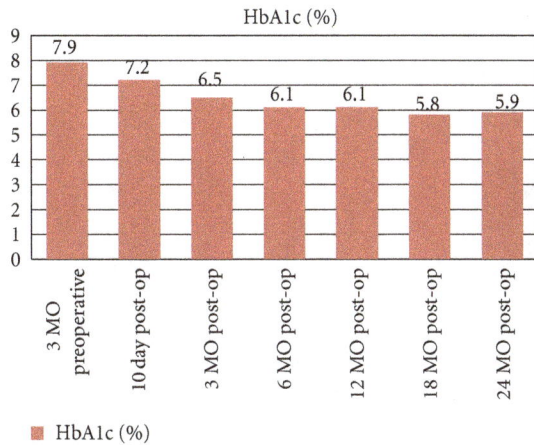

FIGURE 3: Patient's HbA1C levels 3 months preoperatively through 24 months postoperatively.

remission of their type 2 diabetes mellitus [8]. The patient in our case review had complete resolution of her T2DM within six months of her surgery and neither required oral hypoglycemic nor insulin therapy after postoperative day 10. Her HbA1c values achieved percentages of 6.1 at 6 months and 5.9 at her 2-year followup (Figure 3).

Currently, there are few reports on the laparoscopic surgical treatment of patients with T2DM and a BMI lower than 35. The first report was by DePaula et al. in 2008. In his retrospective cohort study DePaula found that "weight loss was not a reliable predictor of (T2DM) resolution or glucose control" in postgastrectomy patients. He reported 39 patients with a BMI less than 35 who underwent either a laparoscopic ileal interposition procedure associated with a sleeve gastrectomy or a laparoscopic ileal interposition procedure associated with a diverted sleeve gastrectomy. The inclusion criteria for the study specified T2DM patients whose disease had been diagnosed for at least 3 years; documentation of HbA1c exceeding 7.5% for at least 3 months; stable weight, defined as no significant change (>3%) over the 3 months before enrollment; evidence of stable treatment with oral hypoglycemic therapy or insulin for at least 12 months. All patients had a BMI less than 35 kg/m^2. In fact, the mean BMI was 30.1 kg/m^2. Of the 39 patients included in the study, 86.9% achieved adequate glycemic control defined as a HbA1c <7% during a mean follow-up period of 7 months [8]. One significant finding in this paper was that zero patients required insulin therapy postoperatively. DePaula also reported that the mean percentage of weight loss was 22% and the mean postoperative BMI was 24.9 kg/m^2. The remarkable findings of adequate glucose control, independent of weight loss, led DePaula to conclude that gastrectomy seemed to be a promising procedure for the control of T2DM.

Caloric restriction, weight loss, and hormonal as well as anatomical changes are some of the major explanations offered as possible mechanisms for improvement in glucose metabolism following surgery. However, the rapid improvement of DM after RYGB counters the argument for weight loss and caloric restriction as these methods require time to achieve proper glycemic control [2]. Instead, hormonal changes driven by anatomical rearrangement appear to be a more likely theory [3]. In T2DM, the effects of the incretin hormones, gastric inhibitory peptide (GIP) and glucagon like peptide (GLP), are impaired. GIP enhances the early phase (0–20 min) insulin response to glucose. In addition, GLP enhances both the early and late phases (20–120 min) of the response of insulin to glucose. Not only is there insulin resistance in T2DM, but there is also a loss of the early phase insulin secretion leading to persistent hyperglycemia secondary to the inability to suppress both glucagon secretion and hepatic glucose output. Other documented effects of GLP include a proliferative effect on B cells as well as delayed gastric emptying.

Following RYGB, the effects of GLP are enhanced leading to marked improvements in both glucose metabolism as well as insulin resistance [8]. This could explain why our patient had rapid glycemic improvements immediately following surgery.

4. Conclusions

Currently, the role of RYGB as a weight loss procedure in patients with at least one comorbidity is reserved for patients with a BMI of 35 kg/m^2 or greater. However, patients with uncontrolled T2DB with BMIs less than 35 should be considered for RYGB as definitive treatment of their T2DM. The NIH guidelines should be reevaluated to consider RYGB in patients with BMI <35 who have uncontrolled T2DM. More prospective studies for the use of RYGB in patients with BMI less than 35 kg/m^2 with comorbidities should be conducted using larger sample sizes with longer follow-up evaluation to include 2 years.

References

[1] G. Schernthaner and J. M. Morton, "Bariatric surgery in patients with morbid obesity and type 2 diabetes," *Diabetes Care*, vol. 31, pp. 297–302, 2008.

[2] S. Coffin, C. Konduru, M. Schwarcz, and W. Frishman, "Surgical approaches for the prevention and treatment of type 2 diabetes mellitus," *Cardiology in Review*, vol. 17, no. 6, pp. 275–279, 2009.

[3] F. Rubino, "Is type 2 diabetes an operable intestinal disease? A provocative yet reasonable hypothesis," *Diabetes Care*, vol. 31, pp. 290–296, 2008.

[4] H. E. Lebovitz, "Type 2 diabetes mellitus-current therapies and the emergence of surgical options," *Nature Reviews Endocrinology*, vol. 7, no. 7, pp. 408–419, 2011.

[5] S. Kim and W. O. Richards, "Long-term follow-up of the metabolic profiles in obese patients with type 2 diabetes mellitus after roux-en-Y gastric bypass," *Annals of Surgery*, vol. 251, no. 6, pp. 1049–1055, 2010.

[6] F. Rubino and M. Gagner, "Potential of surgery for curing type 2 diabetes mellitus," *Annals of Surgery*, vol. 236, no. 5, pp. 554–559, 2002.

[7] S. S. Shah, J. S. Todkar, P. S. Shah, and D. E. Cummings, "Diabetes remission and reduced cardiovascular risk after gastric bypass in Asian Indians with body mass index <35 kg/m^2," *Surgery for Obesity and Related Diseases*, vol. 6, pp. 332–339, 2010.

[8] A. L. DePaula, A. L. V. Macedo, N. Rassi et al., "Laparoscopic treatment of type 2 diabetes mellitus for patients with a body mass index less than 35," *Surgical Endoscopy and Other Interventional Techniques*, vol. 22, no. 3, pp. 706–716, 2008.

Primary Pneumatosis Intestinalis of Small Bowel

Daniela Berritto,[1] **Raffaello Crincoli,**[2] **Francesca Iacobellis,**[1] **Francesca Iasiello,**[1] **Nunzia Luisa Pizza,**[1] **Francesco Lassandro,**[3] **Lanfranco Musto,**[4] **and Roberto Grassi**[1]

[1] Depatment of Radiology, Second University of Naples, P.za Miraglia 2, 80138 Napoli, Italy

[2] Depatment of Radiology, Ospedale Landofi ASL, Solofra Indirizzo, Via Melito, 83029 Solofra, Italy

[3] Depatment of Radiology, Azienda ospedaliera "V. MONALDI," Via Leonardo Bianchi, 80131 Napoli, Italy

[4] Depatment of Radiology, Ospedale Criscuoli. Via Quadrivio, Sant'Angelo dei Lombardi, 83054 Avellino, Italy

Correspondence should be addressed to Daniela Berritto; berritto.daniela@gmail.com

Academic Editor: Carmela De Crea

Pneumatosis intestinalis (PI) is a condition in which multiple gas-filled cysts are located in the bowel wall; it can represent a wide spectrum of diseases and a variety of underlying diagnoses. The present report describes the case of an 86-year-old man with symptomatic primary PI of small bowel treated with surgical approach after periodic episodes of cysts rupture and superimposed inflammation revealed on the basis of a clinical suspicion thanks to abdominal computed tomography. Moreover, after one year of followup, there has been no recurrence of digestive symptoms.

1. Introduction

Pneumatosis intestinalis (PI) is a finding characterized by the presence of gas within the bowel wall [1, 2]. Two main theories have been proposed in the medical literature. A mechanical theory hypothesizes that gas dissects into the bowel wall from either the intestinal lumen or the lungs via the mediastinum due to some mechanism causing increased pressure (i.e., bowel obstruction or emphysema). A bacterial theory proposes that gas-forming bacilli enter the submucosa through mucosal rents or increased mucosal permeability and produce gas within the bowel wall [3, 4].

PI has been classified as primary (idiopathic) and secondary. Primary PI (15%) is generally nonsymptomatic and diagnosis is often occasional. This form is usually located in the colon. Males are more often affected and the age group most affected is between the fourth and sixth decades of life [5].

Secondary PI (85%) has been associated with numerous coexisting disorders of the gastrointestinal tract or the respiratory system, such as chronic obstructive pulmonary disease, intestinal obstruction, ischemic bowel disease, necrotizing enterocolitis in premature infants, immunodeficiency such as AIDS, bacterial and/or viral infection, and drug therapy [6–13]. Morphologically PI may occur in two different types: bubble-like (cysts in intestinal wall), typical of the primary type, and band-like (continuous lines), correlated with secondary PI [14, 15].

We present a rare case of idiopathic bubble like (cystoides) PI of the small bowel.

2. Case Report

An 86-year-old man was admitted to the emergency department presenting with abdominal pain, subobstructive episode, and constipation alternately to diarrhea. His previous medical history revealed a cholecystectomy.

Abdominal examination at admission revealed a diffuse distention and mild rebound tenderness. Laboratory studies revealed unremarkable serum blood count, electrolytes, and liver biochemistry.

Abdominal computed tomography (CT) without intravenous contrast demonstrated some gas-filled cysts within the small bowel wall, not associated with free intraperitoneal air. Based on the CT finding of air within the bowel wall,

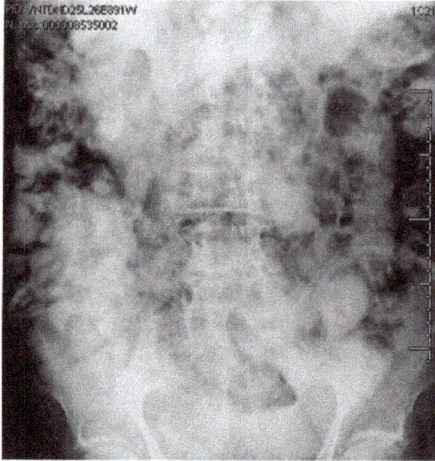

FIGURE 1: Plain abdominal film showing gas in the jejunal wall.

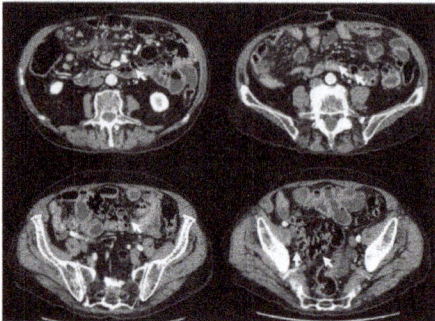

FIGURE 2: Computed tomography showing presence of gas in the intestinal wall (harrows).

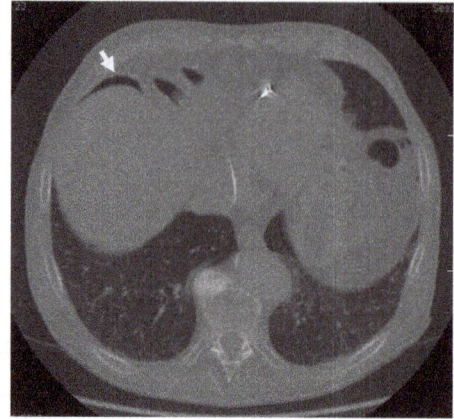

FIGURE 3: Abdominal CT scan showing free intraperitoneal air near the liver.

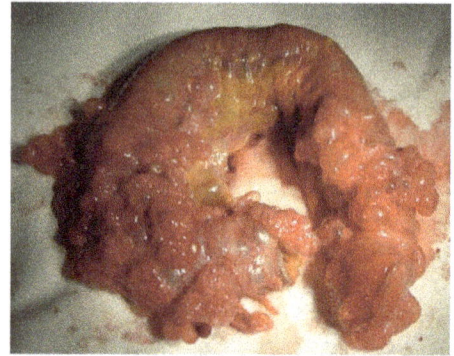

FIGURE 4: Gross appearance of the resected jejunum revealing multiple gas-filled cysts distributed within the bowel wall.

the patient was diagnosed with small bowel PI. The patient was not treated and he was discharged at his own request.

One month later, presenting with a new episode of generalized abdominal pain, the patient underwent abdominal ultrasound (US) and plain abdominal film. The latter showed a large amount of intramural gas within some small bowel loops (Figure 1); US was useless due to intestinal tympanites. Abdominal CT with intravenous contrast administration was performed further to evaluate the pneumatosis and to investigate any possible complications. The scans confirmed the presence of small gas-filled cysts arising from the wall of the jejunum and ileum (Figure 2).

The onset of subobstructive symptoms over the following first month led the patient to repeat abdominal CT examination with intravenous contrast. It demonstrated the presence of small bowel PI with intraperitoneal free air near the liver and in the mesenteric fat due to the rupture of intramural gaseous cysts into the peritoneal cavity (Figure 3). A laparotomy was performed revealing some loops adherent to the parietal peritoneum due to earlier rupture of cysts with superimposed inflammation.

The most prominent affected segment of around 50 cm in length was resected (Figure 4) and lysis of adhesions was performed followed by jejunum resection with a side to side anastomosis.

Histological study revealed cysts located within the subserosa, with giant cells around the cystic wall.

After one year of followup, the patient was still asymptomatic.

3. Discussion

PI is radiologically characterized by cystic or linear collections of gas in the subserosa or submucosa of the gastrointestinal tract [4, 16]. It is an uncommon entity which recently obtained increased attention due to improved radiographic identification.

The first description of pneumatosis cystoides intestinalis was made by Du Vernoin as a postmortem observation [17].

In most cases, PI is an incidental finding, whereas in others PI is secondary to a wide variety of gastrointestinal and nongastrointestinal diseases [18, 19].

Clinically, PI ranges from benign disease, which does not require treatment, to more severe conditions needing oxygen, intravenous hydration, and antibiotics, to a life-threatening entity requiring immediate surgery.

In cases of PI due to benign causes, especially PI associated with pulmonary disease, the patients are usually asymptomatic and often only necessitate conservative therapy. Some patients may have mild abdominal discomfort, which is usually related to the underlying associated medical condition. Physical examination is rarely abnormal unless there are peritoneal signs from intestinal perforation in cases of PI due to life-threatening causes [3, 18, 20, 21].

In our case, the persistence of symptoms, due to inflammatory adhesions subsequent to episodes of asymptomatic rupture of the cysts, has made it necessary for lysis of adhesions. Since the bubbles were limited only to the small bowel, it was possible to perform a preventive partial jejunal and ileal resection in order to prevent further acute episodes.

Endoscopy, barium enema, US, plain abdominal film, and abdominal CT can be supportive in diagnosing PI.

In our case endoscopy was not performed due to the location of cysts into the small intestine, such as for barium enema. However, regarding the latter some authors have warned that PI could be confused with intestinal polyposis on barium enema, as they have very similar appearance [2, 22–26].

US can also be used to detect PI [27–29]. This technique is more commonly applied to the pediatric patient in whom avoidance of ionizing radiation is preferred but in most cases it is hampered by the presence of tympanites, as in our case. PI seen on US has been described as linear or focal echogenic areas within the bowel wall. It can also appear as a continuous echogenic ring in the bowel wall [29–31].

Plain abdominal film can be useful in identification of PI but it is more recommended for the study of complications, such as the pneumoperitoneum that is detectable on erect chest radiography by the presence of subdiaphragmatic air or by the evidence of air pockets on supine plain abdominal film [32].

CT has greater sensitivity in diagnosing PI than plain abdominal film or US since it can distinguish PI from intraluminal air or submucosal fat [18, 22–26].

The ability to study the bowel wall in the coronal, sagittal, and axial planes may allow a more confident diagnosis of PI and portal venous gas. Because CT is more sensitive than plain abdominal film in detecting PI, it can be used to clarify ambiguous radiographic findings and also to search for potential causes. On both plain abdominal film and CT, PI usually appears as a low-density linear or bubbly pattern of gas in the bowel wall. It can be a combination of both linear and bubbly bowel-wall gas. There also may be circular collections of gas in the bowel wall. CT has also been shown to be more sensitive than plain abdominal film in detection of some complications like portal and portomesenteric gas or the presence of pneumoperitoneum detected even with 1-2 mL of free intraperitoneal air [33].

In our case, CT allowed to identify complications consisting of intraperitoneal free air near the liver and in the mesenteric fat, without signs of portomesenteric air. On CT scans we recognized a typical primary cystoids pattern characterized from segmental distribution of the radiolucent clusters along the bowel wall and cysts with a variable diameter between 5 and 30 mm and margins clearly identifiable [34] but with an uncommon small bowel localization.

CT is the most appropriate tool to localize the PI and to make differential diagnosis between primary PI and secondary PI basing on the shape of lesions.

The secondary forms usually have a different feature than idiopathic, showing a linear radiolucency within the wall of the gastrointestinal tract, parallel to the intraluminal gas. Sometimes the aspect can be fine bubble or mist [34].

Currently, there is no consensus on the appropriate management of PI. Since PI can represent a wide range of pathology, it is in itself not diagnostic of any certain condition. The variety of presentations of PI highlights the fact that clinicians should interpret radiographic findings in concert with the current clinical scenario in order to ensure a correct diagnosis and to guide one toward a suitable management. Around 50% of patients with PI can be successfully managed nonoperatively [35].

The idiopathic PI does not require surgical intervention in itself since some lesions disappear spontaneously within months or years [36], unless the breaking of bubbles occurs followed by periodic inflammatory episodes and adhesions with subobstruction as in our case.

Identification of cases in which laparotomy can be avoided, or deferred, is important in order to prevent unnecessary surgery with its associated morbidity and financial costs.

In conclusion the authors emphasize the role of TC in the localization of lesions and identification of PI pattern; the meticulous integration of the appearance on abdominal CT scan, the laboratory data, and clinical presentations permit clinicians to suspect the onset of complications and to distinguish benign from life-threatening PI and to decide whether or not urgent surgical intervention is necessary.

References

[1] G. H. Micklefield, H. D. Kuntz, and B. May, "Pneumatosis cystoides intestinalis: case reports and review of the literature," *Materia Medica Polona*, vol. 22, no. 2, pp. 70–72, 1990.

[2] S. D. St Peter, M. A. Abbas, and K. A. Kelly, "The spectrum of pneumatosis intestinalis," *Archives of Surgery*, vol. 138, no. 1, pp. 68–75, 2003.

[3] S. Galandiuk and V. W. Fazio, "Pneumatosis cystoides intestinalis: a review of the literature," *Diseases of the Colon and Rectum*, vol. 29, no. 5, pp. 358–363, 1986.

[4] B. L. Pear, "Pneumatosis intestinalis: a review," *Radiology*, vol. 207, no. 1, pp. 13–20, 1998.

[5] L. G. Koss, "Abdominal gas cysts (pneumatosis cystoides intestinorum hominis); an analysis with a report of a case and a critical review of the literature," *A. M. A. Archives of Pathology*, vol. 53, pp. 523–549, 1952.

[6] F. I. Luks, M. A. Chung, M. L. Brandt et al., "Pneumatosis and pneumoperitoneum in chronic idiopathic intestinal pseudoobstruction," *Journal of Pediatric Surgery*, vol. 26, no. 12, pp. 1384–1386, 1991.

[7] C. G. Schulze, U. Blum, and K. Haag, "Hepatic portal venous gas imaging modalities and clinical significance," *Acta Radiologica*, vol. 36, no. 4, pp. 377–380, 1995.

[8] J. G. Rabinowitz and R. L. Siegle, "Changing clinical and roentgenographic patterns of necrotizing enterocolitis," *American Journal of Roentgenology*, vol. 126, no. 3, pp. 560–566, 1976.

[9] B. J. Wood, P. N. Kumar, C. Cooper, P. M. Silverman, and R. K. Zeman, "Pneumatosis intestinalis in adults with AIDS: clinical significance and imaging findings," *American Journal of Roentgenology*, vol. 165, no. 6, pp. 1387–1390, 1995.

[10] C. E. Yale and E. Balish, "The natural course of Clostridium perfringens—induced pneumatosis cystoides intestinalis," *Journal of Medicine*, vol. 23, no. 3-4, pp. 279–288, 1992.

[11] G. P. M. Manues, W. J. de Boer, E. van der Jagt, A. F. Meinesz, J. J. Menzelaar, and W. van der Bij, "Pneumatosis intestinalis and active cytomegaloviral infection after lung transplantation. Groningen Lung Transplant Group," *Chest*, vol. 105, no. 3, pp. 929–930, 1994.

[12] L. E. Shindelman, S. A. Geller, N. Wisch, and J. J. Bauer, "Pneumatosis cystoides intestinalis: a complication of systemic chemotherapy," *American Journal of Gastroenterology*, vol. 75, no. 4, pp. 270–274, 1981.

[13] S. Hashimoto, H. Saitoh, K. Wada et al., "Pneumatosis cystoides intestinalis after chemotherapy for hematological malignancies: report of 4 cases," *Internal Medicine*, vol. 34, no. 3, pp. 212–215, 1995.

[14] P. Soyer, S. Martin-Grivaud, M. Boudiaf et al., "Linear or bubbly: a pictorial review of CT features of intestinal pneumatosis in adults," *Journal de Radiologie*, vol. 89, no. 12, pp. 1907–1920, 2008.

[15] T. Ochiai, T. Igri, Y. Kumagai, M. Iida, and S. Yamazaki, "Education and imaging. Gastrointestinal: massive portal venous gas and pneumatosis intestinalis.," *Journal of gastroenterology and hepatology*, vol. 25, no. 6, p. 1178, 2010.

[16] R. Voboril, "Pneumatosis cystoides intestinalis—a review," *Acta Medica*, vol. 44, no. 3, pp. 89–92, 2001.

[17] A. Sahin, "Pnömatosis kistoides intestinalis," *Dirim*, vol. 82, no. 2, pp. 343–349, 2007.

[18] S. J. Knechtle, A. M. Davidoff, and R. P. Rice, "Pneumatosis intestinalis. Surgical management and clinical outcome," *Annals of Surgery*, vol. 212, no. 2, pp. 160–166, 1990.

[19] G. Gagliardi, I. W. Thompson, M. J. Hershman, A. Forbes, P. R. Hawley, and I. C. Talbot, "Pneumatosis coli: a proposed pathogenesis based on study of 25 cases and review of the literature," *International Journal of Colorectal Disease*, vol. 11, no. 3, pp. 111–118, 1996.

[20] J. G. Keene, "Pneumatosis cystoides intestinalis and intramural intestinal gas," *The Journal of Emergency Medicine*, vol. 7, no. 6, pp. 645–650, 1989.

[21] Y. Heng, M. D. Schuffler, R. C. Haggitt, and C. A. Rohrmann, "Pneumatosis intestinalis: a review," *American Journal of Gastroenterology*, vol. 90, no. 10, pp. 1747–1758, 1995.

[22] A. J. Greenstein, S. Q. Nguyen, A. Berlin et al., "Pneumatosis intestinalis in adults: management, surgical indications, and risk factors for mortality," *Journal of Gastrointestinal Surgery*, vol. 11, no. 10, pp. 1268–1274, 2007.

[23] L. M. Ho, E. K. Paulson, and W. M. Thompson, "Pneumatosis intestinalis in the adult: benign to life-threatening causes," *American Journal of Roentgenology*, vol. 188, no. 6, pp. 1604–1613, 2007.

[24] D. Zhang, D. Weltman, and A. Baykal, "Portal vein gas and colonic pneumatosis after enema, with spontaneous resolution," *The American Journal of Roentgenology*, vol. 173, no. 4, pp. 1140–1141, 1999.

[25] A. L. Smit, B. Lamme, J. W. C. Gratama, W. H. Bouma, P. E. Spronk, and J. H. Rommes, "Pneumatosis intestinalis; no disease, but a symptom," *Nederlands Tijdschrift voor Geneeskunde*, vol. 152, no. 31, pp. 1705–1709, 2008.

[26] J. Theisen, P. Juhnke, H. J. Stein, and J. R. Siewert, "Pneumatosis cystoides intestinalis coli.," *Surgical endoscopy*, vol. 17, no. 1, pp. 157–158, 2003.

[27] F. S. Vernacchia, R. B. Jeffrey, F. C. Laing, and V. W. Wing, "Sonographic recognition of pneumatosis intestinalis," *American Journal of Roentgenology*, vol. 145, no. 1, pp. 51–52, 1985.

[28] E. M. Danse, B. E. van Beers, A. Gilles, and L. Jacquet, "Sonographic detection of intestinal pneumatosis," *European Journal of Ultrasound*, vol. 11, no. 3, pp. 201–203, 2000.

[29] D. Soboleski, P. Chait, B. Shuckett, and P. Silberg, "Sonographic diagnosis of systenaic venous gas in a patient with pneumatosis intestinalis," *Pediatric Radiology*, vol. 25, no. 6, pp. 480–481, 1995.

[30] M. Sato, H. Ishida, K. Konno et al., "Sonography of pneumatosis cystoides intestinalis," *Abdominal Imaging*, vol. 24, no. 6, pp. 559–561, 1999.

[31] M. J. Goske, J. R. Goldblum, K. E. Applegate, C. S. Mitchell, and D. Bardo, "The "circle sign": a new sonographic sign of pneumatosis intestinalis—clinical, pathologic and experimental findings," *Pediatric Radiology*, vol. 29, no. 7, pp. 530–535, 1999.

[32] R. Grassi, R. di Mizio, A. Pinto, A. Cioffi, L. Romano, and A. Rotondo, "Sixty-one consecutive patients with gastrointestinal perforation: comparison of conventional radiology, ultrasonography, and computerized tomography, in terms of the timing of the study," *Radiologia Medica*, vol. 91, no. 6, pp. 747–755, 1996.

[33] E. Schröpfer and T. Meyer, "Surgical aspects of pneumatosis cystoides intestinalis: two case reports," *Cases Journal*, vol. 2, no. 8, article 6452, 2009.

[34] S. J. Knechtle, A. M. Davidoff, and R. P. Rice, "Pneumatosis intestinalis. Surgical management and clinical outcome," *Annals of Surgery*, vol. 212, no. 2, pp. 160–165, 1990.

[35] M. S. Morris, A. C. Gee, S. D. Cho et al., "Management and outcome of pneumatosis intestinalis," *The American Journal of Surgery*, vol. 195, no. 5, pp. 679–683, 2008.

[36] C.-H. Liu, H. H. Chen, and W.-T. Huang, "Primary pneumotosis cystoides intestinalis," *Chang Gung Medical Journal*, vol. 26, no. 2, pp. 144–147, 2003.

3

Repair of a Post-Hepatectomy Posterior Sectoral Duct Injury Secondary to Anomalous Bile Duct Anatomy using a Novel Combined Surgical-Interventional Radiologic Approach

Beth-Ann Shanker,[1] Oliver S. Eng,[1] Vyacheslav Gendel,[2] John Nosher,[2] and Darren R. Carpizo[3]

[1] Department of Surgery, Rutgers-Robert Wood Johnson Medical School, New Brunswick, NJ 08903, USA
[2] Division of Interventional Radiology, Department of Radiology, Rutgers-Robert Wood Johnson Medical School, New Brunswick, NJ 08903, USA
[3] Division of Surgical Oncology, Department of Surgery, Rutgers Cancer Institute of New Jersey, Rutgers-Robert Wood Johnson Medical School, New Brunswick, NJ 08903, USA

Correspondence should be addressed to Darren R. Carpizo; carpizdr@cinj.rutgers.edu

Academic Editors: C. Barnett, G. Lal, G. Rallis, G. Santori, and F. Turégano

A 64-year-old woman with a completely transected posterior sectoral duct following extended hepatectomy underwent a combined operative procedure with interventional radiology and surgery to restore biliary-enteric drainage. The anterior and posterior sectoral ducts were identified, and catheters were inserted into both systems. The posterior sectoral catheter was placed intraoperatively through a preoperatively placed sheath, and a new tunnel was created through the regenerated liver surface. Biliary-enteric anastomoses were created over the stents.

1. Introduction

Bile leakage following hepatectomy is a common and sometimes challenging clinical problem with incidences ranging from 3% to 15% [1–4]. Biliary leaks (or fistulas as sometimes called) predispose the patient to significant morbidity, which includes infectious complications due to bacterial contamination of the collecting bile, nutritional depletion, and electrolyte derangement in cases of high-volume leaks (>200 mL/day) secondary to the loss of enterohepatic circulation of bile. Extended left hepatectomy, central bisegmentectomy, and resection of the caudate lobe have a higher incidence of bile leakage as a result of damaging bile ducts from the caudate lobe and anomalous bile duct anatomy [5, 6].

Biliary leaks due to anomalous bile duct anatomy are some of the most challenging to manage, as they are often categorized as total or "complete" fistulae, which means they have no communication with the remaining biliary-enteric system. These fistulae will often not resolve without operative intervention. Once control of a complete fistula is obtained by placement of a percutaneous catheter to drain the relevant bile duct, cholangiography is necessary to define the area of liver that is involved. Surgical management choices are resection of the involved area of liver versus a biliary-enteric drainage procedure. In cases of major hepatectomy for malignancy, resection as a management option is often not feasible, as the patient cannot spare further loss of liver parenchyma; thus, biliary-enteric drainage is necessary. This operation poses significant technical challenges due to difficulties in localizing the site of the anomalous duct in the cut liver surface.

Here we describe successful management of a patient with a complete biliary fistula involving the right posterior sectoral

(a)

(b)

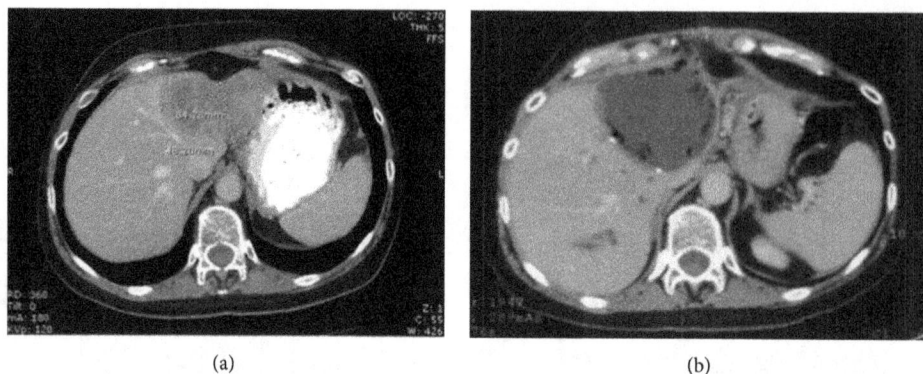

FIGURE 1: Preoperative and postoperative CT scan of patient. (a) preoperative CT scan of this patient demonstrating a large metastatic breast cancer tumor (8.4 × 4.6 cm) located in the left hemiliver abutting the middle hepatic vein. An extended left hepatectomy including caudate lobectomy was performed with negative margins. (b) CT scan performed two weeks after hepatectomy demonstrating a large biloma located in the post-hepatectomy bed.

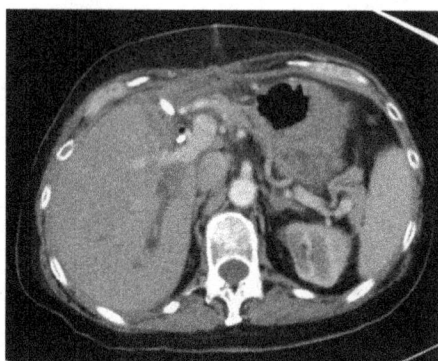

FIGURE 2: Isolated dilated right posterior sectoral duct. CT scan demonstrating dilated right posterior duct after adequate drainage of the biloma. Note the anterior ductal system is decompressed.

FIGURE 3: Post-hepatectomy ERCP. Post-hepatectomy ERCP demonstrating extravasation of contrast (black arrow) from the confluence of the right hepatic duct and left hepatic duct stumps.

duct using a novel combined surgical and interventional radiologic approach.

2. Case Report

A 64-year-old woman was referred to our clinic with a 9 cm left liver mass, biopsy proven to be consistent with metastatic breast cancer, Figure 1(a). The patient had a 17-year history of metastatic invasive ductal carcinoma of the left breast to the small bowel and liver. Over a span of several years, she underwent multiple small bowel resections before developing a solitary left liver metastasis. Over time, it was observed that her tumor biology was unusual not only for its temporal nature (slow progression), but also its location (small bowel) for progression. Due to this unusual nature, as well as the fairly rapid growth of her liver tumor, resection was considered her best treatment option by a multidisciplinary group of oncologists.

An extended left hepatectomy including caudate lobe resection and cholecystectomy was performed. The parenchymal transection in the area of segments 4b/5 went down to the bifurcation of the right and left pedicles in order to

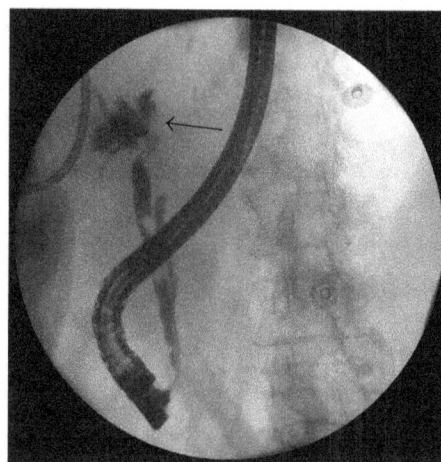

gain adequate tumor clearance. The left hepatic duct was divided separately with an endovascular stapler very close to the bifurcation of the right and left portal pedicles. During the operation, there were no immediate complications, including bile leak. The estimated blood loss was 150 mL, and the patient was discharged on the fourth postoperative day.

On postoperative day 15, she was admitted with abdominal pain, fevers, an elevated total bilirubin, and leukocytosis. CT scan demonstrated a collection in the hepatic fossa (Figure 1(b)), as well as a dilated right posterior bile duct (Figure 2). A percutaneous 10 Fr Felima pigtail drain was placed (Boston Scientific, Natick, MA) to drain the biloma. She then underwent endoscopic retrograde cholangiopancreatography (ERCP), where it appeared on cholangiogram that she had a leak from the left hepatic duct stump (Figure 3). A biliary endostent was inserted with the tip in the right anterior sectoral ductal system in an attempt to occlude the left hepatic duct stump. In followup, she was noted to continue to have a high amount of bilious output from

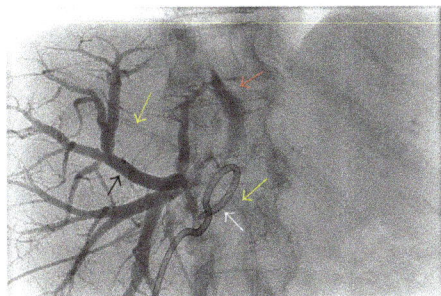

FIGURE 4: Confirmation of anomalous biliary anatomy. Transhepatic cholangiogram. Yellow arrows show endoscopic placed stent in right anterior sectoral duct. There is no contrast in the anterior sectoral duct or its branches. Black arrows show contrast in the posterior sectoral duct and filling of posterior duct and branches. White arrow shows extrahepatic pigtail placed catheter. Red arrow shows extravasation of bile. This cholangiogram demonstrates that the anterior and posterior ducts are not in continuity.

the percutaneous drain, indicating an uncontrolled leak. Two weeks later, a transhepatic cholangiogram was performed through a catheter in the right posterior sectoral ductal system. This cholangiogram demonstrated that the right anterior sectoral duct containing the endoscopic stent was not in continuity with the posterior sectoral duct. The posterior duct was draining through the cut liver surface (Figure 4). We concluded there was anomalous biliary anatomy with the right posterior sectoral duct draining into the left hepatic duct. An external catheter was placed in this posterior duct. Over time, the percutaneous abdominal catheter stopped draining, indicating complete control of the fistula. The patient's sepsis was controlled and she recovered. The cut edge of the liver surface at the site of the transected posterior sectoral duct eventually sclerosed, making the catheter in the posterior sectoral duct no longer in communication with the abdominal cavity. A second operation to restore her biliary system and provide enteric drainage would be necessary. However, this operation posed a significant technical challenge to locate this aberrant duct in a reoperative field. It was decided that a combined interventional surgical approach would be necessary to identify the biliary anatomy intra-abdominally, create a new tract through the regenerated liver surface, and provide a stent to facilitate a new enteric anastomosis.

2.1. Combined Surgical and Interventional Radiologic Approach. The tip of the catheter that was left in the right posterior sectoral duct was not placed in the extrahepatic space of the cut liver surface but rather was pulled into the liver, so we anticipated that this bile duct would have fibrosed in the several month period of time between operations. This would make it nearly impossible to find at reoperation. To facilitate identifying this catheter in the operating room, we first had the catheter injected with contrast in the interventional radiology department on the morning of surgery in an attempt to advance the catheter into the extrahepatic space. This no longer revealed an

extravasation of contrast as when the catheter was initially placed, thus indicating there was no communication of the catheter with the peritoneal cavity. Next, the patient was moved to the operating room, where we performed an exploratory laparotomy; however, the sheath containing the posterior sectoral catheter was left in place to allow further manipulation in the operating room. At operation, we appreciated a large amount of fibrosis around the liver in the area of her previous biliary abscess. Next, the anterior biliary duct endostent was identified by palpation. Dissection around the anterior biliary duct led to the finding of a disruption of this duct at the confluence. This represented site of the leak of the left hepatic ductal stump was initially detected in Figure 4.

We next searched for the posterior sectoral catheter but could not identify or palpate it. This was expected. At this point, the interventional radiology team came into the operating room to provide fluoroscopic guidance for the location of the biliary catheter in the posterior duct. This revealed that the distance between the tip of the catheter and the cut liver surfaces was approximately 2-3 cm likely from regenerated liver. To traverse this distance, a tunnel would need to be made. Using the posterior sheath, we then placed a 16-gauge Colapinto needle with a 9 Fr Sheath (Cook Medical Inc., Bloomington, IN) and tunneled this out into the extrahepatic space, (Figure 5(a)). Using the same catheter system, we tunneled a catheter into the anterior ductal system retrograde from the duct orifice through the parenchyma and out the abdominal wall. We had two internal/external biliary catheters in both the anterior and posterior sectoral systems, (Figure 5(b)). We then fashioned a roux limb of jejunum and performed two separate anastomoses over these stents using interrupted sutures of 5-0 polydioxanone (PDS). The anterior anastomosis was a true hepaticojejunostomy with duct sewn to bowel; however, the posterior sectoral anastomosis was from the jejunum to a layer of fibrous tissue overlying the regenerated liver surface. As this was not a true hepaticojejunostomy, we buttressed this anastomosis using interrupted sutures of 3-0 PDS. The patient tolerated the procedure well and was discharged home on postoperative day 6.

In followup, the anterior internal-external biliary drain was removed after 4 weeks. The posterior internal-external drain was exchanged after 12 weeks for a permanent internal stent, which was composed of two overlapping SMART stents 14 mm × 6 cm and 14 mm × 4 cm (Cordis, Miami Lakes, FL, Figure 6) across the biliary enteric anastomosis. This was done to prevent future closing of the tract between the posterior sectoral duct and the jejunum that would likely happen, as there was approximately two centimeters of liver tissue not lined by biliary epithelium.

3. Discussion

The association of major hepatectomy with increased bile leaks is well established in the literature [2, 6–8]. Left hepatectomy has been shown to be an independent risk factor for bile leaks [8]. Left hepatectomy and trisectionectomy with

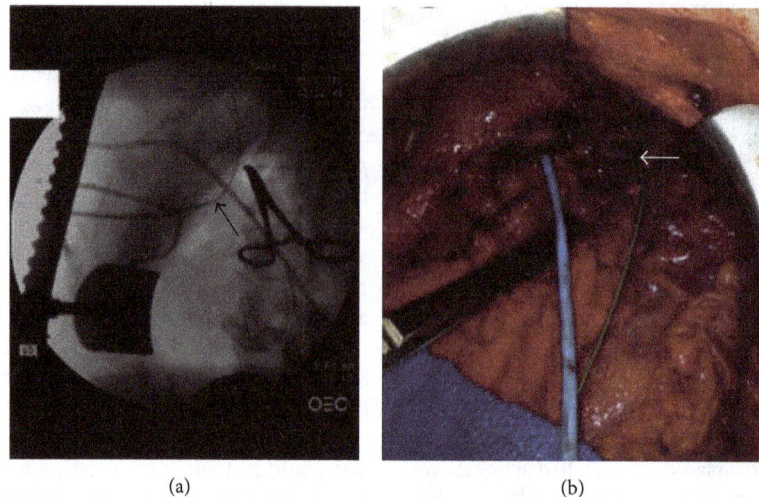

(a)   (b)

FIGURE 5: Intraoperative radiographically guided tunneling of biliary catheters. (a) Intraoperative radiograph showing interventional radiologist tunneling 16 gauge Colapinto needle through the previously placed posterior sectoral sheath (Cook Medical Inc, Bloomington, In). A guidewire traversing regenerated liver into the peritoneal cavity is demonstrated (arrow). (b) Operative field view with a catheter in the anterior ductal system inserted retrograde from the bile duct and out the liver surface and abdominal wall (arrow) and the posterior catheter inserted from an outside-in direction.

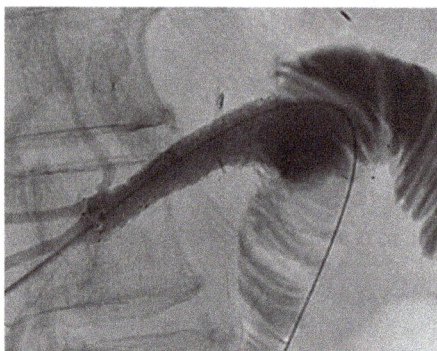

FIGURE 6: Biliary stenting of posterior sectoral anastomosis. Twelve weeks after operation to restore biliary-enteric drainage, interventional radiology placed overlapping SMART stents (Cordis, Miami Lakes, FL) across the posterior sectoral biliary-enteric anastomosis to prevent fibrosis of the tract not lined by bile duct epithelium.

caudate lobe resection have challenging technical aspects including identification of the border between the caudate lobe and the right posterior section and the dividing line of the intrahepatic bile ducts [7]. Benzoni et al. examined their surgical complications in 134 patients with liver resections secondary to hepatocellular carcinoma (HCC) and 153 patients with liver resections secondary to metastasis. They found a significantly higher rate of bile leaks in patients after major hepatectomy, left hepatectomy, trisegmentectomy, and bisegmentectomy [2]. The majority of these bile leaks seal spontaneously, as these are considered "partial" leaks because they remain in communication with the remaining biliary-enteric system. In a retrospective review of 363 hepatectomies for cancer, Tanaka et al. reported an overall leak rate of 7.2% (26/363) with the majority (18/26, 69%) sealing within two weeks. Eight patients required some type of intervention,

with two of the eight requiring reoperation. Neither required reresection or biliary bypass [6].

Infrequently, a bile leak is considered a "complete" biliary leak/fistula, in which a segment or sector is completely separated from the remaining biliary-enteric system. These complete leaks/fistulas are often the result of aberrant hepatic ductal anatomy, most commonly when the right posterior sectoral duct drains via the left hepatic duct and the patient undergoes a left hepatectomy, as in this case. The classification of aberrant duct anatomy is well established (Figure 7), although the incidence of these types varies depending on studies of cadavers or imaging studies [9, 10]. The majority of the aberrant types involve the right system and its configuration with the common hepatic duct or left hepatic duct. The incidence of the type in this case in which the right posterior sectoral duct drains directly into the left hepatic duct before it joins the right anterior sectoral duct to form the common hepatic duct varies from 4–19% [5, 11, 12]. When a leak occurs after hepatectomy due to aberrant ductal anatomy such as this, it must be managed either by resection of the involved segment(s) or a biliary-enteric drainage procedure. Another option is to allow the involved liver to atrophy due to chronic cholestasis, but this can lead to septic complications of cholangitis. Biliary-enteric drainage is technically challenging, as one must locate the aberrant duct at the cut liver surface. Given the frequency of these variants, it is surprising that there is neither literature documenting the frequency of these types of leaks, nor the any description of their operative management.

Obviously, the best strategy for this problem is to avoid it altogether, which would require cholangiography being performed on all major hepatic resections, if not all left or extended left hepatic resections. Endoscopic or percutaneous cholangiography involves another procedure that carries its own set of potential complications. Only until recently have

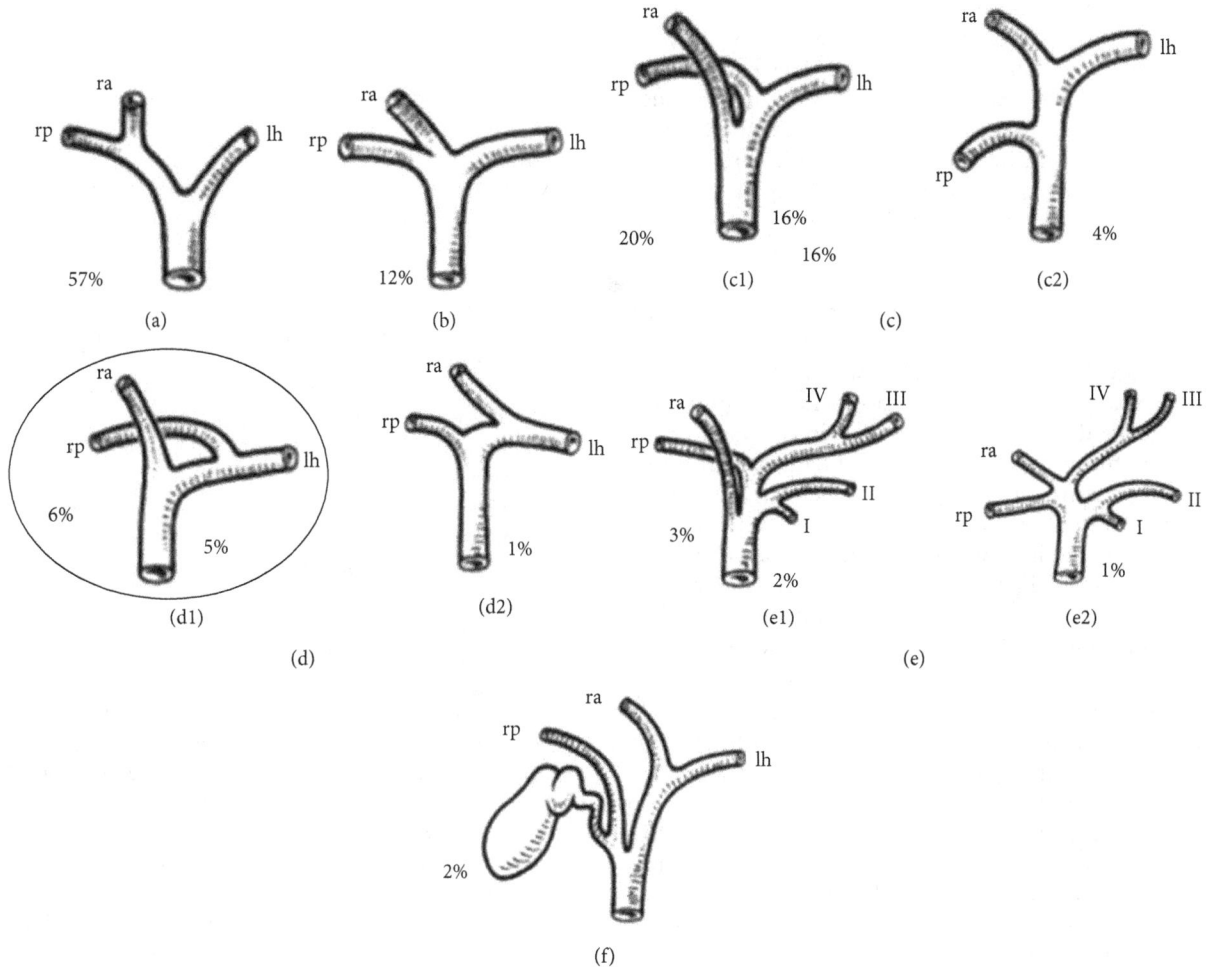

FIGURE 7: Normal hepatic duct anatomy and common variations (Couinaud 1957). (a) Typical anatomy. (b) Triple confluence. (c1) Right anterior draining into common hepatic duct. (c2) Right posterior duct drainage into common hepatic duct. (d) Right sectoral duct into the left hepatic ductal system. Red circle indicates the anatomy of the patient in this study. (e) Absence of confluence. (f) Absence of right hepatic duct. Drainage of right posterior duct into the cystic duct. The circled image corresponds to the biliary anatomy of this patient. Adapted and with permission to publish from Surgery of Liver, Biliary tract, and Pancreas, L. H. Blumgart editor. (2007, Saunders Elsevier: Philadelphia page 44).

improvements in MR cholangiography made it possible to potentially anticipate this problem preoperatively. A growing body of research in the arena of living donor liver transplantation (LDLT) has studied biliary anatomy since donor safety is of particular concern. Approximately 250 cases of LDLT are performed yearly, with a range of 2.4% to 5.3% experiencing biliary complications. Preoperative evaluation had included magnetic resonance cholangiography (MRC) and computed tomography cholangiography (CTC). Conventional MRC may fail to delineate normal intrahepatic ducts because of a poor signal to noise ratio and limited spatial resolution. Wang et al. reviewed the recent literature on image evaluation of bile ducts. They found in a study of 111 LDLT donors that MRC accurately portrayed the anatomy of the biliary system in 88.3% of the subjects. CTC was found to be concordant with surgical findings in 23/24 LDLT patients for right liver donors. Overall, the studies on preoperative MRC and CTC are fairly limited, and in the realm of LDLT, surgeons typically rely on intraoperative cholangiography [13].

Taketomi et al. established an imaging and technical protocol in 2005 to define biliary anatomy and reduce the percentage of biliary leaks in LDLT. Despite preoperative CT cholangiography, they routinely obtained intraoperative cholangiograms after 2005, in addition to making other technical changes. They report a significant decrease in bile leaks since the introduction of their protocol [14]. However, these intraoperative cholangiograms are also limited by a two-dimensional representation of biliary anatomy [13].

The fact that the rate of biliary complications and leaks has not changed over the past decade indicates that preoperative imaging, intraoperative cholangiography, and the use of sealants are still limited in their ability to detect aberrant anatomy and prevent leaks. The management of biliary leaks is well studied in patients after laparoscopic and open cholecystectomy. In this setting, multidisciplinary approaches to manage such complications have been well described between the gastroenterologists and the surgeons. For cystic stump leaks, ERCP is successful as a tool for both diagnosis and therapeutic management with stent placement [4]. Yet, even in the cases of injury during cholecystectomy, aberrant anatomy of the right posterior duct has made it impossible to identify the leak via ERCP if the injured duct is not in communication with the main bile channels. These injuries require definitive management with a roux-en-Y hepaticojejunostomy [15]. Jarnagin and Blumgart reviewed operative repair of bile duct injuries involving the hepatic duct confluence [16]. Prior to any attempt at operative repair, they advocated for percutaneous transhepatic cholangiography to define the injury, angiography if there is concern for vascular injury, drainage of fluid, and biliary decompression if patients are septic. The fundamental principles cited for biliary reconstruction at the confluence include identification of healthy bile duct mucosa, roux-en-Y anastomosis 70 cm proximal to the enteroenterostomy, and a direct mucosa to mucosa anastomosis. In our particular patient, identifying healthy mucosa of the anterior and posterior sectoral ducts was challenging in the dense fibrotic and regenerate hepatic tissue. The combined procedure with interventional radiology and intraoperative fluoroscopy and placement of new biliary catheters allowed us to identify these ducts so that an adequate biliary-enteric anastomosis was performed.

In summary, we describe a novel combined approach in which interventional radiology combined with surgery leads to a successful repair of an aberrant right posterior sectoral duct following extended left hepatectomy. While interventional radiologists and hepatobiliary surgeons often work closely in hepatobiliary units, this is the first time that a surgical biliary bypass procedure has been described as a combined procedure with interventional radiology. Surprisingly there are no reports of techniques to overcome the problem of repairing a complete biliary fistula involving a transected duct at the edge of transection of the liver parenchyma after-hepatectomy. Due to the regeneration of liver tissue at the cut surface, it is impossible to surgically drain without the assistance of interventional radiology.

It might be possible to anticipate this anomalous anatomy through preoperative MR Cholangiography. This raises another issue of what to do if an aberrant posterior sectoral duct is revealed by preoperative MR cholangiography. It might be very difficult to locate such a duct during parenchymal transection even when armed with such knowledge preoperatively. In such a situation, we would advocate a combined surgical and interventional approach as we have described, where the patients have a catheter placed into the posterior sectoral duct preoperatively and advanced into the left hepatic ductal system, such that this duct can easily be located during parenchymal transection and an anastomosis can be made with a roux limb of jejunum. At this time, we would advocate routine MR cholangiography for any extended left hepatic resection.

References

[1] N. Babel, S. V. Sakpal, P. Paragi, J. Wellen, S. Feldman, and R. S. Chamberlain, "Iatrogenic bile duct injury associated with anomalies of the right hepatic sectoral ducts: a misunderstood and underappreciated problem," *HPB Surgery*, vol. 2009, Article ID 153269, 4 pages, 2009.

[2] E. Benzoni, A. Cojutti, D. Lorenzin et al., "Liver resective surgery: a multivariate analysis of postoperative outcome and complication," *Langenbeck's Archives of Surgery*, vol. 392, no. 1, pp. 45–54, 2007.

[3] K. Shimada, T. Sano, Y. Sakamoto, and T. Kosuge, "Safety and effectiveness of left hepatic trisegmentectomy for hilar cholangiocarcinoma," *World Journal of Surgery*, vol. 29, no. 6, pp. 723–727, 2005.

[4] N. Doctor, J. S. Dooley, R. Dick, A. Watkinson, K. Rolles, and B. R. Davidson, "Multidisciplinary approach to biliary complications of laparoscopic cholecystectomy," *The British Journal of Surgery*, vol. 85, no. 5, pp. 627–632, 1998.

[5] R. Mizumoto and H. Suzuki, "Surgical anatomy of the hepatic hilum with special reference to the caudate lobe," *World Journal of Surgery*, vol. 12, no. 1, pp. 2–10, 1988.

[6] S. Tanaka, K. Hirohashi, H. Tanaka et al., "Incidence and management of bile leakage after hepatic resection for malignant hepatic tumors," *Journal of the American College of Surgeons*, vol. 195, no. 4, pp. 484–489, 2002.

[7] K. Uesaka, "Left hepatectomy or left trisectionectomy with resection of the caudate lobe and extrahepatic bile duct for hilar cholangiocarcinoma (with video)," *Journal of Hepato-Biliary-Pancreatic Sciences*, vol. 19, no. 3, pp. 195–202, 2012.

[8] Y. Yamashita, T. Hamatsu, T. Rikimaru et al., "Bile leakage after hepatic resection," *Annals of Surgery*, vol. 233, no. 1, pp. 45–50, 2001.

[9] C. U. Corvera, W. R. Jarnagin, and L. H. Blumgart, *Surgery of the Liver, Biliary Tract and Pancreas*, edited by L. H. Blumgart, Saunders, Elsevier, Philadelphia, Pa, USA, 2007.

[10] W. Wiesner, K. J. Mortelé, J. N. Glickman, H. Ji, and P. R. Ros, "Pneumatosis intestinalis and portomesenteric venous gas in intestinal ischemia: correlation of CT findings with severity of ischemia and clinical outcome," *The American Journal of Roentgenology*, vol. 177, no. 6, pp. 1319–1323, 2001.

[11] G. S. Gazelle, M. J. Lee, and P. R. Mueller, "Cholangiographic segmental anatomy of the liver," *Radiographics*, vol. 14, no. 5, pp. 1005–1013, 1994.

[12] S. G. Puente and G. C. Bannura, "Radiological anatomy of the biliary tract: variations and congenital abnormalities," *World Journal of Surgery*, vol. 7, no. 2, pp. 271–276, 1983.

[13] S. F. Wang, Z. Y. Huang, and X. P. Chen, "Biliary complications after living donor liver transplantation," *Liver Transplantation*, vol. 17, no. 10, pp. 1127–1136, 2011.

[14] A. Taketomi, K. Morita, T. Toshima et al., "Living donor hepatectomies with procedures to prevent biliary complications," *Journal of the American College of Surgeons*, vol. 211, no. 4, pp. 456–464, 2010.

[15] K. D. Lillemoe, J. A. Petrofski, M. A. Choti, A. C. Venbrux, and J. L. Cameron, "Isolated right segmental hepatic duct injury: a diagnostic and therapeutic challenge," *Journal of Gastrointestinal Surgery*, vol. 4, no. 2, pp. 168–177, 2000.

[16] W. R. Jarnagin and L. H. Blumgart, "Operative repair of bile duct injuries involving the hepatic duct confluence," *Archives of Surgery*, vol. 134, no. 7, pp. 769–775, 1999.

4

Total Esophageal Avulsion at the Esophagogastric Junction after Blunt Trauma

Ibrahim Uygun, Selcuk Otcu, Bahattin Aydogdu, Mehmet Hanifi Okur, and Mehmet Serif Arslan

Department of Pediatric Surgery, Medical Faculty of Dicle University, 21280 Diyarbakir, Turkey

Correspondence should be addressed to Ibrahim Uygun; iuygun@hotmail.com

Academic Editors: S. Bhatt, N. A. Chowdri, R. Hasan, H. Imura, and F. Marchal

Total avulsion and transection of the esophagus at the esophagogastric junction are very rare after blunt trauma, and their management is challenging. Here, we present the case of a boy with this injury. To date, only two cases have been reported in children. One was treated successfully and the other died. The initial emergency operation should aim to save the life and native esophagus. Therefore, a primary or early thoracal end esophagostomy with gastrostomy should be performed, while primary repair should not be.

1. Introduction

The frequency of traumatic esophageal injures varies by country. However, they occur in <1% of all traumatic injuries but are associated with a significant risk of morbidity and mortality (6%–70%) [1, 2]. The outcome of esophageal injuries is determined by several factors that increase the risk of complications and death. A delay in diagnostic studies to determine the presence of these injuries and the difficulty identifying these injuries, particularly when other life-threatening injuries are present, can be problematic [1, 2]. Late surgical intervention for esophageal injuries is the most important determinant of the high rates of mortality and morbidity [1, 2].

Total avulsion and transection of the esophagus at the esophagogastric junction are very rare after blunt trauma, and their management its challenging. To-date, only two cases have been reported in children [3, 4]. Here, we present the case of a boy with this injury.

2. Case Report

A 12-year-old boy was admitted to the emergency department due to a bicycle accident. A car had hit him 30 min previously. He was in hypovolemic shock (Glasgow coma score 10), and he had an acute abdomen with abdominal distention.

An emergency thoracoabdominal computerized tomography with intravenous contrast agent showed laceration of the spleen (grade V), intra-abdominal massive free fluid with free air, active intraperitoneal bleeding, mediastinal massive free air, and multiple pubic fractures (Figure 1). He underwent an emergency exploratory laparotomy. During the operation, we discovered massive intra-abdominal blood with gastric contents (food particles, chips, etc.) and a splenic laceration with active bleeding. Thus, a splenectomy was performed. The stomach was ruptured on the anterior corporeal wall at approximately 8 cm, and the stomach was totally free. A total esophageal avulsion at the esophagogastric junction and active bleeding from the esophageal hiatus were identified. The avulsed distal esophageal end was ragged (tassel-like) and had retracted into the mediastinum. Gastric contents were present in the mediastinum. No other intra-abdominal injuries were noted. After the bleeding was controlled and washed out, the gastric rupture was repaired. An esophagogastrostomy at the site of the avulsion was carried out over a nasogastric tube after mobilizing the esophageal distal end. Two drains were inserted: one into the lower abdomen and the other into the mediastinum at the esophagogastric junction. After the operation, he was mechanically ventilated for 24 hours. He was fed on postoperative day four via a nasojejunal tube, because there was no discharge from the drains. Nevertheless, he was operated on for a second time for

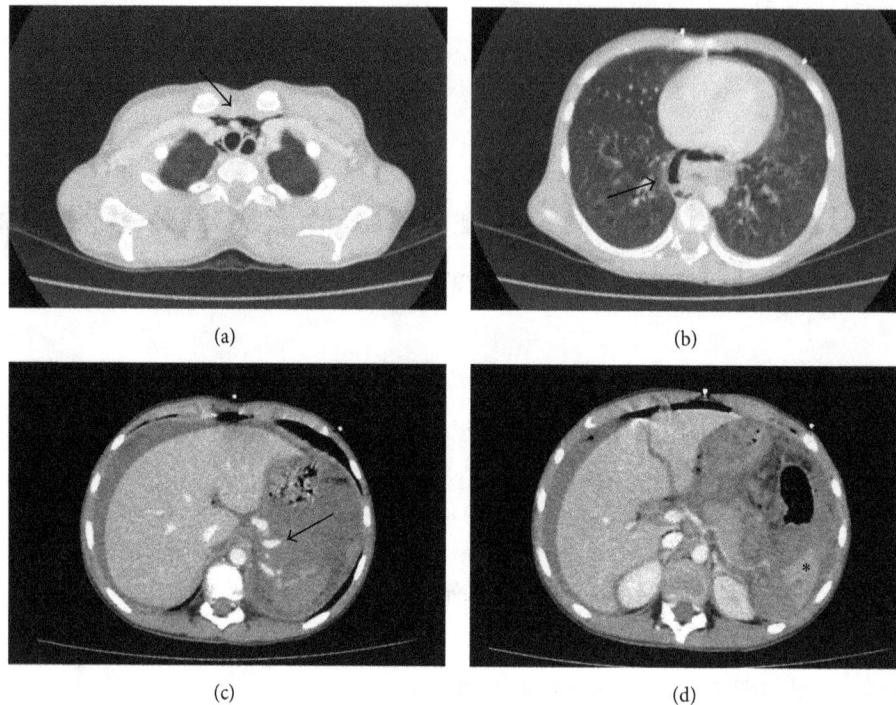

FIGURE 1: Thoracoabdominal emergency computerized tomography. (a) and (b) Mediastinal massive free air (arrows). (c) and (d) Laceration of the spleen (asterisk), massive intra-abdominal free fluid with free air, and active intraperitoneal bleeding (arrow).

a thoracotomy due to uncontrolled mediastinitis signs (severe fever, tachypnea, and tachycardia) on postoperative day 13, and mediastinitis due to an esophagogastric anastomotic leakage was identified. A mediastinal tube thoracostomy drainage and esophageal repair were performed. However, the esophageal leakage and severe mediastinitis could not be controlled by several sequential interventions (esophageal end closure and gastrostomy, cervical loop esophagostomy, and esophageal stapling with a stapler). Esophageal leakage of saliva and mediastinal discharge continued, from which bacteria (Acinetobacter baumannii, Cedecea lapagei, and Tatumella ptyseos) were isolated. These were suppressed successfully with broad-spectrum antibiotics such as cefoperazone-sulbactam, linezolid, and tigecycline. The patient was fed fully via the gastrostomy. Finally, right lateral cervical end esophagostomy was performed. Subsequently, he improved quickly and was discharged uneventful with esophagostomy and gastrostomy. Six months after the accident, a gastric pullup was performed to replace the esophagus. A postoperative anastomotic leakage was treated medically with antibiotics, tube thoracostomy, and nasojejunal feeding, and he was discharged uneventful. After esophageal replacement surgery, he is well and can swallow solid food without dysphagia at the two-year followup (Figure 2).

3. Discussion

Esophageal injuries are rare because the elasticity, mobility, and secluded position of the esophagus protect it from blunt trauma; however, if injured, management of an esophageal injury is a challenge for the surgeon [1, 2]. Esophageal leakage is the main problem, as it may cause mediastinitis, pneumonia, sepsis, or death [1, 2]. Treatment of esophageal leakage after failure of an anastomosis and iatrogenic perforation is mostly medical, but after traumatic injury, it is mostly surgical [1, 2]. Saliva and gastric acid contents may leak after opening the esophagus. If the diagnosis is delayed, fluid and solid food may leak. Early treatment is the most important factor for morbidity and mortality due to esophageal damage [1, 2]. However, management of a total avulsion and transection of the esophagus at the esophagogastric junction is very challenging for the surgeon even if it is diagnosed early. Data are insufficient, as only two cases of transection of the esophagus at the esophagogastric junction by blunt trauma have been reported in children [3, 4].

In the first case reported by Barrie et al. in 1961, a 13-year-old girl sustained a fall on the left chest and abdomen [3]. Primary reconstruction was performed by esophagogastrostomy through separate abdominal and thoracic incisions. Hypotension, hyperthermia, and renal shutdown developed postoperatively, and she died four days after the injury. The esophageal reconstruction was intact at autopsy. The authors questioned the advisability of a prolonged primary reconstruction versus a shorter exclusion operation that carried the disadvantage of a cervical esophagostomy [3].

In the second case reported by Miller in 1968, a 13-year-old boy was in a truck accident and was operated on via an extended laparothoracotomy [4]. After a left mediastinal and thoracal washout, the authors closed the proximal end of the esophagus rather than risk the chance of an anastomotic leakage from a primary esophagogastric reconstruction; thus,

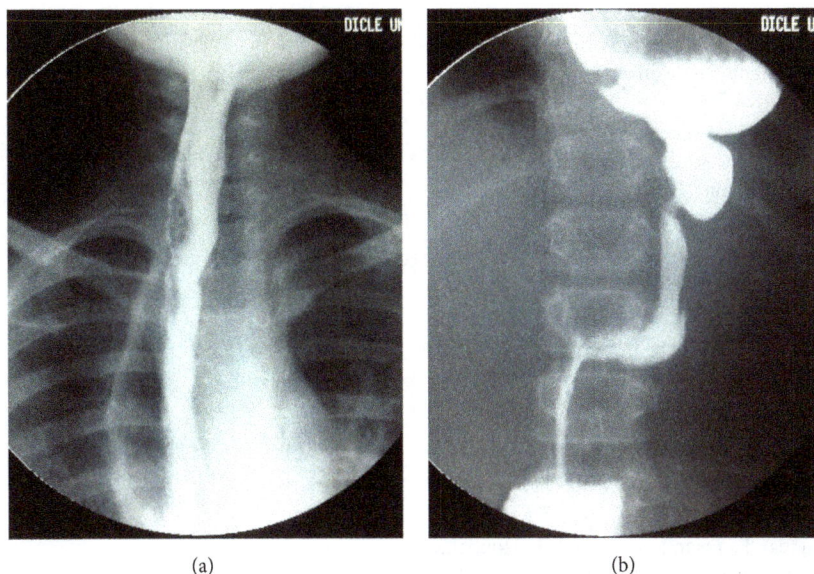

(a)   (b)

FIGURE 2: Barium swallow study after a gastric pull-up procedure. (a) Cervical esophagogastrostomy and stomach in the mediastinum. (b) Pylorus and duodenum in the abdomen.

a cervical double-barrel esophagostomy to defunctionalize the thoracic esophageal segment was performed. However, purulent discharge from the posterior mediastinal tube drain continued for six weeks, and the patient developed recurrent suppurative mediastinitis. Then, an esophagography showed free communication of the distal end of the esophagus with the mediastinum, which was believed to be the source of the recurrent mediastinal contamination. He recovered promptly after an esophagectomy. Esophageal replacement surgery was conducted using the terminal ileum and right colon. A minimal leak at the proximal anastomosis closed after one week. Finally, he was well. This was the first reported case of recovery from an esophageal avulsion [4].

In our case, we tried to save the life and the esophagus. But, we could not save all of the native esophagus. We did insert effective drains into the abdomen and mediastinum and a feeding tube such as nasojejunal tube or gastrostomy/gastrojejunal tube to supply energy. An esophagogastrostomy or closure of the proximal end of the esophagus to save the esophagus has been tried, but all failed. The infection caused by the contamination and presence of food particles in the mediastinum, even if they were washed out, was the most important factor. Infection impairs wound healing and also tissue damage, necrosis, and loss of the end of avulsed organs. Tissue-loss-induced tension from the anastomosis causes leakage, which leads to infection. Additionally, esophageal mucosal secretions are important. Because the esophagus always secretes mucosal secretion, which collects in the esophageal pouch when the esophagus is closed blindly, even if the saliva is stopped using cervical loop or a double-barrel esophagostomy [4, 5]. The collection of secretions in the esophageal pouch causes infection and leakage [4]. Furthermore, esophageal motility together with the secretions opens the closure in the esophagus as in our case and in the second case reported by Miller [4].

Mediastinitis caused by esophageal leakage is the most important reason for death after esophageal injury and must be prevented or controlled [1, 2]. Therefore, a primary or early thoracal end esophagostomy should be performed to save the life and as much as possible the native esophagus, but primary repair should not be attempted in cases of the total esophageal avulsion at the esophagogastric junction [4].

Antibiotic-resistant bacterial nosocomial infections are a major problem, particularly for patients with prolonged hospitalization in the intensive care unit. *A. baumannii* is the most significant nosocomial infection agent in our country and in our hospital [6]. It was isolated from the mediastinal discharge and was susceptible to cefoperazone/sulbactam, piperacillin/tazobactam, and tigecycline only but was uniformly resistant to other antimicrobial agents. Interestingly, *C. lapagei* and *T. ptyseos*, which are very uncommon agents, were also isolated and were susceptible to cefoperazone/sulbactam [7, 8].

Managing a total avulsion and transection of the esophagus at the esophagogastric junction after blunt trauma is challenging for the surgeon. The initial emergency operation should aim to save the life and native esophagus. Therefore, a primary or early thoracal end esophagostomy with gastrostomy should be performed, while primary repair should not be.

Disclosure

The authors have indicated that they have no financial relationships relevant to this paper to disclose.

References

[1] R. J. Skipworth, O. M. McBride, J. J. Kerssens, and S. Paterson-Brown, "Esophagogastric Trauma in Scotland," *World Journal of Surgery*, vol. 36, pp. 1779–1784, 2012.

[2] J. A. Asensio, S. Chahwan, W. Forno et al., "Penetrating esophageal injuries: Multicenter Study of the American Association for the Surgery of Trauma," *Journal of Trauma*, vol. 50, no. 2, pp. 289–296, 2001.

[3] J. Barrie, R. Sarrazin, and J. Bonnet-Eymard, "Traumatic rupture of the abdominal esophagus," *Mémoires Académie de Chirurgie*, vol. 87, pp. 662–667, 1961.

[4] D. R. Miller, "Transection of the esophagus at the esophagogastric junction by blunt trauma. Report of a case," *Journal of Trauma*, vol. 8, no. 6, pp. 1105–1110, 1968.

[5] S. Abdulnour-Nakhoul, N. L. Nakhoul, S. A. Wheeler, P. Wang, E. R. Swenson, and R. C. Orlando, "HCO_3^- secretion in the esophageal submocosal glands," *American Journal of Physiology*, vol. 288, no. 4, pp. G736–G744, 2005.

[6] S. Hosoglu, M. Hascuhadar, E. Yasar, S. Uslu, and B. Aldudak, "Control of an Acinetobacter baumannii outbreak in a neonatal ICU without suspension of service: a devastating outbreak in Diyarbakir, Turkey," *Infection*, vol. 40, pp. 11–18, 2012.

[7] P. S. G. da Costa, J. M. de Castro Mendes, and G. M. Ribeiro, "Tatumella ptyseos causing severe human infection: report of the first two Brazilian cases," *Brazilian Journal of Infectious Diseases*, vol. 12, no. 5, pp. 442–443, 2008.

[8] G. Yetkin, S. Ay, U. Kayabaş, E. Gedik, N. Gucluer, and A. Caliskan, "A pneumonia case caused by Cedecea Lapagei," *Mikrobiyoloji Bulteni*, vol. 42, no. 4, pp. 681–684, 2008.

5

Successful Treatment of Bleeding Gastric Varices with Splenectomy in a Patient with Splenic, Portal, and Mesenteric Thromboses

Lior Menasherian-Yaccobe,[1] Nathan T. Jaqua,[1] and Patrick Kenny[1,2]

[1] Department of Internal Medicine, Tripler Army Medical Center, 1 Jarrett White Road, Honolulu, HI 96859, USA
[2] Gastroenterology Service, Tripler Army Medical Center, USA

Correspondence should be addressed to Nathan T. Jaqua; nathan.jaqua@gmail.com

Academic Editors: A. Cho and S. S. Kim

A 59-year-old female with a history of multiple splanchnic and portal thromboses treated with warfarin underwent an esophagogastroduodenoscopy for cancer screening, and a polypoid mass was biopsied. One week later, she was admitted with upper gastrointestinal hemorrhage. Her therapeutic coagulopathy was reversed with fresh frozen plasma, and she was transfused with packed red blood cells. An esophagogastroduodenoscopy demonstrated an erosion of a gastric varix without evidence of recent bleeding. Conservative measures failed, and she continued to bleed during her stay. She was not considered a candidate for a shunt procedure; therefore, a splenectomy was performed. Postoperative esophagogastroduodenoscopy demonstrated near complete resolution of gastric varices. One year after discharge on warfarin, there has been no recurrence of hemorrhage. Gastric varices often arise from either portal hypertension or splenic vein thrombosis. Treatment of gastric variceal hemorrhage can be challenging. Transjugular intrahepatic portosystemic shunt is often effective for emergency control in varices secondary to portal hypertension. Splenectomy is the treatment for varices that arise from splenic vein thrombosis. However, treatment of gastric variceal hemorrhage in the context of multiple splanchnic and portal vein thromboses is more complicated. We report splenectomy as a successful treatment of gastric varices in a patient with multiple extrahepatic thromboses.

1. Introduction

Gastric varices are less common than esophageal varices in patients with portal hypertension, occurring in up to 33% of patients [1–3]. Gastric varices are more common in patients with noncirrhotic portal hypertension and extrahepatic portal vein thrombosis, are associated with a lower incidence of bleeding, and have a higher mortality rate than esophageal varices [1–3]. Optimal management of gastric variceal bleeding is debatable, because of lack of data from large randomized controlled trials [3]. We present a case of gastric variceal bleeding caused by prehepatic venous thrombosis from essential thrombocythemia that was successfully treated with therapeutic splenectomy.

2. Case Report

A 59-year-old female with a history of essential thrombocythemia and heterozygous prothrombin gene mutation was hospitalized for abdominal pain. Evaluation revealed portal, superior mesenteric and splenic vein thrombosis, and she was started on warfarin (Figures 1, 2, and 3). She presented two months later with one week of dull epigastric abdominal pain which was worse with movement and food and better with lying down. She also had three days of one to three black and tarry stools daily and progressive fatigue. One week priorly, she underwent esophagogastroduodenoscopy (EGD) to screen for gastric cancer with biopsy of a polypoid mass. The patient had requested the evaluation because of a vague family history of gastric cancer.

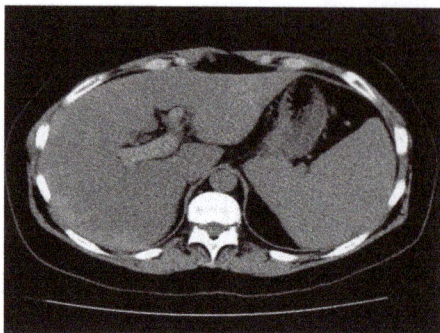

FIGURE 1: CT demonstrating portal thrombosis.

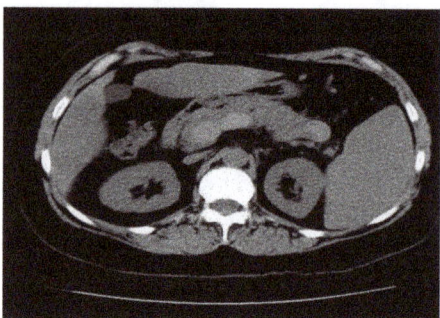

FIGURE 2: CT demonstrating splenic thrombosis.

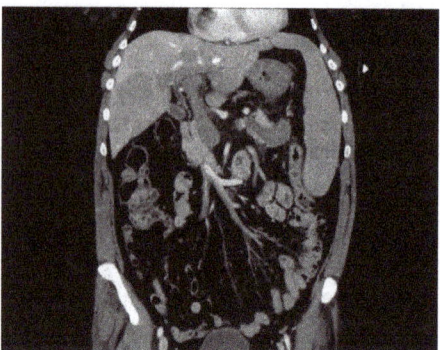

FIGURE 3: Superior mesenteric thrombosis.

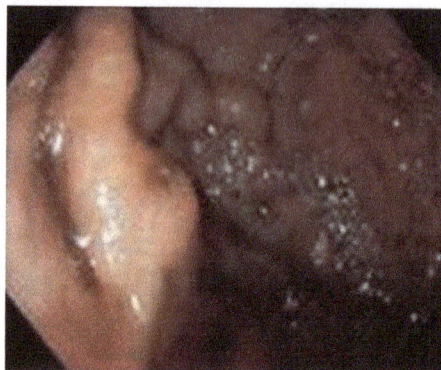

FIGURE 4: EGD demonstrated a gastric varix with erosion.

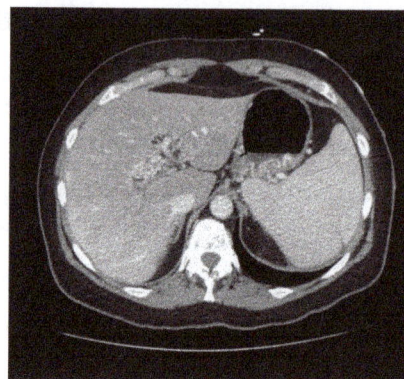

FIGURE 5: CT demonstrated periportal collateral circulation and gastric varices.

Initial vital signs were remarkable for tachycardia with heart rate of 103, but otherwise benign with a blood pressure of 120/78, respiratory rate of 16, temperature of 98.3 F, and oxygen saturation of 98% on room air. Examination revealed no conjunctival pallor, moist mucosal membranes, and no acute distress. Abdominal examination revealed mild tenderness to palpation of the epigastric region, without guarding, rebound, rigidity, or organomegaly; normoactive bowel sounds; and no stigmata of chronic liver disease.

Initial laboratory evaluation revealed hemoglobin of 10.4 g/dL (she had a normal hemoglobin value of 14.6 g/dL eight weeks prior to presentation), white blood cell count of 10.1×10^9/L, a platelet count of 325×10^9/L, prothrombin time (PT) of 33.4 (11.7–14.2 sec), partial thromboplastin time (PTT) of 41 (24–36 sec), and international normalized ratio

(INR) of 3.6 (0.8–1.3). Alanine aminotransferase, aspartate aminotransferase, alkaline phosphatase, total bilirubin, blood urea nitrogen, and creatinine were all within normal limits.

She was admitted and started on pantoprazole with an 80 mg IV bolus followed by a maintenance rate of 8 mg/hour. She was typed and crossed for two units of packed red blood cells and received two units of fresh frozen plasma. Repeated CBC the following morning showed that her hemoglobin decreased from 10.4 to 7.1 g/dL, and she was transfused with two units of PRBC and two more units of FFP. INR following the transfusion was 1.7. EGD revealed isolated fundic varices with an erosion over a moderately large gastric varix (Figure 4). Intravenous octreotide at 50 mcg/hr and propranolol 20 mg orally twice a day were started.

Abdominal computed tomography (CT) showed reduced clot burden within the portal, splenic, and superior mesenteric veins compared to her recent hospitalization; however, she also had new periportal collateral veins and fundic gastric varices (Figure 5). In spite of conservative measures, she continued to bleed with another decrease in hemoglobin to 7.1 g/dL. The patient was transfused one more unit of PRBC and vaccinated for encapsulated organisms, and surgery was consulted. Hand-assisted laparoscopic splenectomy was performed after reviewing all possible options and risks, and benefits were discussed with the patient. Postoperative EGD demonstrated near complete resolution of gastric varices

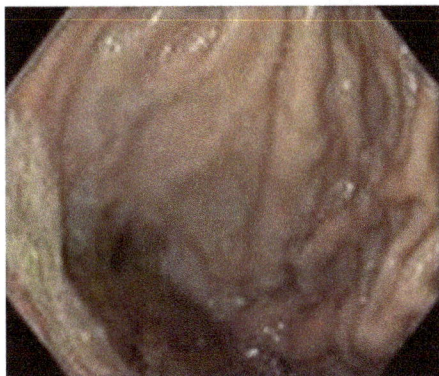

FIGURE 6: Follow-up EGD demonstrated resolution of varices.

(Figure 6). Twelve months after discharge on warfarin, there has been no reported recurrence of hemorrhage. Repeated abdominal CT imaging one year after discharge showed no significant interval change in splenic, portal, and mesenteric veins thromboses. Also, prominent periportal collateral veins as well as prominent veins near the gastric fundus persisted.

3. Discussion

Gastric varices (GV) are generally divided into those that are a result of splenic vein thrombosis (SVT) and those from portal hypertension (cirrhotic or noncirrhotic). SVT usually develops in the context of acute or chronic pancreatitis, pancreatic pseudocyst, or neoplasm [4–7]. However, GV arising from portal hypertension are more common than from SVT [1]. SVT-associated GV tend to present as multiple varices and are often difficult to manage endoscopically because of bleeding recurrence in alternative short gastric connections [4]. For these patients, splenectomy often resolves the varices.

An estimated 30% of cirrhotic patients develop variceal bleeding, and of these, approximately 10% to 20% are gastric varices [8, 9]. Gastric variceal bleeding tends to be more severe and to have greater morbidity and mortality than esophageal variceal bleeding [9]. Fundal varices have accounted for up to 80% of bleeding GV in one series [9].

Fundal varices often appear as serpiginous, vascular structures or may also present as polypoid masses [4]. Fundal varices may present as an acute, active hemorrhage or incidentally discovered varices. Their polypoid appearance has led to errant biopsy in patients without known liver disease or thrombosis [4]. High-risk GV with recent bleeding or bleeding fundal varices are often difficult to treat. Previous studies have shown a high failure rate for acute control and an early rebleeding rate with sclerotherapy [10].

Initial treatment of variceal hemorrhage involves octreotide and balloon tamponade, followed by either surgery or transjugular intrahepatic portosystemic shunt (TIPS). Gastric varices secondary to portal hypertension are often amenable to emergency TIPS for short-term control [11]. In hemorrhage from varices secondary to isolated SVT, splenectomy is the preferred treatment. Splenectomy decompresses

the short gastric vessels by decreasing the inflow from the splenic circulation.

Splenectomy is a known treatment for gastric varices secondary to isolated SVT; however, the presence of multiple thromboses complicates treatment decisions. Our patient was also not a candidate for a shunt procedure. Although the lack of esophageal varices and the transformed portal veins was reassuring, complications of splenectomy in this context may include further thrombosis of the mesenteric system, worsening of the right-sided portal hypertension, and subsequent development of esophageal varices.

4. Conclusion

Gastric variceal bleeding may be caused by portal hypertension or splenic vein thrombosis. In the context of portal hypertension, emergency TIPS is often successful in controlling hemorrhage. Splenectomy is often reserved for patients with isolated splenic vein thrombosis, and in the context of multiple splanchnic and portal thrombosis, treatment is more complicated. We report that splenectomy was a successful treatment for this patient with gastric varices and multivessel extrahepatic thromboses secondary to essential thrombocythemia.

Disclosure

The views expressed in this paper are those of the authors and do not reflect the official policy or position of the Department of the Army, Department of Defense, or the US Government. This work did not receive any specific grant from any funding agency in the public, commercial, or not-for-profit sector.

References

[1] S. K. Sarin, D. Lahoti, S. P. Saxena, N. S. Murthy, and U. K. Makwana, "Prevalence, classification and natural history of gastric varices: a long-term follow-up study in 568 portal hypertension patients," *Hepatology*, vol. 16, no. 6, pp. 1343–1349, 1992.

[2] S. Irani, K. Kowdley, and R. Kozarek, "Gastric varices: an updated review of management," *Journal of Clinical Gastroenterology*, vol. 45, no. 2, pp. 133–148, 2011.

[3] S. K. Sarin and S. Negi, "Management of gastric variceal hemorrhage," *Indian Journal of Gastroenterology*, vol. 25, pp. S25–S28, 2006.

[4] A. M. Al-Osaimi and S. H. Caldwell, "Medical and endoscopic management of gastric varices," *Seminars in Interventional Radiology*, vol. 28, no. 3, pp. 273–282, 2011.

[5] J. P. Sutton, D. Y. Yarborough, and J. T. Richards, "Isolated splenic vein occlusion. Review of literature and report of an additional case," *Archives of Surgery*, vol. 100, no. 5, pp. 623–626, 1970.

[6] G. R. D. Evans, A. E. Yellin, F. A. Weaver, and S. C. Stain, "Sinistral (left-sided) portal hypertension," *American Surgeon*, vol. 56, no. 12, pp. 758–763, 1990.

[7] C. Muhletaler, A. J. Gerlock Jr., V. Goncharenko et al., "Gastric varices secondary to splenic vein occlusion: radiographic diagnosis and clinical significance," *Radiology*, vol. 132, no. 3, pp. 593–598, 1979.

[8] B. M. Ryan, R. W. Stockbrugger, and J. M. Ryan, "A pathophysiologic, gastroenterologic, and radiologic approach to the management of gastric varices," *Gastroenterology*, vol. 126, no. 4, pp. 1175–1189, 2004.

[9] W. Trudeau and T. Prindiville, "Endoscopic injection sclerosis in bleeding gastric varices," *Gastrointestinal Endoscopy*, vol. 32, no. 4, pp. 264–268, 1986.

[10] S. K. Sarin, "Long-term follow-up of gastric variceal sclerotherapy: an eleven-year experience," *Gastrointestinal Endoscopy*, vol. 46, no. 1, pp. 8–14, 1997.

[11] T. N. Chau, D. Patch, Y. W. Chan et al., "'Salvage' transjugular intrahepatic portosystemic shunts: gastric fundal compared with esophageal variceal bleeding," *Gastroenterology*, vol. 114, no. 5, pp. 981–987, 1998.

6

Gastrojejunal Anastomosis Perforation after Gastric Bypass on a Patient with Underlying Pancreatic Cancer

Omar Bellorin,[1] Anna Kundel,[2] Alexander Ramirez-Valderrama,[1] and Armando Castro[1]

[1]Department of General Surgery, New York Hospital Medical Center of Queens/Weill Cornell Medical College, 5645 Main Street, Flushing, NY 11355, USA
[2]Department of Endocrine Surgery, New York University Langone Medical Center, 550 First Avenue, New York, NY 10016, USA

Correspondence should be addressed to Omar Bellorin; omarbellorin@gmail.com

Academic Editor: Muthukumaran Rangarajan

Introduction. We describe a case of gastrojejunal anastomosis perforation after gastric bypass on a patient with underlying pancreatic cancer. *Case Description.* A 54-year-old female with past surgical history of gastric bypass for morbid obesity and recent diagnosis of unresectable pancreatic cancer presents with abdominal pain, peritonitis, and sepsis. Computerized axial tomography scan shows large amount of intraperitoneal free air. The gastric remnant is markedly distended and a large pancreatic head mass is seen. Intraoperative findings were consistent with a perforated ulcer located at the gastrojejunal anastomosis and a distended gastric remnant caused by a pancreatic mass invading and obstructing the second portion of the duodenum. The gastrojejunal perforation was repaired using an omental patch. A gastrostomy for decompression of the remnant was also performed. The patient had a satisfactory postoperative period and was discharged on day 7. *Discussion.* Perforation of the gastrojejunal anastomosis after Roux-en-Y gastric bypass is an unusual complication. There is no correlation between the perforation and the presence of pancreatic cancer. They represent two different conditions that coexisted. The presence of a gastrojejunal perforation made the surgeon aware of the advanced stage of the pancreatic cancer.

1. Introduction

We present a case of a patient with history of pancreatic cancer and Roux-en-Y gastric bypass for morbid obesity who presented with acute abdomen secondary to perforation at the gastrojejunum anastomosis (GJA). The ideology, medical and surgical treatment, surveillance, and complications of GJA ulceration are reviewed. The relationship of obesity and cancer and its implications after gastric bypass is also addressed.

2. Case Description

54-year-old female with past surgical history of antecolic antegastric Roux-en-Y gastric bypass in 2004 and recently diagnosed with unresectable pancreatic cancer status after chemotherapy presents with severe left upper quadrant abdominal pain and left sided chest pain which began 12

hours prior. Her current BMI is 35 and she still receives treatment for hypertension and diabetes. The pain was sudden in onset, sharp, and radiating to left shoulder. She had no previous episodes and had no recent esophagogastroduodenoscopy (EGD). Physical exam reveals tachycardia, tachypnea, hypotension, and left upper quadrant tenderness and guarding consistent with peritonitis. Computerized axial tomography (CAT) of the abdomen shows moderate to large amount of intraperitoneal free air, likely representing bowel perforation. The gastric remnant is markedly distended and the free air is only seen in the upper abdomen (Figure 1). There is a pancreatic mass obstructing the second portion of the duodenum (Figure 2).

The patient was resuscitated with intravenous fluid and given antibiotics and thereafter was brought to the operating room for exploratory laparotomy.

Intraoperative findings were consistent with a perforated ulcer located at the GJA and a distended gastric remnant

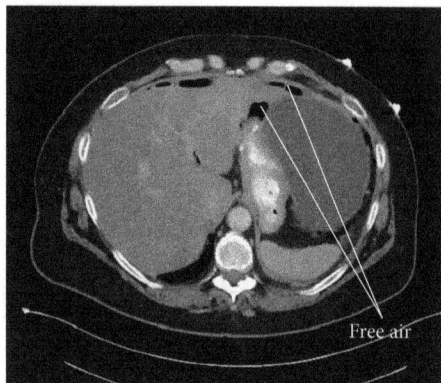

FIGURE 1: CT scan of abdomen showing moderate to large amount of intraperitoneal free air, likely representing bowel perforation.

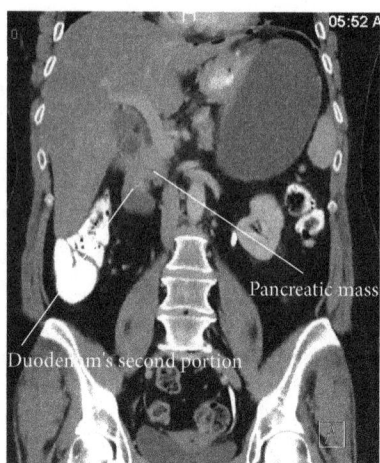

FIGURE 2: CT scan of abdomen demonstrating a pancreatic mass obstructing the second portion of the duodenum.

TABLE 1: Reported incidence of marginal ulceration of GJA after gastric bypass.

Author	Incidence of GJA ulceration (%)
Suggs et al. [1]	6.3
Higa et al. [12]	1.4
Gonzalez et al. [2]	0
Luján et al. [13]	3.4
DeMaria et al. [14]	5.1
Kligman et al. [3]	0.6
Schwartz et al. [4]	0.8
MacLean et al. [15]	16

caused by a pancreatic mass invading and obstructing the second portion of the duodenum. The abdominal cavity was thoroughly washed and the GJA perforation was repaired using an omental patch (Graham's). A gastrostomy for decompression of the remnant was also performed. The patient had a satisfactory postoperative period and was discharged on day 7.

3. Discussion

Patients with gastric bypass may experience a wide variety of complications that can be classified as acute or chronic. Marginal ulcers of the GJA usually represent a chronic complication that the bariatric surgeon encounters frequently.

The reported incidence of marginal ulceration of GJA after gastric bypass varies widely, ranging from 0 to 16% (Table 1). The risk factors for ulceration are smoking, use of nonsteroidal anti-inflammatory drugs (NSAIDs) and steroids, stress, recent surgery, and the presence of gastrogastric fistulas. Higher incidence has been reported in patients who underwent gastric bypass using circular staplers for the construction of the GJA as opposed to a linear stapler [1–4].

The use of nonabsorbable sutures in the GJA is also associated with marginal ulceration [5]. The presence of *Helicobacter pylori* may additionally play a role in the development of marginal ulcers. Schirmer et al. [6] described a 2.4% incidence of marginal ulcers in patients who underwent treatment for *Helicobacter pylori* preoperatively compared to those who did not (6.8%).

The majority of these ulcers can be treated medically. However, a subset of patients will have intractable disease requiring surgery for definitive management as the last resort. Patients with marginal ulcers are primarily medically treated with H2 blockers or proton pump inhibitors. Sucralfate is also added as well as smoking cessation and substitution of ulcerogenic medications. An upper gastrointestinal study is advised if a gastrogastric fistula is suspected and/or patients show no improvement after medical management. There is no consensus on the length of treatment, but the majority of bariatric surgeons choose a minimum of two to three months' regimen followed by an upper endoscopy for confirmation of resolution. Some surgeons advocate the endoscopic removal of nonabsorbable sutures, if present [5].

Clinically the symptoms suggestive of marginal ulceration include, but are not limited to, upper abdominal pain or progressive upper abdominal discomfort and intolerance of food and upper gastrointestinal bleed. Intractability is generally defined as persistence of symptoms after 3 months of medical treatment. Patel et al. [7] reported 39 patients with intractable marginal ulcers whose primary signs and symptoms included chronic abdominal pain (66.6%), GI bleeding (20.5%), stomal obstruction (10.2%), and perforation (2.5%). A minority of these patients will present with an acute abdomen similar to the patient we presented, and free perforation of the ulcer must be ruled out. Perforation of GJA ulcers is uncommon; the incidence ranges from 0.25 to 1% [7–10]. The risk factors for perforation are the same as for ulceration; however, smoking, history of recent surgery, and NSAIDs and steroids use are the common denominator in this particular situation [11]. They represent a life-threatening condition with a mortality rate of 10% [11].

Patients with perforation of a GJA ulcer need aggressive fluid resuscitation and prompt initiation of antibiotic therapy prior to any urgent surgical management. The definitive approach can be performed via open surgery or laparoscopy and consists of primary repair of the ulcer and omental patch along with a thorough washout of the abdominal cavity. A gastrostomy for feeding purposes should be performed as well. Large perforations not amenable to primary and patch repair may require revision of the gastrojejunal anastomosis.

The decision to use laparoscopic approach depended solely on the surgeon's expertise and confidence in advanced laparoscopy. There are several studies comparing open versus laparoscopic repair of perforated peptic ulcers that have demonstrated better outcomes in the laparoscopic group [16, 17]. Shorter hospital stay, reduced wound pain, and earlier return to normal activities are the main advantages. Kalaiselvan et al. [11] reported a series of 10 patients presented with perforated GJA ulcers. All patients were treated with abdominal washout, primary closure of the perforation, and omental patch. Five patients were operated on by general surgeons via an open approach and 5 underwent laparoscopic repair by bariatric surgeons. The laparoscopic group experienced lower morbidity, no mortality, and shorter hospital stay compared to those who underwent open surgery.

Postoperatively, these patients should have a reduction of risk factors, prolonged H2 blockers/proton pump inhibitors regimen, and eradication of *Helicobacter pylori* on those tested positive.

Also an upper endoscopy 3 months after the procedure to assess the GJA is recommended.

Obesity and cancer are strongly related. In the United States, approximately 85,000 new cases of patients with cancer per year are related to obesity [18]. Studies have found that an increase of body mass index by 5 kg/m^2 is associated with a 10% higher cancer-related mortality. On the other hand, patients who undergo bariatric surgery have a lower incidence of cancer and a decrease in cancer-related mortality. This is presumably related to weight loss as demonstrated by Adams et al. [19] in a 12.5-year mean follow-up study of patients who underwent gastric bypass surgery compared to severely obese controls.

Early detection and treatment of cancer in patients undergoing bariatric surgery may also play a role. These patients undergo comprehensive gastrointestinal, pulmonary, and cardiovascular workup preoperatively that is not performed routinely in the general population. Moreover, the stomach remnant after gastric bypass will no longer be conveniently accessible, thus making the preoperative assessment of the upper gastrointestinal tract even more important. Zeni et al. [20] reported the presence of Barrett's esophagus in preoperative EGD to be 1.3%, GIST in 0.7%, gastric polyps in 5%, and *Helicobacter pylori*-associated gastritis and duodenitis in 27% and 6%, respectively. This extensive workup may result in early cancer diagnosis and is possibly part of the reason why patients undergoing obesity surgery have a lower cancer-related mortality.

Once a gastric bypass for obesity is performed, access to the gastric remnant and the biliary tree becomes complicated. There is no standard recommendation for a routine assessment of the gastric remnant after gastric bypass. Although technically difficult, double balloon enteroscopy is a feasible way to assess the duodenum and the residual stomach when the patient experiences symptoms that warrants further

workup. Ultrasound or CT guided percutaneous gastrostomy and subsequent gastroscopy are another option. Combined laparoscopy-endoscopy can be used as last resort for diagnosis and treatment.

This anatomic exclusion certainly may result in a delayed diagnosis and treatment of a gastric/duodenal/pancreatic/periampular cancer. A locally advanced pancreatic mass in a patient who has undergone a gastric bypass may result in gastric outlet obstruction of the remaining stomach, which may lead to gastric distention, isquemia, and eventual perforation of the gastric remnant. A decompressive gastrostomy of the remnant is the treatment of choice to avoid this complication.

4. Conclusion

Perforation of the GJA after Roux-en-Y gastric bypass is an unusual complication. There is no correlation between the perforation and the presence of pancreatic cancer. They represent two different conditions that coexisted. The presence of a gastrojejunal perforation made the surgeon aware of the advanced stage of the pancreatic cancer that otherwise would have remained undetected for longer time. Overall the approach performed on the presented patient corresponds to the standard and the current literature. The laparoscopic approach by an experienced surgeon may afford the patient the advantages of minimally invasive surgery.

References

[1] W. J. Suggs, W. Kouli, M. Lupovici, W. Y. Chau, and R. E. Brolin, "Complications at gastrojejunostomy after laparoscopic Roux-en-Y gastric bypass: comparison between 21- and 25 mm circular staplers," *Surgery for Obesity and Related Diseases*, vol. 3, no. 5, pp. 508–514, 2007.

[2] R. Gonzalez, E. Lin, K. R. Venkatesh, S. P. Bowers, and C. D. Smith, "Gastrojejunostomy during laparoscopic gastric bypass," *Archives of Surgery*, vol. 138, no. 2, pp. 181–184, 2003.

[3] M. D. Kligman, C. Thomas, and J. Saxe, "Effect of the learning curve on the early outcomes of laparoscopic Roux-en-Y gastric bypass," *American Surgeon*, vol. 69, no. 4, pp. 304–309, 2003.

[4] M. L. Schwartz, R. L. Drew, R. W. Roiger, S. R. Ketover, and M. Chazin-Caldie, "Stenosis of the gastroenterostomy after laparoscopic gastric bypass," *Obesity Surgery*, vol. 14, no. 4, pp. 484–491, 2004.

[5] B. C. Sacks, S. G. Mattar, F. G. Qureshi et al., "Incidence of marginal ulcers and the use of absorbable anastomotic sutures in laparoscopic Roux-en-Y gastric bypass," *Surgery for Obesity and Related Diseases*, vol. 2, no. 1, pp. 11–16, 2006.

[6] B. Schirmer, C. Erenoglu, and A. Miller, "Flexible endoscopy in the management of patients undergoing Roux-en-Y gastric bypass," *Obesity Surgery*, vol. 12, no. 5, pp. 634–638, 2002.

[7] R. A. Patel, R. E. Brolin, and A. Gandhi, "Revisional operations for marginal ulcer after Roux-en-Y gastric bypass," *Surgery for Obesity and Related Diseases*, vol. 5, no. 3, pp. 317–322, 2009.

[8] M. Lublin, M. McCoy, and D. J. Waldrep, "Perforating marginal ulcers after laparoscopic gastric bypass," *Surgical Endoscopy and Other Interventional Techniques*, vol. 20, no. 1, pp. 51–54, 2006.

[9] A. M. C. Macgregor, N. E. Pickens, and E. K. Thoburn, "Perforated peptic ulcer following gastric bypass for obesity," *American Surgeon*, vol. 65, no. 3, pp. 222–225, 1999.

[10] E. L. Felix, J. Kettelle, E. Mobley, and D. Swartz, "Perforated marginal ulcers after laparoscopic gastric bypass," *Surgical Endoscopy*, vol. 22, no. 10, pp. 2128–2132, 2008.

[11] R. Kalaiselvan, G. Exarchos, N. Hamza, and B. J. Ammori, "Incidence of perforated gastrojejunal anastomotic ulcers after laparoscopic gastric bypass for morbid obesity and role of laparoscopy in their management," *Surgery for Obesity and Related Diseases*, vol. 8, no. 4, pp. 423–428, 2012.

[12] K. D. Higa, K. B. Boone, and T. Ho, "Complications of the laparoscopic Roux-en-Y gastric bypass: 1,040 patients—what have we learned?" *Obesity Surgery*, vol. 10, no. 6, pp. 509–513, 2000.

[13] J. A. Luján, M. D. Frutos, Q. Hernández, J. R. Cuenca, G. Valero, and P. Parrilla, "Experience with the circular stapler for the gastrojejunostomy in laparoscopic gastric bypass (350 cases)," *Obesity Surgery*, vol. 15, no. 8, pp. 1096–1102, 2005.

[14] E. J. DeMaria, H. J. Sugerman, J. M. Kellum, J. G. Meador, and L. G. Wolfe, "Results of 281 consecutive total laparoscopic Roux-en-Y gastric bypasses to treat morbid obesity," *Annals of Surgery*, vol. 235, no. 5, pp. 640–647, 2002.

[15] L. D. MacLean, B. M. Rhode, C. Nohr, S. Katz, and A. P. H. McLean, "Stomal ulcer after gastric bypass," *Journal of the American College of Surgeons*, vol. 185, no. 1, pp. 1–7, 1997.

[16] W. T. Siu, H. T. Leong, B. K. B. Law et al., "Laparoscopic repair for perforated peptic ulcer: a randomized controlled trial," *Annals of Surgery*, vol. 235, no. 3, pp. 313–319, 2002.

[17] V. Minutolo, G. Gagliano, C. Rinzivillo et al., "Laparoscopic surgical treatment of perforated duodenal ulcer," *Chirurgia italiana*, vol. 61, no. 3, pp. 309–313, 2009.

[18] K. Basen-Engquist and M. Chang, "Obesity and cancer risk: recent review and evidence," *Current Oncology Reports*, vol. 13, no. 1, pp. 71–76, 2011.

[19] T. D. Adams, A. M. Stroup, R. E. Gress et al., "Cancer incidence and mortality after gastric bypass surgery," *Obesity*, vol. 17, no. 4, pp. 796–802, 2009.

[20] T. M. Zeni, C. T. Frantzides, C. Mahr et al., "Value of preoperative upper endoscopy in patients undergoing laparoscopic gastric bypass," *Obesity Surgery*, vol. 16, no. 2, pp. 142–146, 2006.

7

A Pleural Solitary Fibrous Tumor, Multiple Gastrointestinal Stromal Tumors, Moyamoya Disease, and Hyperparathyroidism in a Patient Associated with NF1

Yoko Yamamoto,[1] Ken Kodama,[1] Shigekazu Yokoyama,[2] Masashi Takeda,[3] and Shintaro Michishita[4]

[1]Department of Thoracic Surgery, Yao Municipal Hospital, Yao City, Osaka 581-0069, Japan
[2]Department of Gastroenterological Surgery, Yao Municipal Hospital, Yao City, Osaka 581-0069, Japan
[3]Department of Pathology, Yao Municipal Hospital, Yao City, Osaka 581-0069, Japan
[4]Department of Breast and Endocrine Surgery, Osaka University, Osaka 565-0871, Japan

Correspondence should be addressed to Yoko Yamamoto; yokes615@yahoo.co.jp

Academic Editor: Geeta Lal

Neurofibromatosis type 1 (NF1), also called von Recklinghausen's disease, is a multisystemic disease caused by an alteration of the NF1 gene, a tumor suppressor located on the long arm of chromosome 17 (17q11.2). Loss of the gene function, due to a point mutation, leads to an increase in cell proliferation and the development of several tumors. We report a 60-year-old female patient manifesting hypercalcemia due to hyperparathyroidism, a solitary fibrous tumor (SFT) of the pleura, multiple gastrointestinal stromal tumors (GISTs), and moyamoya disease associated with NF1. The SFT and GISTs were removed by staged operations. Then, hypercalcemia was successfully controlled after resection of the parathyroid adenoma. Based on a literature review, these combinations have never been reported, and the relevant literature is briefly discussed.

1. Introduction

Neurofibromatosis type 1 (NF1) is an autosomal dominant inherited disease characterized by café-au-lait spots and multiple dermal neurofibromatosis. This condition is also known as von Recklinghausen's disease. NF1 is caused by mutation of the NF1 gene, which spans over 350 kb of genomic DNA on chromosome 17q11.2. The protein encoded by the NF1 gene is neurofibromin, which is a member of the GTPase-activating protein (GAP) family of Ras regulatory proteins.

NF1 is also associated with several tumors. Some reports have described the association of NF1 and GISTs, which are the most common mesenchymal neoplasms of the gastrointestinal tract. In many cases of NF1, multiple GISTs predominantly involve the small intestine. On the other hand, a solitary fibrous tumor (SFT) is a rare spindle cell neoplasm, usually occurring in the pleura. The association between an SFT and NF1 has not been elucidated. Moyamoya disease, which is a cerebrovascular disease of unknown cause, is also rarely seen in NF1 patients.

The association of NF1 and primary hyperparathyroidism is also described as a rare entity. This association supports the hypothesis that it is one of the variant types of multiendocrine neoplasia (MEN) syndrome.

Here, we report the results of treating an NF1 patient with the coexistence of multiple GISTs of the gastrointestinal tract, SFT of the pleura, hyperparathyroidism, and moyamoya disease.

2. Case

In August, 2013, a 60-year-old Japanese female consulted her primary physician for melena. Her laboratory tests showed anemia and hypercalcemia. Whole body computed tomography (CT) performed at that time showed an anterior mediastinal nodule, and an abdominal tumor was detected

(a)   (b)

(c)

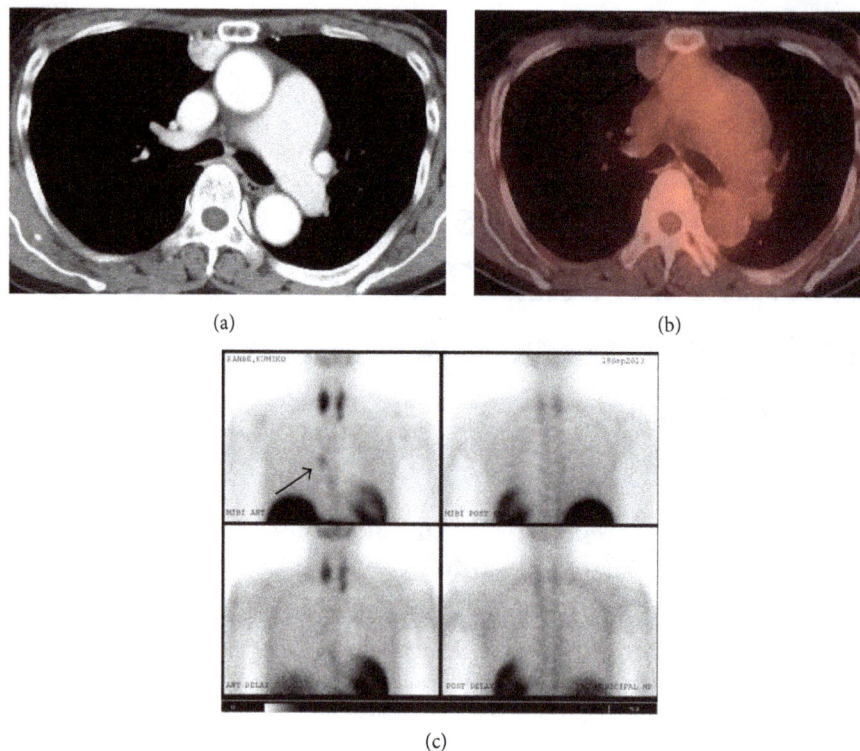

FIGURE 1: Mediastinal nodule (arrow). (a) CT revealed the presence of a 20 mm nodule in the anterior mediastinum. (b) PET-CT imaging revealed FDG uptake in the nodule. (c) Tc 99m MIBI scan showing an intense focus in the anterior mediastinum.

concomitantly. Then, she was referred to our hospital for further investigation.

Physical examination revealed café-au-lait spots as well as multiple skin nodules distributed over her entire body and Lisch nodules on her eyes, thus showing typical features of NF1. Her two daughters were positive for similar skin findings, but there was no evidence of familial MEN syndrome.

Laboratory tests showed a serum calcium level of 11.8 mg/dL (normal range: 8.6–10.1), a phosphorus level of 2.4 mg/dL (normal range: 2.5–4.5), and a plasma intact parathyroid hormone (PTH) level of 427.2 pg/mL (normal range: <65.0), and a diagnosis of primary hyperparathyroidism was made. No tumor markers were elevated.

Her chest CT revealed the presence of a 20 mm nodule in the anterior mediastinum adjacent to the right pleura (Figure 1(a)). The nodule showed no invasion to the surrounding structures. Abdominal CT revealed a 40 mm, well-circumscribed, firm, and well-enhanced mass adjacent to the upper jejunum (Figure 2(a)). Positron emission tomography (PET) revealed focal FDG uptake (standard uptake value (SUV) max, 4.2) in the abdominal mass (Figure 2(b)) but not mediastinal nodule (Figure 1(b)). Tc 99m MIBI parathyroid scintigraphy demonstrated an intense focus in the anterior mediastinum (Figure 1(c)). Thus, the mediastinal nodule was diagnosed as an ectopic parathyroid adenoma. Magnetic resonance imaging (MRI) of the abdomen demonstrated the mass showing a low signal intensity in T1-weighted images and intermediate signal intensity in a T2-weighted image.

Both gastroscopic and colonoscopic examinations were within their normal limit. Endoscopic ultrasonography (EUS) demonstrated that the internal echo of the main lesion was slightly heterogeneous and separated from the pancreas. Spindle cells were verified by EUS-fine needle aspiration (EUS-FNA) cytology. Based on these findings, the abdominal tumor was suspected to be a GIST.

Further examinations using MRI were conducted to investigate the clinical manifestations of NF1. As a result, brain MRI revealed no brain tumor. On the other hand, MR angiography showed occlusion of the bilateral internal carotid artery (ICA) and the absence of the anterior and middle cerebral arteries with multiple tiny basal collateral arteries (Figure 3). These findings are consistent with moyamoya disease.

Initially, we attempted resection of the anterior mediastinal nodule diagnosed with ectopic parathyroid adenoma to control her hypercalcemia. We resected the nodule with hemithymus through a median sternotomy. However, after the operation, the serum calcium level was not decreased. Based on permanent section histology (Figure 4(a)), the tumor was composed of a solid, unorganized proliferation of spindle cells with small and mildly irregular nuclei. No significant necrosis was seen. Immunohistochemistry examination shows positive reactivity for c-Kit (Figure 4(b)), CD34 (Figure 4(c)), bcl-2, and STAT6, but it shows negative result for AE1/3, S-100 protein, and SMA. The Ki-67 labeling index was irregularly expressed, exhibiting positivity in up to

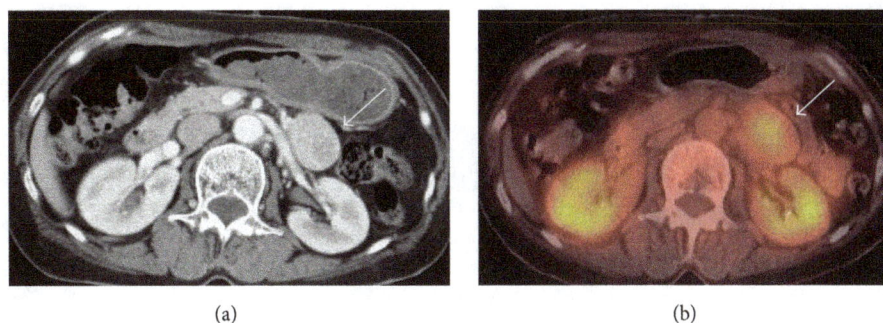

FIGURE 2: Abdominal mass (arrow). (a) CT revealed a 40 mm, well-circumscribed, firm, and well-enhanced mass adjacent to the upper jejunum. (b) PET-CT imaging showing the abdominal mass with an SUV max of 4.2.

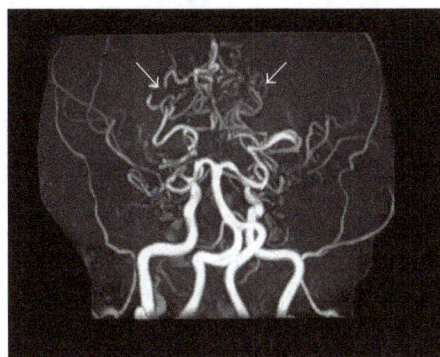

FIGURE 3: MR angiography confirmed occlusion of the bilateral internal carotid artery (ICA) and the absence of the anterior and middle cerebral arteries with multiple tiny basal collateral arteries (arrows).

about 5% of neoplastic cell. There was neither cell invasion in the thymus nor evidence of malignancy. Pathologically, the tumor was diagnosed as a benign SFT of the pleura based on the above findings. Her postoperative course was uneventful. She was discharged with no complications under medical control of hypercalcemia.

Three months after the first operation, she received a laparotomy under a clinical diagnosis of GIST of the upper jejunum. The operative findings showed multiple mucosal tumors in the stomach, 2nd portion of the duodenum, distal to the ligament of Treitz, and in the upper part of the jejunum. During the operation, we found 9 tumors, and all of them were removed. These tumors showed an extramural growth pattern, the main tumor measured 35 mm in diameter distal to the ligament of Treitz and the other tumors were less than 10 mm. Histological examination (Figure 4(d)) showed that the tumors were highly cellular and composed of spindle-shaped cells arising in the proper muscle layer of the gastrointestinal wall. No significant necrosis was seen. The overlying mucosa was intact. Immunohistochemically, the tumors were strongly stained positive for c-Kit (Figure 4(e)) and CD34 (Figure 4(f)), whereas S-100 and SMA were negative. The Ki-67 labeling index was less than 2-3%. The postoperative course after the second operation was also uneventful, and she was discharged with no complications.

Four months after the second operation, we performed MIBI scintigraphy again. The second time, MIBI scintigraphy revealed focal uptake in the left lower pole of thyroid gland and neck ultrasound showed solid nodule in the left lower pole of thyroid gland. She subsequently underwent parathyroidectomy to control hypercalcemia. The pathological diagnosis was parathyroid adenoma. After the operation, the value of serum Ca rapidly decreased to within the normal range. She showed a favorable condition 14 months after the first surgery without symptoms.

3. Discussion

The NF1 occurs in about 1 in 3,000–3,500 births, and it can be familial with an autosomal inheritance pattern. In addition to cutaneous café-au-lait spots and multiple neurofibromas, various accompanying lesions are known to occur in the eyes, bone, central nerves, and endocrine system [1, 2]. Gastrointestinal abnormalities in NF1 patients have been reported to occur in up to 10–25% of patients, including mesenchymal neoplasms, neuroendocrine tumors of the duodenum, hyperplasia of intestinal neural tissues, and other gastrointestinal neoplasms [3]. The overall rate of NF1 among GIST patients can reach up to 6% [4]. GISTs originate from the intestinal cells of Cajal (ICC). They are often found in patients with anemia, constipation or obstruction, and palpation of a tumor. Making an early diagnosis of a GIST is important due to the risk of malignancy and hemorrhagic-obstructive complications. GISTs can be better defined on

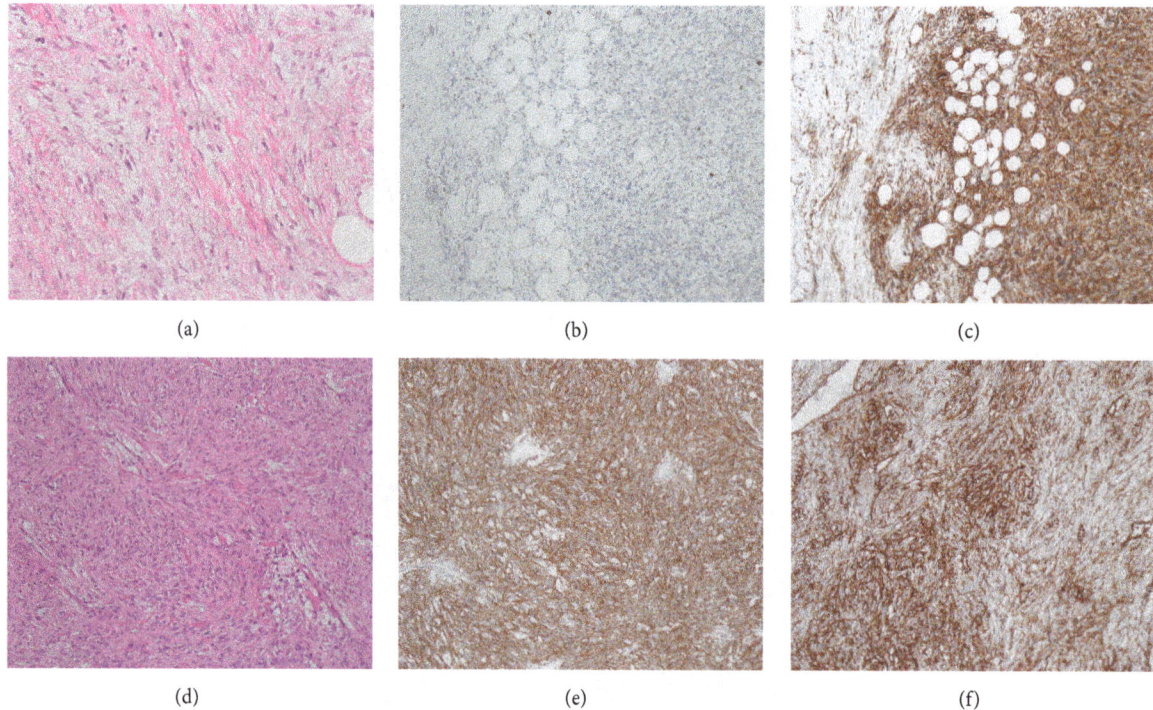

(a)　　　　　　　　　　　　　　(b)　　　　　　　　　　　　　　(c)

(d)　　　　　　　　　　　　　　(e)　　　　　　　　　　　　　　(f)

FIGURE 4: Histologic findings. A SFT composed of a solid unorganized proliferation of spindle cells with small and mildly irregular nuclei (a) (hematoxylin and eosin; ×40), which showed the absence of c-Kit (b) and the presence of CD34 (c) markers on immunohistochemical staining (×20). A GIST composed of spindle-shaped cells with marked cellularity (d) (hematoxylin and eosin; ×40), which showed the presence of c-Kit (e) and CD34 (f) markers on immunohistochemical staining (×20).

immunohistochemical examination: positive activity for c-Kit and CD34 and negative activity for S-100 [5]. GISTs are the most common mesenchymal neoplasms of the gastrointestinal tract and they have been described in association with NF1. The incidence of GISTs in NF1 patients varies from 3.9 to 25% [4]. The majority of GISTs in NF1 patients were reported to be multicentric and mainly localized in the jejunum, as in the present case, and these tumors were not associated with malignancy, suggesting a favorable long-term prognosis, which is rarely observed in sporadic GISTs. Surgical resection remains the mainstay of treatment and offers the only chance for cure [6, 7]. Adjuvant chemotherapy or radiotherapy had not been proven to be effective [6].

A solitary fibrous tumor (SFT) is an uncommon mesenchymal neoplasm that arises primarily from the pleura. Currently, SFTs are immunohistochemically characterized by negative activity for cytokeratin, suggestive of an epithelial origin, and by positive reactivity for CD34, suggestive of a mesenchymal origin, and they are considered to arise from undifferentiated mesenchymal cells in the subpleural connective tissue. The major difference between GISTs and SFTs was strong c-Kit immunoexpression in all GISTs and the absence of this expression in all SFTs [5]. Recently, a recurrent gene fusion NAB2-STAT6 has been identified as molecular hallmark. Molecular detection of the fusion gene and immunohistochemical expression of nuclear STAT6 can be helpful in diagnosing SFT [8]. Adequate therapy consists of complete resection. Histopathologically, SFTs are classified

into benign and malignant forms. The cell density, necrosis, number of mitotic figures, and cell atypia indicate malignancy [9]. Although surgical resection is the treatment rule for pleural SFTs, many SFTs were reported to recur even if they had been diagnosed as benign [10]. Thus, SFTs require complete surgical resection and careful long-term follow-up even if benign. According to our search, the association between SFTs and NF1 has been reported only once before in the English language literature. Conzo et al. firstly described a right suprarenal SFT in a patient with NF1. However, NF1 gene mutation has not been investigated systematically in SFT cases, and the available evidence in the literature is insufficient [11]. Our case is the second reported case of the coexistence of NF1 and SFT. In our case, SFT mimicked the appearance of ectopic parathyroid adenoma based on the finding of Tc-99m MIBI parathyroid scintigraphy. Tc-99m MIBI, a lipophilic cationic molecule which was initially used for cardiac imaging, showed uptake in the mitochondria and cytoplasm of parathyroid tissue. The distribution of Tc-99m MIBI is proportional to blood flow and mitochondrial activity. The sensitivity and positive predictive values of Tc-99m MIBI are 82.1 and 93%, respectively. False uptake of Tc-99m MIBI has been documented in benign and malignant tissues with a high mitochondrial content. Most cases of false-positive Tc-99m MIBI involve thyroid disease. However, other tissues, such as lung, brain, and bone, and carcinoid tumors, lymphoma and thymoma, can also produce false-positive results [12].

Moyamoya disease is characterized by progressive stenosis or occlusion at the distal ends of the bilateral carotid arteries that may subsequently progress to their major branches. The clinical findings present with neurological symptoms, whereas ischemic stroke develops in young adults and subarachnoid hemorrhage develops in older patients in moyamoya disease. Most cases are asymptomatic, as in our present case. The prevalence of moyamoya disease in NF1 patients is estimated at 0.6%, among more than one hundred cases reported in pediatric patients [2, 13]. The gene abnormality has been detected in chromosome 17q25.2, which is in close proximity to the NF1 gene on chromosome 17q11.2. There are several reports concerning the association of moyamoya disease and NF1, which could be explained by the close proximity of genes on chromosome 17 [14].

A combination of hyperparathyroidism and NF1 is also a rare phenomenon. Although some NF1 patients who developed primary hyperparathyroidism have been reported in the literature, the pathogenesis of parathyroid adenoma in NF1 patients has not been yet elucidated, but multiple endocrine adenoma and a genetic link have been suggested. Daly et al. reported that their patients' conditions resembled Sipple's syndrome in that they had both parathyroid adenoma and neurofibromatosis, which suggested the tumors to be genetically linked [15]. Gkaliagkousi et al. described a case with a clinically and genetically established NF1 diagnosis and clinically established MEN2A diagnosis, but genetic testing for MEN2A was negative [16]. Also, there are several case reports in which NF1 was combined not only with the presence of parathyroid neoplasms, but also with other neoplastic disorders [17]. This association supports the hypothesis of a variant of MEN syndrome.

NF1 has been reported to be associated with a number of neoplasms; however, to the best of our knowledge, the coexistence of NF1, SFT, GIST, and moyamoya disease has not been previously reported. Therefore, this case is likely to be the first reported case to involve the coexistence of all four conditions. Further studies are needed to elucidate the association between these rare but interesting conditions. In conclusion, we encountered pleural SFT, multiple GISTs, moyamoya disease, and hyperparathyroidism in a patient with NF1.

References

[1] S. A. Rasmussen and J. M. Friedman, "NF1 gene and neurofibromatosis," *American Journal of Epidemiology*, vol. 151, no. 1, pp. 33–40, 2000.

[2] J. M. Friedman, J. Arbiter, J. A. Epstein et al., "Cardiovascular disease in neurofibromatosis 1: report of the NF1 Cardiovascular Task Force," *Genetics in Medicine*, vol. 4, no. 3, pp. 105–111, 2002.

[3] C. E. Fuller and G. T. Williams, "Gastrointestinal manifestations of type 1 neurofibromatosis (von Recklinghausen's disease)," *Histopathology*, vol. 19, no. 1, pp. 1–11, 1991.

[4] M. Miettinen, J. F. Fetsch, L. H. Sobin, and J. Lasota, "Gastrointestinal stromal tumors in patients with neurofibromatosis 1: a clinicopathologic and molecular genetic study of 45 cases," *American Journal of Surgical Pathology*, vol. 30, no. 1, pp. 90–96, 2006.

[5] V. B. Shidham, M. Chivukula, D. Gupta, R. N. Rao, and R. Komorowski, "Immunohistochemical comparison of gastrointestinal stromal tumor and solitary fibrous tumor," *Archives of Pathology and Laboratory Medicine*, vol. 126, no. 10, pp. 1189–1192, 2002.

[6] K. Hirashima, H. Takamori, M. Hirota et al., "Multiple gastrointestinal stromal tumors in neurofibromatosis type 1: report of a case," *Surgery Today*, vol. 39, no. 11, pp. 979–983, 2009.

[7] J. A. Giuly, R. Picand, D. Giuly, B. Monges, and R. Nguyen-Cat, "Von Recklinghausen disease and gastrointestinal stromal tumors," *American Journal of Surgery*, vol. 185, no. 1, pp. 86–87, 2003.

[8] D. M. England, L. Hochholer, and M. J. McCarthy, "Localized benign and malignant fibrous tumors of pleura. A clinicopathologic review of 223 cases," *The American Journal of Surgical Pathology*, vol. 13, no. 8, pp. 640–658, 1989.

[9] R. Vogels, M. Vlenterie, Y. Versleijen-Jonkers et al., "Solitary fibrous tumor—clinicopathologic, immunohistochemical and molecular analysis of 28 cases," *Diagnostic Pathology*, vol. 9, article 224, 2014.

[10] M. de Perrot, A.-M. Kurt, J. H. Robert, B. Borisch, and A. Spiliopoulos, "Clinical behavior of solitary fibrous tumors of the pleura," *Annals of Thoracic Surgery*, vol. 67, no. 5, pp. 1456–1459, 1999.

[11] G. Conzo, E. Tartaglia, C. Gambardella et al., "Suprarenal solitary fibrous tumor associated with a NF1 gene mutation mimicking a kidney neoplasm: implications for surgical management," *World Journal of Surgical Oncology*, vol. 12, article 87, 2014.

[12] L. C. Cunningham, J.-G. Yu, K. Shilo et al., "Thymoma and parathyroid adenoma: false-positive imaging and intriguing laboratory test results," *JAMA Otolaryngology—Head and Neck Surgery*, vol. 140, no. 4, pp. 369–373, 2014.

[13] E. Vargiami, E. Sapountzi, D. Samakovitis et al., "Moyamoya syndrome and neurofibromatosis type 1," *Italian Journal of Pediatrics*, vol. 40, article 59, 2014.

[14] T. Yamauchi, M. Tada, K. Houkin et al., "Linkage of familial moyamoya disease (spontaneous occlusion of the circle of Willis) to chromosome 17q25," *Stroke*, vol. 31, pp. 930–935, 2000.

[15] D. Daly, M. Kaye, and R. L. Estrada, "Neurofibromatosis and hyperparathyroidism: a new syndrome?" *Canadian Medical Association Journal*, vol. 103, no. 3, pp. 258–259, 1970.

[16] E. Gkaliagkousi, Z. Erlic, K. Petidis et al., "Neurofibromatosis type 1: should we screen for other genetic syndromes? A case report of co-existence with multiple endocrine neoplasia 2A," *European Journal of Clinical Investigation*, vol. 39, no. 9, pp. 828–832, 2009.

[17] A. E. Altinova, F. Toruner, A. R. Cimen et al., "The association of neurofibromatosis, bilateral pheochromocytoma and primary hyperparathyroidism," *Experimental and Clinical Endocrinology and Diabetes*, vol. 115, no. 7, pp. 468–470, 2007.

8

Successful Treatment of Persistent Postcholecystectomy Bile Leak using Percutaneous Cystic Duct Coiling

Vinay Rai,[1] Akin Beckley,[1] Anna Fabre,[2] and Charles F. Bellows[1]

[1]*Department of Surgery, University of New Mexico, Albuquerque, NM 87131, USA*
[2]*Department of Radiology, University of New Mexico, Albuquerque, NM 87131, USA*

Correspondence should be addressed to Vinay Rai; vkrai@salud.unm.edu

Academic Editor: Muthukumaran Rangarajan

Laparoscopic cholecystectomy is one of the most commonly performed operations worldwide. Cystic duct is the most common site of bile leak after cholecystectomy. The treatment of choice is usually conservative. Using sufficient percutaneous drainage of the biloma cavity and endoscopic retrograde cholangiography (ERCP) with sphincterotomy and/or stenting, the cure rate of bile leaks is greater than 90%. In very rare cases, all of these measures remain unsuccessful. We report a technique for the successful treatment of persistent cystic duct leak. After failed ERCP and stenting, bile leak was treated by coiling the cystic duct through a drain tract. This technique is safe and effective and helps avoid the morbidity of reoperation.

1. Introduction

Cystic duct leak is the commonest biliary complication of cholecystectomy [1, 2]. Frequency of cystic duct leak ranges from 0.07 to 0.63% in large series [3]. Endoscopy with sphincterotomy and stenting is the first line of treatment with a success rate greater than 90% [2]. If this option fails, reoperation with ligation or reclipping of cystic duct has been described [4]. However, this is associated with high morbidity and mortality.

We present a case report of a patient who underwent urgent subtotal cholecystectomy complicated by the development of a persistent, controlled bile leak. This was successfully managed using a novel technique by coiling the cystic duct through the drain tract. This case demonstrates an alternative option to treat this complication of cholecystectomy and avoid a high-risk operation.

2. Case Presentation

A 54-year-old morbidly obese female with COPD, diabetes, hypertension, anxiety, and depression presented with right upper quadrant pain, leukocytosis, and fever. Ultrasound confirmed acute cholecystitis. Bile duct was of normal size and liver function tests were normal.

Patient was taken to the operating room for an urgent laparoscopic cholecystectomy. However, upon visualization, gallbladder was gangrenous and conversion to an open subtotal cholecystectomy became necessary due to inability to safely dissect inflammatory adhesions and failure to clearly delineate the anatomy. The gallbladder remnant was closed and a Jackson-Pratt drain was placed in the gallbladder fossa.

The patient initially did well but, on the second postoperative day, a significant amount of bile was noticed in the drain. An endoscopic retrograde cholangiopancreatography (ERCP) was performed and revealed a bile leak from the cystic duct (Figure 1). Biliary sphincterotomy was performed and a 10-French × 7 cm plastic CBD stent placed. The patient did well and was discharged home on POD 5 with JP drain left in place.

During her follow-up visits, persistent leakage of bile was noted despite clinical return to baseline health status. At 8 weeks another ERCP was performed which confirmed an ongoing bile leak from the cystic duct stump. Consequently, the original stent was replaced by a fully covered temporary 10 × 60 millimeter metal CBD stent (Figure 2).

As the bile leak persisted, treatment options were discussed with gastroenterologist and interventional radiologist. Surgical option was also considered as the last resort.

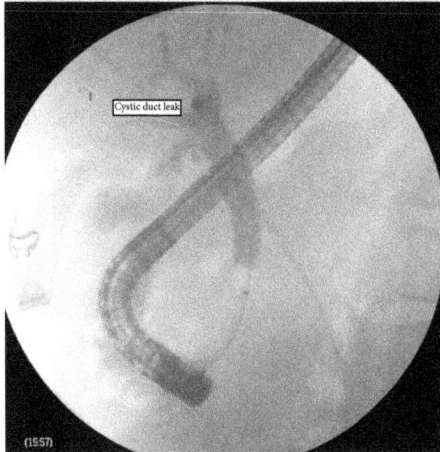

FIGURE 1: ERCP: bile leak from cystic duct.

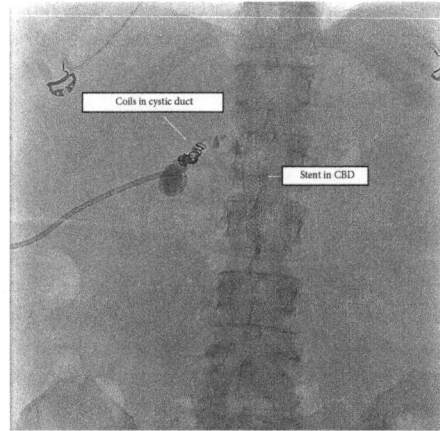

FIGURE 2: Stent in common bile duct.

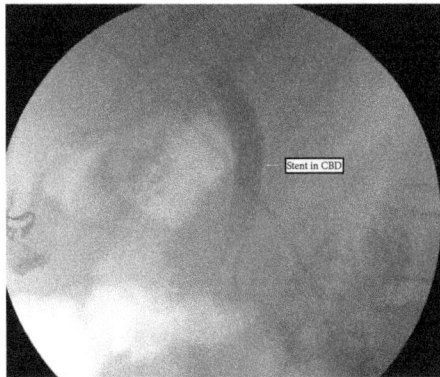

FIGURE 3: Coiling the cystic duct.

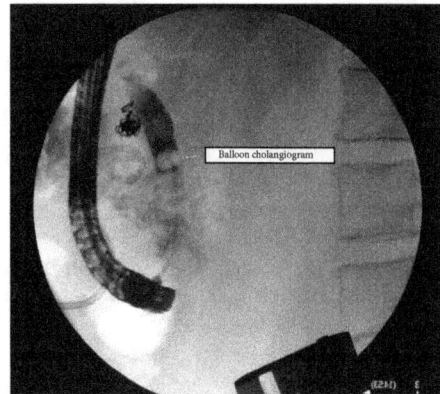

FIGURE 4: ERCP: occlusive cholangiogram with no leak.

After discussion (5 weeks from last ERCP), the tract was accessed by interventional radiologist. Contrast study showed that the covered stent was not covering the origin of the cystic duct. The cystic duct was coiled with total of 5 Tornado embolization coils (Cook Medical) (6–8 mm) (Figure 3). Follow-up cholangiogram demonstrates interval decrease in patency of the cystic duct. A pigtail drain was adjacent to the cystic duct.

The pigtail drain was clamped after the bile drainage stopped at 1-week follow-up. On subsequent ERCP done 2 weeks later, occlusion cholangiogram revealed no evidence of bile leak (Figure 4) and the stent and drain were removed. The patient was seen 4 months later with no further biliary complications.

3. Discussion

Laparoscopic cholecystectomy is one of the most commonly performed operations in the world. Bile leak from the cystic duct stump remains a significant complication of this operation [1, 2]. Bile peritonitis, subhepatic abscesses, bile duct stricture, and perihepatic inflammation leading to fibrosis have all been associated with bile leaks [3].

Endoscopic treatment at ERCP with stent and sphincterotomy is usually the first line of treatment with success rate greater than 90% [2, 5]. The median time for resolution of the leak was 3 days (range 1–39 days) [5]. Kaffes and colleagues [5] reported that stent insertion alone for postcholecystectomy bile leak is superior to sphincterotomy alone, because fewer patients required additional intervention (particularly surgery) to control the leak.

If these strategies fail, high-risk surgery (22%–37% morbidity and 3%–18% mortality) is one option [6]. Other options reported include injection of glue or coils either via endoscope or transhepatically.

Seewald et al. [7] reported their experience with endoscopic occlusion of cystic duct for bile leakage with injection of cyanoacrylate glue in 9 patients; two of them had bile leak after cholecystectomy. Other authors have also reported successful endoscopic glue injection for cystic duct leak [6]. Combination of cyanoacrylate glue and angiographic coils has also been deployed via endoscope at ERCP to resolve cystic duct leak after failed operations [8]. Percutaneous trans hepatic deployment of Hydrocoil into the cystic duct stump has been reported as well [9].

In the case presented, we used coiling of cystic duct with success to avoid operation in a patient with significant comorbidities including morbid obesity and COPD with continued smoking. To our knowledge, only another case of trans catheter cystic duct coiling has been reported in the published literature [10].

4. Conclusion

Trans catheter coiling of cystic duct for bile leak from cystic stump is an innovative technique, which can help avoid high-risk reoperation in patients, many of whom have significant comorbidities as in our patient. This technique can only be used in patients who have well-established drain tract.

References

[1] K. H. Kim and T. N. Kim, "Endoscopic management of bile leakage after cholecystectomy: a single-center experience for 12 years," *Clinical Endoscopy*, vol. 47, no. 3, pp. 248–253, 2014.

[2] I. A. A. Shaikh, H. Thomas, K. Joga, A. I. Amin, and T. Daniel, "Post-cholecystectomy cystic duct stump leak: a preventable morbidity," *Journal of Digestive Diseases*, vol. 10, no. 3, pp. 207–212, 2009.

[3] S. Eisenstein, A. J. Greenstein, U. Kim, and C. M. Divino, "Cystic duct stump leaks after the learning curve," *Archives of Surgery*, vol. 143, no. 12, pp. 1178–1183, 2008.

[4] M. S. Woods, J. L. Shellito, G. S. Santoscoy et al., "Cystic duct leaks in laparoscopic cholecystectomy," *The American Journal of Surgery*, vol. 168, no. 6, pp. 560–565, 1994.

[5] A. J. Kaffes, L. Hourigan, N. De Luca, K. Byth, S. J. Williams, and M. J. Bourke, "Impact of endoscopic intervention in 100 patients with suspected postcholecystectomy bile leak," *Gastrointestinal Endoscopy*, vol. 61, no. 2, pp. 269–275, 2005.

[6] G. Wright, V. Jairath, M. Reynolds, and R. G. Shidrawi, "Endoscopic glue injection for persistent biliary leakage," *Gastrointestinal Endoscopy*, vol. 70, no. 6, pp. 1279–1281, 2009.

[7] S. Seewald, S. Groth, P. V. J. Sriram et al., "Endoscopic treatment of biliary leakage with n-butyl-2 cyanoacrylate," *Gastrointestinal Endoscopy*, vol. 56, no. 6, pp. 916–919, 2002.

[8] E. K. Ganguly, K. E. Najarian, J. A. Vecchio, and P. L. Moses, "Endoscopic occlusion of cystic duct using N-butyl cyanoacrylate for postoperative bile leakage," *Digestive Endoscopy*, vol. 22, no. 4, pp. 348–350, 2010.

[9] T. Doshi, A. Mojtahedi, G. K. Goswami, R. T. Andrews, B. Godke, and K. Valji, "Persistent cystic duct stump leak managed with hydrocoil embolization," *Cardiovascular and Interventional Radiology*, vol. 32, no. 2, pp. 394–396, 2009.

[10] H. Berger, M. Weinzierl, E.-S. Neville, and E. Pratschke, "Percutaneous transcatheter occlusion of cystic duct stump in postcholecystectomy bile leakage," *Gastrointestinal Radiology*, vol. 14, no. 4, pp. 334–336, 1989.

9

Intestinal Malrotation: A Rare Cause of Small Intestinal Obstruction

Mesut Sipahi,[1] **Kasim Caglayan,**[1] **Ergin Arslan,**[1]
Mustafa Fatih Erkoc,[2] **and Faruk Onder Aytekin**[1]

[1] *Department of General Surgery, School of Medicine, Bozok University, 66100 Yozgat, Turkey*
[2] *Department of Radiology, School of Medicine, Bozok University, 66100 Yozgat, Turkey*

Correspondence should be addressed to Mesut Sipahi; sipahi@dr.com

Academic Editor: Boris Kirshtein

Background. The diagnosis of intestinal malrotation is established by the age of 1 year in most cases, and the condition is seldom seen in adults. In this paper, a patient with small intestinal malrotation-type intraperitoneal hernia who underwent surgery at an older age because of intestinal obstruction is presented. *Case.* A 73-year-old patient who presented with acute intestinal obstruction underwent surgery as treatment. Distended jejunum and ileum loops surrounded by a peritoneal sac and located between the stomach and transverse colon were determined. The terminal ileum had entered into the transverse mesocolon from the right lower part, resulting in kinking and subsequent segmentary obstruction. The obstruction was relieved, and the small intestines were placed into their normal position in the abdominal cavity. *Conclusion.* Small intestinal malrotations are rare causes of intestinal obstructions in adults. The appropriate treatment in these patients is placement of the intestines in their normal positions.

1. Introduction

Intestinal malrotation is a congenital disorder caused by rotation of the intestines during foetal development. Embryological development and anatomical variations were described in 1923 by Dott [1]. The intestines start to grow in the fourth week of gestation. Physiological herniation occurs in the umbilical cord causing it to rotate in an anticlockwise direction. The hernia is reduced in the 10th week of gestation, and the caecum settles in its normal right bottom position at the 12th week [2]. Intestinal malrotation is a disorder resulting from the lack of foetal intestinal physiological rotation [3]. There is often a fibrous band called Ladd's band that prevent the rotation of the intestines. Intestinal malrotations comprise various anatomic anomalies ranging from complete nonrotation to normal positioning [4, 5]. Intestinal malrotations are named according to anatomical variations such as incomplete rotation, mixed rotation, atypical malrotation, and variants of malrotation [6]. They can be categorised into two groups: typical and atypical malrotation based on the position of the ligament of Treitz according to the right and left of the midline, respectively [4]. Intestinal malrotations

occur in approximately 0.2% of all births. Symptoms usually occur in the early weeks of life, and the malrotations are generally diagnosed during this period. More than 40% of intestinal malrotations are diagnosed within 1 week after birth and 75–85% within 1 year after birth [6]. Although the precise incidence of intestinal malrotation is unknown, it is estimated that it occurs between the rates of 0.0001% and 0.19% in adults [3]. Generally, intestinal malrotation is incidentally determined in adults due to its asymptomatic or nonspecific presentation with mild symptoms. In the present paper, we present a case of an elderly patient with intestinal malrotation-type intraperitoneal hernia. The colon was rotated normally, but all of the intraperitoneal small intestines were placed in the lesser sac.

2. Case Report

A 73-year-old female patient was referred to our department with abdominal pain, swelling, constipation, nausea, and vomiting for 2 days. She had hypertension for 10 years, chronic obstructive pulmonary disease for 6 years, and type 2

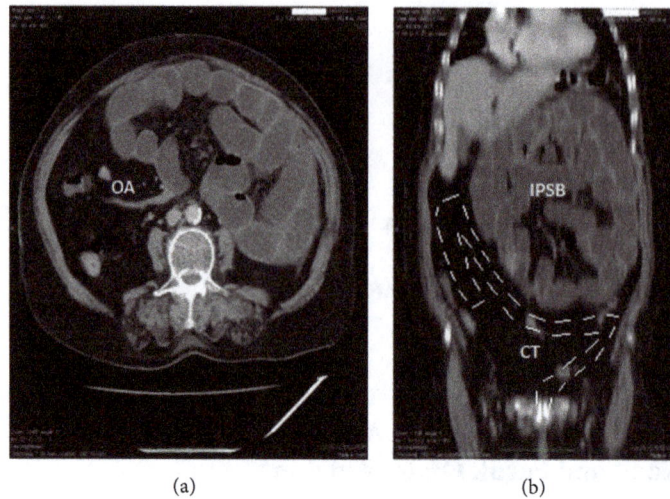

(a)   (b)

FIGURE 1: CT images demonstrating intestinal malrotation. On axial image (a), obstructed area (OA) indicates the obstructed part of terminal ileum. On coronal (b) image intraperitoneal small bowel (IPSB) is indicated in upper abdomen. Colon trace (CT) is oriented with (-) symbol.

diabetes mellitus for 4 years in her medical history. She had no history of abdominal surgery, trauma, jaundice, rectal bleeding, and weight loss. On physical examination, abdominal distension, tinkling, and increased bowel sounds were observed. There was generalised abdominal tenderness, guarding was positive, and rebound was negative. The ampulla was found to be empty on digital rectal examination. In laboratory tests, the leukocyte count was 12,500 K/μL (normal range: 4.6–10.2 K/μL), and the blood glucose level was determined to be 150 mg/dL. Other biochemical tests were within normal limits. Air-fluid levels localised in the upper left quadrant were determined by abdominal X-ray. Ultrasonography could not be performed because of dense intestinal gas. On abdominal tomography, small intestinal segments were observed to be dilated in the left quadrant and distal part of ileum; colon segments were collapsed (Figure 1). The patient underwent surgery with the diagnosis of acute intestinal obstruction. There was no free abdominal fluid at the exploration. The colon was observed in the normal position with lower right localisation of the caecum. The small intestines were palpated under the gastrocolic ligament, which was then opened. The intestines were located in the lesser sac surrounded by a sac, which was opened (Figure 2). The intestines were in a dilated position, and intestinal perfusion was normal. No space-occupying lesion was found. The terminal ileum had entered into the right lower part of the transverse mesocolon (right side of the middle colic artery) and was obstructed there. No cohesiveness or input-output section similar to herniation was found in this transition area. This area was similar to the right localisation ligament of Treitz. After the obstruction, the ileum moved 4 cm further and was joined to the caecum (Figure 3). It is defined as intraperitoneal hernia form of intestinal malrotation [7]. No other small intestinal part in the abdominal cavity except this 4 cm ileum segment was noted. There was no possibility of internal herniation at the point where the terminal ileum passed through the transverse mesocolon. Therefore, it was

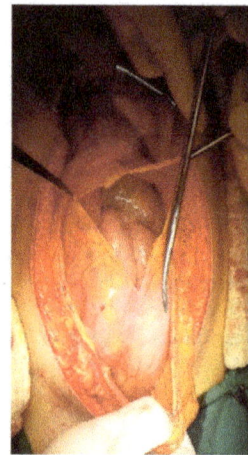

FIGURE 2: Small intestines located in lesser sac and the surrounding sac.

thought that congenital malrotation caused an obstruction in this case. The obstruction was opened by widening the hole through which the ileum passed in the transverse mesocolon. The intestines were pulled from this aperture to the normal position in the abdominal cavity. The defect in the mesocolon was covered with sutures. The patient started to ingest food orally on the third postoperative day, and she was discharged uneventfully on the fifth day. There was no complaint at the first-month follow-up. The complaint of swelling that had occurred repeatedly for the last 2 years also disappeared.

3. Discussion

The intestines are classified into three groups based on the origin of the arterial supplies: foregut, midgut, and hindgut. The duodenum, ileum, jejunum, caecum, and ascending colon constituting two-thirds of the proximal part of the

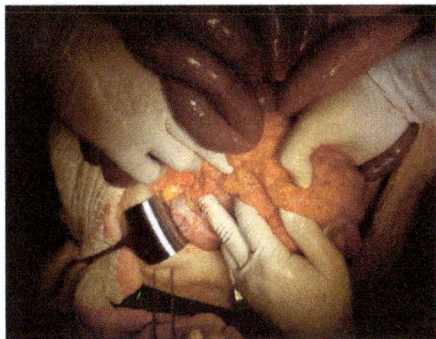

FIGURE 3: The place where terminal ileum comes out of transverse mesocolon.

transverse colon are supplied from the superior mesenteric artery (SMA). Intestinal rotation is completed within 4–12 weeks of intrauterine life. The rapid prolongation of the intestine and physiologic herniation into the umbilical cord occurs in the fifth week, a 270° anticlockwise rotation along the SMA axis and the return of herniation back into the abdominal cavity occur in the 10th week, and the location of the caecum in the right lower quadrant are completed in the 12th week [8]. The variations between the normal rotation and failure of the intestines to rotate due to any malfunction in this process are known as malrotations [6]. Although malrotation is a disease in which small intestines located in the right abdominal quadrant and the colon and caecum located in the left quadrant are generally unrotated owing to the bands and adherences [9]. There are several types of malrotation: diversity of anatomic configurations, ranging from a not-quite normal intestinal position to complete nonrotation [7]. The intermediate forms are known as atypical malrotations [6]. The most common variations are nonrotation, reverse fixation, and malrotation [5]. We described that our case was a type intraperitoneal hernia.

The symptoms in newborn infants are intestinal obstruction findings, such as bilious vomiting [10]. Malrotation is generally determined incidentally in adults because it often progresses asymptomatically or with nonspecific mild symptoms. Patients may have crampy abdominal pain, nausea, or bilious vomiting symptoms [5]. Therefore, complete or partial small bowel obstruction and vascular occlusion may develop [11]. The incidence of intestinal malrotation was found to be 0.2% when incidentally found in imaging studies performed for other reasons [3]. The rate of malrotation in autopsies is estimated to be 1 in 6,000. Typical malrotation is a paediatric surgical disease with well-known diagnostic and treatment aspects. Ladd's procedure is the choice of treatment, consisting of volvulus reduction, separation of the abdominal peritoneal bands, and placing of the small intestines in the right quadrant and caecum in the left quadrant of the abdomen [12]. By contrast, atypical malrotation is not a well-defined condition [6]. Asymptomatic cases are often seen in adults explored for other reasons. However, intestinal malrotation is a rare cause of intestinal obstruction in adults. Establishing a diagnosis before the operation is difficult because the symptoms are nonspecific, and malrotation is a rarely seen condition.

Infants and children are diagnosed largely through upper gastrointestinal contrast studies [7]. Adults are diagnosed using various imaging modalities, including upper gastrointestinal contrast studies, barium enema, plain abdominal radiography, computed tomography (CT), and ultrasonography. In adults, plain abdominal radiography may show abnormal localisation of the intestine. Abdominal CT can show clearly bowel settlements and the position of SMA. Surgery for incidentally detected asymptomatic cases is controversial because of the risk of volvulus and obstruction. However, surgery is recommended for patients with intestinal obstruction [5]. Ladd's procedure in nonrotation can be applied with success laparoscopically with a short hospital stay and early recovery benefits [13]. The procedure involves reduction of the volvulus, if present, division of the abnormal peritoneal bands (Ladd's bands), placement of the small bowel to the right of the abdomen and caecum to the left, and appendectomy. We believe that, in other variants of malrotation, considering the volvulus, ischaemia, internal herniation, and obstruction possibilities, as well as case-based surgery (adhesion lyses and placement of the organs more closely to normal anatomy), would be appropriate.

4. Conclusion

Intestinal malrotation is not only a newborn disease. Surgeons may encounter malrotations that, in rare cases, can lead to obstruction in adults. In these cases, treating the obstruction and placing the intestines as close as possible to their normal anatomical position may be an appropriate surgical approach.

References

[1] N. M. Dott, "Anomalies of intestinal rotation: their embryology and surgical aspects: with report of five cases," British Journal of Surgery, vol. 11, no. 42, pp. 251–286, 1923.

[2] A. K. Wanjari, A. J. Deshmukh, P. S. Tayde, and Y. Lonkar, "Midgut malrotation with chronic abdominal pain," North American Journal of Medical Sciences, vol. 4, no. 4, pp. 196–198, 2012.

[3] O. F. Emanuwa, A. A. Ayantunde, and T. W. Davies, "Midgut malrotation first presenting as acute bowel obstruction in adulthood: a case report and literature review," World Journal of Emergency Surgery, vol. 6, no. 1, article 22, 2011.

[4] J. R. Mehall, J. C. Chandler, R. L. Mehall, R. J. Jackson, C. W. Wagner, and S. D. Smith, "Management of typical and atypical intestinal malrotation," Journal of Pediatric Surgery, vol. 37, no. 8, pp. 1169–1172, 2002.

[5] G. Vaos and E. P. Misiakos, "Congenital anomalies of the gastrointestinal tract diagnosed in adulthood-diagnosis and management," Journal of Gastrointestinal Surgery, vol. 14, no. 5, pp. 916–925, 2010.

[6] M. R. McVay, E. R. Kokoska, R. J. Jackson, and S. D. Smith, "The changing spectrum of intestinal malrotation: diagnosis and management," *The American Journal of Surgery*, vol. 194, no. 6, pp. 712–719, 2007.

[7] S. A. Kapfer and J. F. Rappold, "Intestinal malrotation-not just the pediatric surgeon's problem," *Journal of the American College of Surgeons*, vol. 199, no. 4, pp. 628–635, 2004.

[8] V. Martin and C. Shaw-Smith, "Review of genetic factors in intestinal malrotation," *Pediatric Surgery International*, vol. 26, no. 8, pp. 769–781, 2010.

[9] P. J. Pickhardt and S. Bhalla, "Intestinal malrotation in adolescents and adults: spectrum of clinical and imaging features," *The American Journal of Roentgenology*, vol. 179, no. 6, pp. 1429–1435, 2002.

[10] H. C. Lee, S. S. Pickard, S. Sridhar, and S. Dutta, "Intestinal malrotation and catastrophic volvulus in infancy," *The Journal of Emergency Medicine*, vol. 43, no. 1, pp. e49–e51, 2012.

[11] T. Berrocal, M. Lamas, J. Gutiérrez, I. Torres, C. Prieto, and M. L. Del Hoyo, "Congenital anomalies of the small intestine, colon, and rectum," *Radiographics*, vol. 19, no. 5, pp. 1219–1236, 1999.

[12] T. Kamiyama, F. Fujiyoshi, H. Hamada, M. Nakajo, O. Harada, and Y. Haraguchi, "Left-sided acute appendicitis with intestinal malrotation," *Radiation Medicine: Medical Imaging and Radiation Oncology*, vol. 23, no. 2, pp. 125–127, 2005.

[13] N. E. Seymour and D. K. Andersen, "Laparoscopic treatment of intestinal malrotation in adults," *Journal of the Society of Laparoendoscopic Surgeons*, vol. 9, no. 3, pp. 298–301, 2005.

10

Small Bowel Perforation due to Gossypiboma Caused Acute Abdomen

Tahsin Colak, Tolga Olmez, Ozgur Turkmenoglu, and Ahmet Dag

Department of General Surgery, Medical Faculty, Mersin University, 33079 Mersin, Turkey

Correspondence should be addressed to Tahsin Colak; tcolak@mersin.edu.tr

Academic Editors: A. Cho, D. Mantas, M. Rangarajan, and C. Tunon-de-Lara

Gossypiboma, an infrequent surgical complication, is a mass lesion due to a retained surgical sponge surrounded by foreign body reaction. In this case report, we describe gossypiboma in the abdominal cavity which was detected 14 months after the hysterectomy due to acute abdominal pain. Gossypiboma was diagnosed by computed tomography (CT). The CT findings were a rounded mass with a dense central part and an enhancing wall. In explorative laparotomy, small bowel loops were seen to be perforated due to inflammation of long standing gossypiboma. Jejunal resection with end-to-end anastomosis was performed. The patient was discharged whithout complication. This case was presented to point to retained foreign body (RFB) complications and we believed that the possibility of a retained foreign body should be considered in the differential diagnosis of who had previous surgery and complained of pain, infection, or palpable mass.

1. Introduction

Retained foreign body (RFB) has been reported after abdominal, thoracic, cardiovascular, orthopedic, and neurosurgical procedures [1]. RFB is a rare condition for both patient and surgeon that can lead to very serious consequences after abdominal surgery. Gossypiboma can cause serious complications such as intra-abdominal abscess in the early stages. But it might remain asymptomatic for many years. Some imaging modalities including plain radiography, ultrasonography (USG), computed tomography (CT), and magnetic resonance imaging (MRI) may help to have exact diagnosis [2]. Surgery is the recommended treatment option in these cases. Gossypiboma, in patients with a diagnosis of intra-abdominal mass and had previous history of surgery, should be considered in the differential diagnosis, even if it is a rare condition. The appropriate surgical intervention should be planned as soon as possible due to legal and medical problems. The present case had emergency hysterectomy 14 months ago and suffered from mild intermittent abdominal pain only since to present acute abdominal syndrome and was admitted to hospital. The aim of present case was to draw attention to the complication of RFB.

2. Case Presentation

A 38-year-old woman with 27.3 BMI needed an emergency caesarean section in the fourth delivery 14 months ago in public hospital. After caesarean section, the surgeons had to perform hysterectomy due to continued bleeding. Medical record revealed no postoperative complication and the patient was discharged after one week from the hospital. In the follow up, the patient suffered sometimes from mild intermittent abdominal pain only. However, the surgeons did not perform advanced examinations and the problem was explained with postoperative adhesions. The patient was satisfied with surgeons' statements and did not continue the followup. But, after 13 months of operation, mild intermittent abdominal pain was converted to mild abdominal colic and the patient felt discomfort. Hence, last week before admittance to hospital, intermittent fever, which reached up to 39°C, and severe abdominal colic emerged. The patient was admitted to emergency department with above mentioned symptoms. Physical and laboratory examinations showed that the blood pressure was 100/80 mmHg, pulse was 110/min, body temperature was 38.5°C, WBC was $6.3 \times 10^3/\mu L$, and CRP was 241 mg/L. Abdominal USG shows a mass in pelvic

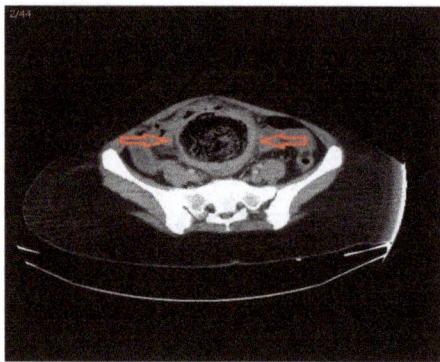

FIGURE 1: Abdominal CT scan revealed intra-abdominal mass—gossypiboma.

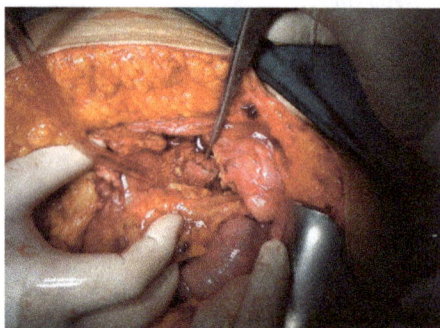

FIGURE 2: Exploratory laparotomy revealed an encapsulated sponge surrounded by omentum.

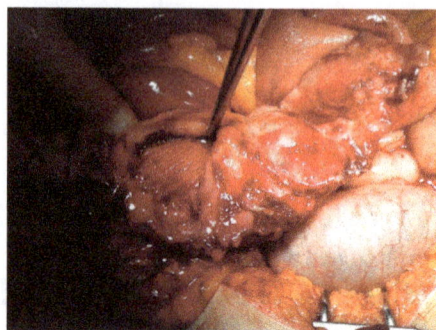

FIGURE 3: Perforation area on small bowel.

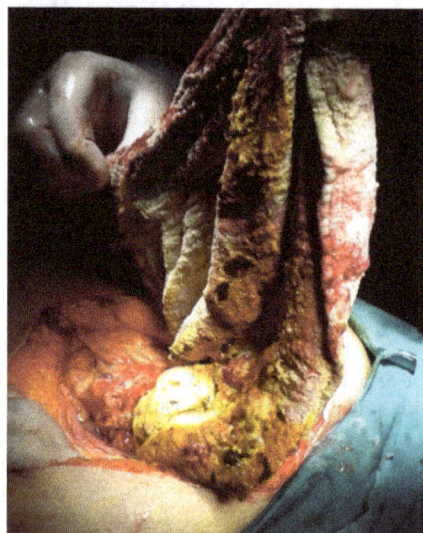

FIGURE 4: Surgical specimen (gossypiboma).

area, but the source is not certain. CT demonstrated that a mass (15×13 cm) with a dense central part and an enhancing wall (gossypiboma) was located in the pelvic area (Figure 1). The patient underwent emergency surgery and exploratory laparotomy shows that an encapsulated abdominal compression is surrounded by omentum (Figures 2 and 3). Retained abdominal sponge caused perforation of jejunum at the 50 cm below the ligament of Treitz and was surrounded by intestinal content, which caused regional contamination (Figure 4). After removal of abdominal sponge, adhesiolysis and segmental small bowel resection with end-to-end anastomosis were performed. The abdominal cavity was irrigated with 8–10 L saline and three abdominal drains were inserted. Bowel sound was begun and serous drainage content decreased to 50 mL in postoperative day (POD) 2. The patient tolerated the solid diet at POD 3. Drains were taken at POD 5 and CRP decreased up to 15. The patient was discharged at POD 7 due to patient feeling good enough. The patient was still well in one-week and one-month followup.

3. Discussion

The reported incidence of retained surgical sponge is one per 1,000–15,000 abdominal operations [3]. Incidence of gossypiboma is low in developed countries due to the advanced operation room conditions and radiological techniques. A surgical sponge can be retained after any surgery but most

commonly after hysterectomy, appendectomy, and cholecystectomy. Persistent wound infection, unexplained pain, and fever in the postoperative period should lead one to suspect a retained foreign body. This condition is often underestimated, because case numbers are calculated only on the basis of malpractice claims. Reason of nonreporting of occurrences is the fear of medicolegal repercussions [4]. Patients are often asymptomatic and not detected for a long time. In fact, many cases were discovered to have a retained surgical sponge more than 30 years after the initial surgery [5]. Some of patients present with abdominal mass or subacute intestinal obstruction. They may rarely result in fistula, perforation, or even extrusion per anus. In our case, the patient had also a gynecological operation 14 months ago and she had intermittent abdominal pain only. The main signs and symptoms are pain/irritation (42%), palpable mass (27%), and fever (12%) [2].

The retained surgical sponge triggers two biological responses named as aseptic fibrinous responses due to foreign body granuloma or exudative reaction leading to abscess formation [6]. The most common detection methods were computed tomography (61%), plain radiography (35%), and ultrasound (34%). So, the first diagnostic modality to rule it out should be a computed tomography scan. MRI features can be confusing because the radio-opaque marker is not magnetic or paramagnetic [7]. Intense acoustic collection in operation area or the mass can be shown by USG. If sponge contains radio-opaque marker, it can be seen in direct X-ray. The universal guideline which was stated by the American College of Surgeons in October 2005 strictly recommended that radio-opaque sponges should only be used, and accurate sponge counts should be performed before the procedure, and before and after closure of the abdomen.

Migration of retained sponge into bowel is rare but does occur when compared to abscess formation and occur as a result of inflammation of the intestinal wall that evolves to necrosis [8]. In our case, a large surgical sponge caused intestinal perforation 14 months after surgery.

Operation under emergency conditions, involvement of more than the surgical team in the operation, change in assistant staff during operation, increased BMI, volume loss, number of surgeons, and female gender are all risk factors for RFB [3]. Irrespective of the rarity of reports, operating teams should take care to count swabs used in all procedures. Surgeons should develop a habit of performing a brief but thorough routine postoperative wound and cavity exploration prior to wound closure [4]. Treatment of gossypiboma is the surgical removal usually through the previous operative site, but endoscopic or laparoscopic approaches may be attempted [9].

As a result, Gossypiboma is usually asymptomatic, has nonspecific radiological findings, and is a rare condition. These situations might delay the diagnosis. Also, a gossypiboma can cause complications such as perforation and adhesion to the adjacent structures. In order to avoid gossypiboma, the surgeons should comply with recommended statement on the prevention of retained foreign bodies after surgery. Atypical abdominal pain should be kept in mind since the gossypiboma even out of operation for a long time can be passed.

References

[1] F. W. Abdul-Karim, J. Benevenia, M. N. Pathria, and J. T. Makley, "Case report 736: retained surgical sponge (gossypiboma) with a foreign body reaction and remote and organizing hematoma," Skeletal Radiology, vol. 21, no. 7, pp. 466–470, 1992.

[2] M. K. Malhotra, "Migratory surgical gossypiboma-cause of iatrogenic perforation: case report with review of literature," Nigeria Journal of Surgery, vol. 18, no. 1, pp. 27–29, 2012.

[3] A. A. Gawande, D. M. Studdert, E. J. Orav, T. A. Brennan, and M. J. Zinner, "Risk factors for retained instruments and sponges after surgery," The New England Journal of Medicine, vol. 348, no. 3, pp. 229–235, 2003.

[4] M. E. Asuquo, N. Ogbu, J. Udosen et al., "Acute abdomen from gossypiboma: a case series and review of literature," Nigerian Journal of Surgical Research, vol. 8, no. 3-4, pp. 174–176, 2006.

[5] Y. Zantvoord, R. M. F. van der Weiden, and M. H. A. van Hooff, "Transmural migration of retained surgical sponges a systematic review," Obstetrical and Gynecological Survey, vol. 63, no. 7, pp. 465–471, 2008.

[6] V. C. Gibbs, F. D. Coakley, and H. D. Reines, "Preventable errors in the operating room: retained foreign bodies after surgery—part I," Current Problems in Surgery, vol. 44, no. 5, pp. 281–337, 2007.

[7] A. Aminiam, "Gossypiboma: a case report," Cases Journal, vol. 1, no. 1, p. 220, 2008.

[8] C. S. Silva, M. R. Caetano, E. A. W. Silva, L. Falco, and E. F. C. Murta, "Complete migration of retained surgical sponge into ileum without sign of open intestinal wall," Archives of Gynecology and Obstetrics, vol. 265, no. 2, pp. 103–104, 2001.

[9] T. Karahasanoglu, E. Unal, K. Memisoglu, I. Sahinler, and G. Atkovar, "Laparoscopic removal of a retained surgical instrument," Journal of Laparoendoscopic and Advanced Surgical Techniques A, vol. 14, no. 4, pp. 241–243, 2004.

11

Insulinoma-Induced Hypoglycemia in a Patient with Insulinoma after Gastrojejunostomy for Prepyloric Ulcer

Yavuz Savas Koca,[1] **Bünyamin Aydın,**[2] **Tugba Koca,**[3]
Mustafa Tevfik Bülbül,[1] **and Mehmet Numan Tamer**[2]

[1]*Department of General Surgery, School of Medicine, Suleyman Demirel University, 32200 Isparta, Turkey*
[2]*Division of Endocrinology and Metabolism, Department of Internal Medicine, School of Medicine, Suleyman Demirel University,*
32200 Isparta, Turkey
[3]*Department of Pediatric Gastroenterology, Hepatology and Nutrition, School of Medicine, Suleyman Demirel University,*
32200 Isparta, Turkey

Correspondence should be addressed to Yavuz Savas Koca; yavuzsavaskoca@gmail.com

Academic Editor: Akihiro Cho

Hyperinsulinism due to dumping syndrome following gastric surgery is an uncommon condition. It is specified with hypoglycemic attacks. However, linking symptoms to dumping syndrome in each patient to whom gastric surgery was performed leads to inappropriate diagnosis and therapy. Insulinoma and other causes that give rise to hyperinsulinemia should not be ignored and these diagnoses should be excluded. In this paper, 71-year-old male patient who was followed up for 2 years with a false conclusion of dumping syndrome and operated on due to insulinoma diagnosed at endoscopic ultrasonography is presented in the light of the literature.

1. Introduction

Hypoglycemia is a clinical syndrome that is characterized by adrenergic activation and neuroglycopenic symptoms due to the decrease in plasma glucose level. Hypoglycemia whether or not be insulin-mediated. In cases that are assumed to be healthy, the most frequent causes of hypoglycemia are drugs, insulinoma, islet cell hyperplasia/nesidioblastosis, and factitious hypoglycemia due to surreptitious administration of insulin or sulfonylureas. Though history is important for diagnosis, signs and symptoms are nonspecific. Dumping syndrome may occur in hypoglycemic patients who have a history of gastric surgery.

Hypoglycemia that is related to endogenous hyperinsulinemia is rarely seen. Pancreatic islet cell adenomas with autonomous insulin production, commonly termed as insulinoma, are rare gastropancreatic neuroendocrine tumours (NETs) with an estimated incidence of 1 or 4 per million [1].

We, herein, report a patient who underwent gastrojejunostomy for duodenal ulcer and then developed symptomatic hypoglycemia because of insulinoma.

2. Case Report

A 71-years-old male admitted to emergency department complaining of fatigue, sweating, and unconsciousness. He had admitted to different centers for nearly 1 year with similar complaints. He had undergone antrectomy + loop gastrojejunostomy operation 2 years ago because of gastric outlet obstruction due to prepyloric gastric ulcer and shortly after the surgery, complaints started. In clinics where he had admitted with these complaints, various examinations such as computed tomography (CT) and abdominal ultrasound (US) were performed; all were in normal ranges and no pathology was observed except a minimal fall in blood glucose. The clinical diagnosis was dumping syndrome, and the patient was discharged with diet recommendations. As a result, in a clinic he admitted 1 week ago, an operation was planned for dumping syndrome. In our emergency department, blood glucose was 55 mg/dL, and he was hospitalized. Physical examination revealed that he was slightly overweight, his body mass index (BMI) was 29 kg/m^2, blood pressure was 130/85 mm/Hg, and heart rate was 110/min.

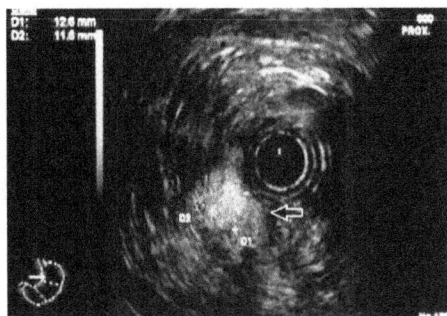

FIGURE 1: Endoscopic ultrasound image of a 12.5 × 11.6 mm hypoechoic mass located at pancreatic head.

He had an operation scar from xyphoid till lower umbilicus due to previous gastric surgery. In biochemical analysis, results of complete blood count, liver function tests, and renal function tests were normal. Adrenocorticotropic hormone was 14.7 pg/mL (0–46); cortisol, 17.8 μg/dL (2.32–19.52); total testosterone, 602 ng/dL; thyroid-stimulating hormone, 1.45 mIU/L (0.34–4.2); free thyroxine, 9 pg/mL (11–23); and free triiodothyronine, 2.91 pg/mL (2.5–3.9). His complaints were more severe in the morning when he wakes up, became more severe before meals with hunger, and eased with ingesting food. Before gastric surgery, he also had several deteriorations and then, it was considered as a hypoglycemic attack since he had no gastric passage. An endoscopic ultrasound was performed because the symptoms did not correlate with dumping syndrome and no pancreatic mass had been observed in pancreas by various imaging methods. Currently, a mass of 12.5 × 11.6 mm is seen in head of pancreas (Figure 1). This mass was first considered as insulinoma and a 72-hour extended fasting test was performed. In the 6th hour of the test, sweating and palpitation were observed and blood glucose was 37 mg/dL. After taking blood for C peptide and insulin, 1 mg glucagon was given subcutaneously. Blood glucose was measured at the 10th, 20th, and 30th minutes and the test was completed. Insulin was 44.6 μU/Ml ($N < 25$); C-peptide, 3.6 ng/mL (0.9–7.1); and blood glucose, 55 mg/dL, 74 mg/dL, and 82 mg/dL at the 10th, 20th, and 30th minutes, respectively. A mass was extracted from pancreas with an enucleation method during operation. Histopathological examination revealed an insulinoma (well-differentiated neuroendocrine tumor). The patient was discharged at the postoperative 6th day without complication. The complaints did not recur at postoperative first and third months.

3. Discussion

Since signs are not specific, insulinoma can be diagnosed rather later. Clinically, symptoms of hypoglycemia belong to two groups as adrenergic (anxiety, irritability, tremor, sweating, feeling of hunger, palpitations, angina, etc.) and neuroglycopenic symptoms (dizziness, confusion, fatigue, headache, difficulty in speaking, difficulty in concentration, epilepsy, coma, temporary hemiplegia, etc.) [2]. Neuroglycopenic symptoms are observed frequently in insulinoma

because extended hypoglycemia downregulates counterregulatory responses. Cases with behavioral disorders and psychiatric signs similar to our case have been reported [3]. Symptoms start several years before diagnosis; time to diagnosis is between 10 days to 20 years and patients may be followed up and treated with false diagnosis [1]. The case we present has admitted many times to different clinics and followed up with a diagnosis of dumping syndrome and could be correctly diagnosed only after 2 years.

Late dumping syndrome is a common delayed complication of bariatric surgery characterized by reactive hypoglycemia secondary to postprandial insulin surge. Symptoms such as weakness, sweating, and dizziness appear 2-3 hours after meals and occur a few months after surgery. Symptoms usually improve after a few months with dietary modifications. We moved away from diagnosis of dumping syndrome observing that the patient who had an operation before 2 years got no benefit from dietary modification.

Hyperinsulinemia with symptomatic hypoglycemia and relief of symptoms with glucose supply suggest insulinoma (Whipple triad) [1]. As in our case, hypoglycemia commonly presents in the fasting state, with the patient complaining of symptoms on waking in the morning. There is an excess weight in a quarter of cases resulting from overnutrition due to hypoglycemia symptoms [4]. Our case had a BMI of 29 kg/m^2 and was considered overweighed. With extended (72 hours) fasting test, a biochemical diagnosis can be made in 95% of cases. Insulin (μU/mL)/plasma glucose (mg/dL) (>0.27) or glucose/insulin ratio and insulin/c-peptide ratio might help in diagnosis.

Diagnosis is difficult since it is a rare condition and, also, does not have unique symptoms; symptoms are intermittent, show alterations between patients, and, more importantly, have different presentations from time to time in the same patient.

After biochemical diagnosis of insulinoma, the lesion needs to be localized. Because of high false positive and negative rates, imaging methods should not be used for diagnostic purposes. The most frequently used methods to localize pancreatic endocrine tumors are IV and oral contrast-enhanced dynamic abdominal CT. The accuracy of CT in determining primary islet cell tumors changes between 35 and 85% [5]. The aim of imaging methods in insulinoma is to determine tumor localization and evaluate metastasis. Although insulinoma has a characteristic image in CT and magnetic resonance imaging (MRI), its sensitivity is low (33–64% and 40–90%, resp.) [6]. The sensitivity of imaging methods is higher in tumors >2 cm. For the reason that tumor size was <2 cm in our case, it could not be localized with noninvasive methods.

Endoscopic US is the most sensitive test (84–93%) compared with tests such as somatostatin receptor scintigraphy, US, spiral CT, MRI, and angiography [7]. As in our case, noninvasive methods such as US and MRI are performed firstly. However, EUS can be used in cases when tumor could not be detected.

Selective arterial calcium stimulation test is an invasive dynamic test that shows tumor localization. If tumor could not be detected despite all investigations, intraoperative US and palpation are recommended [8].

Insulinoma, although rare, can lead to severe morbidity and mortality if not treated. Particularly, in cases presenting with neuroglycopenic symptoms, it should be taken into consideration in hypoglycemia etiology. The diagnosis is biochemical, but preoperative localization methods increase operation success and, also, enable less aggressive surgical procedures.

Acknowledgment

The authors would like to thank Altug Senol for his contribution.

References

[1] A. Janez, "Insulinoma causing liver metastases 15 years after initial surgery, accompanied by glomerulonephritis," *Case Reports in Endocrinology*, vol. 2012, Article ID 168671, 3 pages, 2012.

[2] S. Vig, M. Lewis, K. J. Foster, and A. Stacey-Clear, "Lessons to be learned: a case study approach insulinoma presenting as a change in personality," *The Journal of the Royal Society for the Promotion of Health*, vol. 121, no. 1, pp. 56–61, 2001.

[3] S. Ebady, M. Arami, and E. Kucheki, "A case of insulinoma with neuropsychiatric symptoms and cerebral infarction," *The Internet Journal of Neurology*, vol. 4, no. 2, pp. 1–5, 2005.

[4] M. L. Virally and P. J. Guillausseau, "Hypoglycemia in adults," *Diabetes and Metabolism*, vol. 25, no. 6, pp. 477–490, 1999.

[5] O. Porzio, G. Rossi, A. Biscardi et al., "Insulinoma. Clinical and surgical considerations concerning a case," *Minerva Chirurgic*, vol. 52, no. 3, pp. 289–293, 1997.

[6] S. Miani, M. Boneschi, M. Erba, D. Eusebio, and F. Giordanengo, "Pancreatic insulinomas," *Minerva Chirurgica*, vol. 48, no. 23-24, pp. 1459–1465, 1993.

[7] T. Rösch, C. J. Lightdale, J. F. Botet et al., "Localization of pancreatic endocrine tumors by endoscopic ultrasonography," *The New England Journal of Medicine*, vol. 326, no. 26, pp. 1721–1726, 1992.

[8] K. Azimuddin and R. S. Chamberlain, "The surgical management of pancreatic neuroendocrine tumors," *Surgical Clinics of North America*, vol. 81, no. 3, pp. 511–525, 2001.

12

Unusual Localization of Clostridium Difficile Infection in an Isolated Segment of the Descending Colon in a Critical Care Patient

Evgeni Brotfain, Leonid Koyfman, Amit Frenkel, Jochanan G. Peiser,
Abraham Borer, Benjamin F. Gruenbaum, Alexander Zlotnik, and Moti Klein

*Department of Anesthesiology and Critical Care, Soroka Medical Center, Ben-Gurion University of the Negev,
84105 Beer Sheva, Israel*

Correspondence should be addressed to Evgeni Brotfain, bem1975@gmail.com

Academic Editors: F.-M. Haecker and A. K. Karam

Unrecognized severe pseudomembranous colitis may become life threatening. A typical Clostridium difficile infection is associated with involvement of the colon; however, small bowel disease has also been described. Here, we present a case of a 48-year-old man with Clostridium difficile colitis of an isolated segment in the descending colon treated by a novel catheter intraluminal antibiotic irrigation. The intraluminal antibiotic irrigation was performed through a Foley catheter inserted into the isolated mucus fistula. The patient recovered after three weeks of intraluminal vancomycin (250 mg diluted in 150 ml of normal saline x Q6) and metronidazole (500 mg x Q8). Both antibiotics were given into the mucus fistula over 30 min. The patient was discharged from the unit four weeks after admission. This novel technique, in which the antibiotic was administered through an inserted intraluminal Foley urinary catheter, may be an efficient and safe alternative when conventional routes cannot be implemented.

1. Introduction

Clostridium difficile is a gram-positive, toxin produced, anaerobic microorganism [1]. A simple asymptomatic carrier could rapidly progress to subsequent pseudomembranous colitis and even fulminant toxic megacolon, which is associated with a high mortality rate [2]. Severely ill patients could be detected by an elevated white cell count and fever. This may be followed by an increase in serum creatinine level and hemodynamic instability [2, 3]. A typical Clostridium difficile infection is associated with involvement of the colon [2]; however, small bowel disease has also been described [1, 2]. Initial measures include stopping antibiotic treatment, supportive care, and peroral metronidazole management [3, 4]. Tremendous clinical deterioration and life-threatening gastrointestinal complications might need intensive care management and even emergency surgery. Here, we present a case of Clostridium difficile colitis of an unusual intestinal localization treated by a novel catheter intraluminal antibiotic irrigation.

2. Case Report

A 48-year-old male was admitted to the internal medicine ward with chronic pancytopenia secondary to megaloblastic anemia. He had a past medical history of hypertension, dyslipidemia, and a history of smoking.

Three days after admission, septic bursitis of the right olecranon was diagnosed and the patient was treated by surgical drainage of the abscess and a week-long course of antibiotic therapy (fluoroquinolone and penicillin groups). During the next 72 hours, a high fever and abdominal distention were noted. Free air in the abdomen was shown on urgently performed CT and the patient was transferred to the operating room.

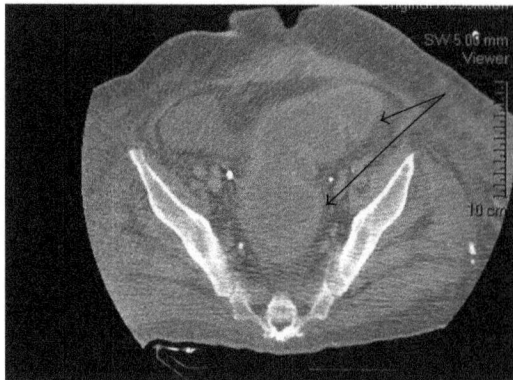

FIGURE 1: CT abdomen of a patient with Clostridium difficile colitis. The image shows dilated descending loop with thickening of wall (see black arrows).

Exploration of the abdomen revealed an ischemic area in the cecum with a perforation. Right hemicolectomy with ileostomy was performed. The remaining large intestine was brought out to the abdominal wall as a mucous fistula at the left upper quadrant.

During the next four days in the intensive care unit, the patient continued to be septic with highly elevated temperatures (39.2°C) and extensive leukocytosis (37000 cells/uL). During this time, intensive supportive management included the administration of vasopressors and broad spectrum antibiotics.

On a detailed workup of sepsis, stool sample cultures for Clostridium difficile toxins from the rectum and end ileostomy were performed. Diagnosis of colitis was made by a positive Clostridium difficile toxin in the rectal sample and was confirmed by CT findings of a thickened, dilated, and distended colonic wall (mucus fistula segment) (Figure 1). Clostridium difficile culture from the ileostomy was negative. Moreover, a pathological examination disclosed cecal perforation, acute peritonitis, and a tubulovillous adenoma in the cecum which was located 3 centimeters distal to the point of perforation. No evidence of colitis was encountered in the removed segment of the right colon.

Infection disease was consulted on how to treat the colonic descending loop. A novel intraluminal antibiotic irrigation through a Foley catheter inserted into the isolated mucus fistula was implemented. The patient recovered after three weeks of intraluminal vancomycin (250 mg diluted in 150 mL of normal saline x Q6) and metronidazole (500 mg x Q8). Both antibiotics were given into the mucus fistula over 30 min. The patient was discharged from the unit four weeks after admission.

3. Discussion

Primary diagnosis of Clostridium difficile colitis is based on the presentation of diarrhea with positive toxin stool cultures. Endoscopic examination may also detect typical macroscopic pseudomembrane findings of the colonic wall.

CT findings can be helpful in confirming the diagnosis, showing thickening, dilation, and potential perforation of the colon [2, 5–7].

This patient presented with classic clinical features of severe Clostridium difficile, marked by a high-grade fever and extensive leukocytosis. However, the perforated caecum had no signs of mucus edema, congestion, or pseudomembrane formation on biopsy and the end-ileostomy Clostridium difficile toxin test was negative.

There was a high level of suspicion of end-ileostomy infection, given a previous history of antibiotic use, which led us to the diagnosis of Clostridium difficile colitis in the isolated descending left colon. Our suspicions were confirmed by a positive Clostridium difficile toxin test from the isolated colon and remarkable CT findings.

This unusual localization of Clostridium difficile infection has been previously described [8–10]. Causey et al. reported three cases of Clostridium difficile enteritis developed after total colectomy [11]. Moreover, it has been recognized in surgical literature as secondary pouchitis of the ileal pouch-anal anastomosis after colorectal surgery. However, in our patient, Clostridium difficile colitis developed only in the isolated colon loop.

Al-Mufarrej et al. described a curious case of a 47-year-old male who developed Clostridium difficile infection in an interposed reconstructed colon after esophagectomy [8]. In addition, Oppermann et al. reported about isolated Clostridium difficile colitis in the ascending colon after transverse colon loop colostomy [12]. The overall collection of cases strongly supports the ability of previously colonized heat-resistant Clostridium difficile spores to convert to vegetative forms, capable of rapidly progressing to severe systemic disease even in isolated segments of the colon.

The challenge of an appropriate route of therapy was elusive. We started to treat our patient in accordance with the well-described guidelines for severe Clostridium difficile. However, oral metronidazole and vancomycin together with metronidazole intravenous therapy were not suitable in our case considering the isolated location. We decided to implement a novel method of administration through a Foley urinary catheter inserted into a mucus fistula end. The rapid improvement of our patient demonstrated that this route of administration could be considered in future cases with a similar presentation.

4. Conclusion

Unrecognized severe pseudomembranous colitis may become life threatening. Unusual localizations must be considered in patients after intestinal resection surgeries. The workup of sepsis in critical illness population should include stool samples from different intestinal sites and also isolated segments of intestine. In the case described, local intraluminal antibiotic therapy was defiant. We present a novel technique, in which the antibiotic was administered through an inserted intraluminal Foley urinary catheter as an efficient and safe alternative when conventional routes cannot be implemented.

Authors' Contribution

Brotfain Evgeni and Koyfman Leonid are equally contributed authors.

References

[1] C. P. Kelly and J. T. LaMont, "Clostridium difficile—more difficult than ever," *New England Journal of Medicine*, vol. 359, no. 18, pp. 1932–1940, 2008.

[2] V. G. Loo, L. Poirier, M. A. Miller et al., "A predominantly clonal multi-institutional outbreak of Clostridium difficile-associated diarrhea with high morbidity and mortality," *New England Journal of Medicine*, vol. 353, no. 23, pp. 2442–2449, 2005.

[3] B. Faris, A. Blackmore, and N. Haboubi, "Review of medical and surgical management of Clostridium difficile infection," *Techniques in Coloproctology*, vol. 14, no. 2, pp. 97–105, 2010.

[4] D. C. Metz, "Clostridium difficile colitis: wash your hands before stopping the proton pump inhibitor," *American Journal of Gastroenterology*, vol. 103, no. 9, pp. 2314–2316, 2008.

[5] M. Zerey, B. L. Paton, A. E. Lincourt, K. S. Gersin, K. W. Kercher, and B. T. Heniford, "The burden of Clostridium difficile in surgical patients in the United States," *Surgical Infections*, vol. 8, no. 6, pp. 557–566, 2007.

[6] S. E. Noblett, M. Welfare, and K. Seymour, "The role of surgery in Clostridium difficile colitis," *BMJ*, vol. 338, p. b1563, 2009.

[7] L. C. McDonald, M. Owings, and D. B. Jernigan, "Clostridium difficile infection in patients discharged from US short-stay hospitals, 1996–2003," *Emerging Infectious Diseases*, vol. 12, no. 3, pp. 409–415, 2006.

[8] F. Al-Mufarrej, M. Margolis, B. Tempesta, E. Strother, and F. Gharagozloo, "Post-esophagectomy pseudomembranous inflammation of the interposed colon," *Surgical Infections*, vol. 11, no. 5, pp. 479–481, 2010.

[9] A. D. Malkan, J. M. Pimiento, S. P. Maloney, J. A. Palesty, and S. J. Scholand, "Unusual manifestations of clostridium difficile infection," *Surgical Infections*, vol. 11, no. 3, pp. 333–337, 2010.

[10] U. Navaneethan and B. Shen, "Secondary pouchitis: those with identifiable etiopathogenetic or triggering factors," *American Journal of Gastroenterology*, vol. 105, no. 1, pp. 51–64, 2010.

[11] M. W. Causey, M. P. Spencer, and S. R. Steele, "Clostridium difficile enteritis after colectomy," *American Surgeon*, vol. 75, no. 12, pp. 1203–1206, 2009.

[12] T. E. Oppermann, W. A. Christopherson, and K. R. Stahlfeld, "Fulminant Clostridium difficile colitis isolated to the ascending colon by a diverting transverse loop colostomy," *American Surgeon*, vol. 75, no. 9, pp. 859–860, 2009.

13

Primary Malignant Melanoma of the Rectum

Kodai Tomioka,[1,2] **Hitoshi Ojima,**[2] **Makoto Sohda,**[2] **Akiko Tanabe,**[2] **Yasuyuki Fukai,**[2] **Akihiko Sano,**[2] **Takahiro Fukuda,**[2] **and Masahiko Murakami**[1]

[1] *Department of Gastroenterological and General Surgery, Showa University Hospital, 1-5-8 Hatanodai, Shinagawa, Tokyo 142-8666, Japan*
[2] *Department of Gastroenterological Surgery, Gunma Prefectural Cancer Center, 617-1 Takabayashi-Nishi, Ota, Gunma 373-8550, Japan*

Correspondence should be addressed to Hitoshi Ojima, hiojima@gunma-cc.jp

Academic Editors: S. Bhatt, P. De Nardi, S. Landen, and M. Picchio

We report two cases of rectal malignant melanomas. The patients were an 84-year-old male and a 66-year-old female who had blood in their stools. They were preoperatively diagnosed with poorly differentiated adenocarcinoma of the rectum. The clinical diagnosis for each was rectal carcinoma at stage IIIc according to the tumor-node-metastasis classification (6th edition), and the patients underwent abdominoperineal resection with dissection of lymph nodes. Pathological examination of the resected specimens revealed a malignant melanoma. Immunohistochemical analysis results were positive for HMB-45 and negative for cytokeratin AE1/AE3, CD45, and synaptophysin. Primary anorectal melanoma is an uncommon and aggressive disease that carries a poor prognosis. Therefore, it is necessary to provide systemic treatment. To improve prognosis, it is important to detect anorectal melanoma at an early stage.

1. Introduction

Anorectal melanoma is an uncommon and aggressive disease. The anorectum is the third most common location of malignant melanoma after the skin and retina. The most common symptom is rectal bleeding, which is often mistaken for bleeding associated with hemorrhoids. Diagnosis is very difficult, and initial diagnosis may be incorrect in 80% of all cases [1, 2]. For patients with anorectal malignant melanoma, treatment strategy includes surgery, chemotherapy, and radiotherapy. However, the tumor tends to be considerably resistant to radiotherapy and shows a poor response to chemotherapy. The choice of wide local excision (WLE) or abdominoperineal resection (APR) is also controversial [3–6]. The prognosis is very poor, with less than 20% survival five years after diagnosis [4, 5, 7]. We present two cases of rectal malignant melanoma with a rapid and fatal course that could not be diagnosed preoperatively.

2. Case Presentation

2.1. Case 1. An 84-year-old male was referred to our hospital with the chief complaint of bloody stool. Digital examination of the rectum revealed a hard mass at the 9 o'clock position. Colonoscopy revealed an irregular surface mass with a diameter of approximately 60 mm, located on the right wall of the lower rectum, 30 mm from the anal verge. Biopsy of the rectal mass was performed, and histopathological examination showed poorly differentiated adenocarcinoma. Computed tomography (CT) showed a thickening of the rectal wall and lymph node swelling of the circumference of an internal iliac artery; however, there was no evidence of distant metastasis (Figure 1(a)). Magnetic resonance imaging (MRI) also showed thickening of the rectal wall and enlarged regional lymph nodes. Diffusion-weighted imaging (DWI) produced a high signal, and ^{18}F-fluorodeoxyglucose positron emission tomographic (FDG-PET) imaging revealed a soft mass with increased accumulation of FDG (Figure 1(b)). The

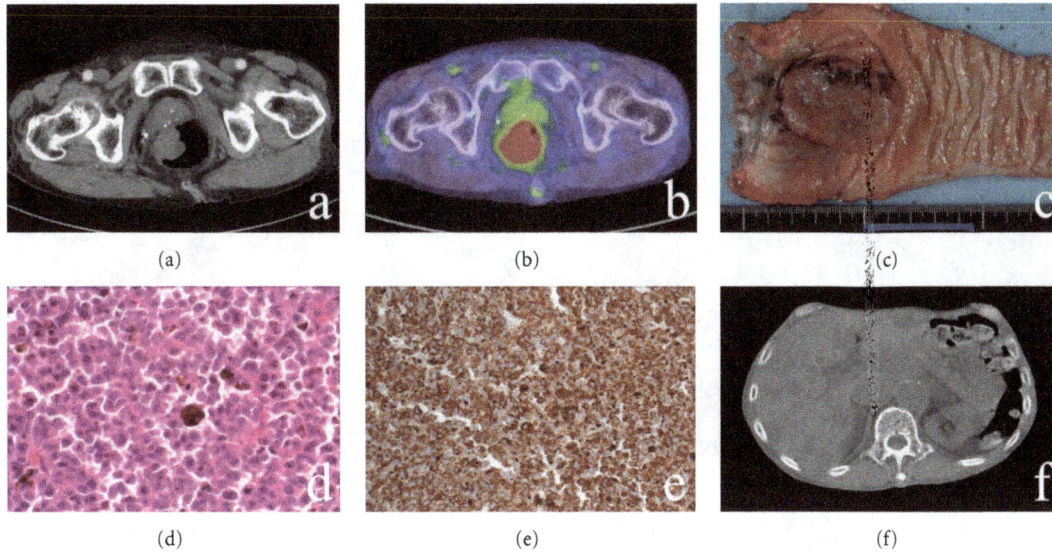

FIGURE 1: Case 1 CT, FDG-PET, MRI, and pathological imaging. (a) CT shows that the tumor into the lumen. (b) FDG-PET shows that increased accumulation of FDG. (c) Macroscopic image of the rectal tumor showing pigmented lesions. (d) Histopathological examination of the rectal specimen showed the nest of melanocytic cells (e.g., HE stain, ×40). (e) Rectal specimen is positive for the expression of HMB-45 (×20). (f) CT shows multiple liver metastases.

standardized uptake value of the main tumor was 19.25. Laboratory data as well as serum carcinoembryonic antigen (CEA) and CA19-9 levels were almost normal.

The clinical diagnosis was rectal carcinoma at stage IIIc according to the tumor-node-metastasis (TNM) classification (6th edition). The patient was treated by abdominoperineal resection (APR) with dissection of lymph nodes. The resected specimen showed some pigmented lesions within the tumor and around the anal verge (Figure 1(c)). Histopathological examination of the specimen showed a pattern of pleomorphic cells with melanin pigmentation of the cytoplasm (Figure 1(d)). Immunohistochemical analysis results were positive for the expression of S-100 protein and HMB-45 (Figure 1(e)) and negative for the expression of cytokeratin AE1/AE3, CD45, and synaptophysin. The final diagnosis was malignant melanoma. The patient was discharged on the 21st postoperative day after an uneventful course. Postoperative adjuvant chemotherapy was not performed because of advanced age.

Three months after the resection, the patient was rehospitalized with a chief complaint of right leg edema and dyspnea. Laboratory data showed liver and renal dysfunction. CT showed multiple liver and right inguinal lymph node metastases (Figure 1(f)). The patient died of hepatic insufficiency three days later.

2.2. Case 2. A 66-year-old female was referred to our hospital with the chief complaint of blood in the stool. Digital examination revealed a hard mass located all around the wall, 1.0 cm from the anal verge. Colonoscopy revealed an irregular surface large mass of approximately 80 mm in diameter located all around the wall of the lower rectum, 10 mm from the anal verge. Histopathological examination showed features of poorly differentiated adenocarcinoma.

CT and MRI revealed an increased density in the perirectal area, rectal wall thickening all-around, and regional lymph node metastases. DWI produced a high signal in the previously described area. Laboratory data as well as CEA and CA19-9 levels were almost normal. The boundary with the vaginal wall was unclear. Under the diagnosis of stage IIIc rectal carcinoma according to the TNM classification (6th edition), we performed an APR with dissection of lymph nodes. Because there was invasion of the vagina, a part of the vagina was also resected at the same time. The resected specimen revealed some pigmented lesions within the tumor and around the anal verge (Figure 2(a)). The patient was discharged on the 31st postoperative day after an uneventful course.

Histopathological examination showed the characteristics of malignant melanoma. Immunohistologically, the results showed positive expression of HMB-45 (Figure 2(b)) and cytokeratin AE1/AE3 and negative expression of S-100 protein, CD45, and synaptophysin. Postoperative adjuvant chemotherapy of dacarbazine (DTIC) was given. Bleeding from the vagina occurred one month after leaving the hospital, and a local recurrence was detected. Two months later, liver, lung, and brain metastases were detected. The chemotherapy appeared to be ineffective in preventing disease progression. The patient died of hepatic insufficiency and disseminated intravascular coagulation six months after the resection.

3. Discussion

Malignant melanoma of the rectum is rare and has very poor prognosis. The incidence has been reported to be 0.4%–3.0% of all malignant melanoma and 0.1%–4.6% of all anorectal malignant tumors [4, 8–10]. Melanomas of the anorectum

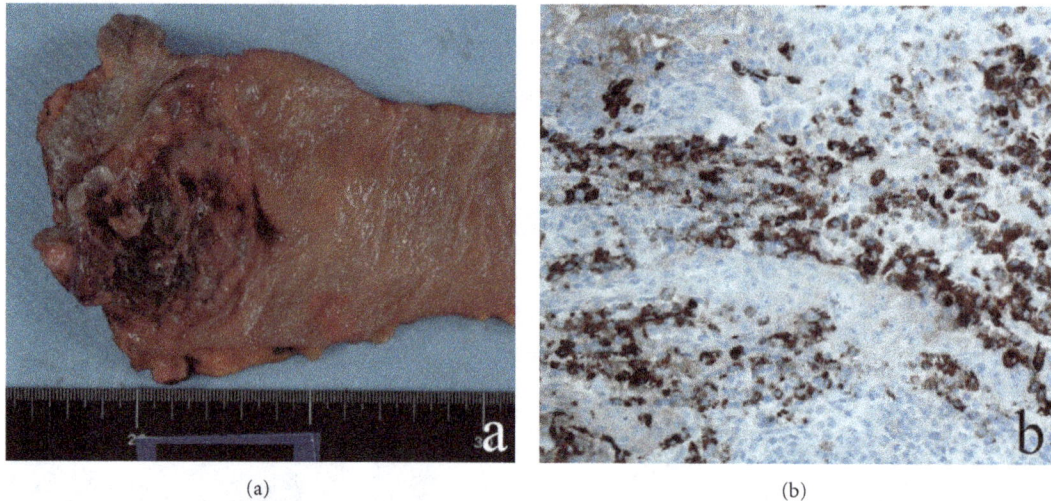

(a)   (b)

FIGURE 2: Case 2 pathological imaging. (a) Macroscopic image of the rectal tumor showing some pigmented lesions. (b) Rectal specimen is positive for the expression of HMB-45 ($\times 20$).

are the third most common after melanomas of the skin and retina. Malignant melanomas occur frequently in the anorectum because of the presence of abundant melanocytes in the mucosa of the anal canal. The reported 5-year overall survival rate is 6%–15% of patients after surgery [4, 5, 7, 11–13]. Several studies have reported cases of long-term survival [14–16]. The main determinants of prognosis are the depth of invasion and stage of the disease [17]. Early-stage detection is important. The tumor has been reported in older patients and women, and the common initial symptoms are rectal bleeding and/or pain. Obvious melanin pigmentation is present in only 20% of patients [18]. Therefore, the symptoms are often confused as those of hemorrhoids. Nonspecific symptoms cause delayed diagnosis, which is also caused by the similarity of histological findings to those of other malignancies. The clinical diagnosis may be incorrect in 80% of all cases [1, 2, 18]. Because of delayed diagnosis and rapid progression, malignant rectal melanomas have been accompanied by distant metastases in 60% of patients at the time of final diagnosis [4, 13]. The two present cases had a chief complaint of rectal bleeding, and clinical diagnosis before surgery was rectal carcinoma. Although curative surgery was performed for these cases, their disease had already advanced to stage IIIb. Preoperative biopsy of the tumors showed poorly differentiated adenocarcinoma, which was different from the final diagnosis. Immunohistochemical studies are useful methods for establishing correct diagnosis, and the diagnoses in our cases were confirmed by the expressions of S-100 protein and HMB-45. In these cases, the final diagnosis was based on immunohistochemical studies.

For anorectal malignant melanoma, multimodality treatments including surgery, chemotherapy, and radiotherapy have been used. Surgery is the main treatment. The surgical procedure varies from WLE to APR. However, the relative benefit of these individual procedures is unclear [5, 19]. In our cases, APR was performed because the preoperative diagnosis was poorly differentiated adenocarcinoma, and

it was possible to perform curative surgery. There are some reports that these surgical therapies have minimal impact on prognosis, but they can have some effect in controlling symptoms or improving the patient's quality of life. Correlation between the depth of invasion and median survival has also been reported [17], and long-term survival is possible after curative surgery [14–16]. Therefore, we should choose surgical procedures according to the tumor stage.

The tumor tends to be quite radiotherapy resistant and shows a poor response to chemotherapy [16]. The role of adjuvant chemotherapy has not been established. The prognosis is poor regardless of any therapies, and the most important predictors of prognosis are disease stage, symptom duration, tumor size, and nodal status [15, 20, 21]. Therefore, early detection of anorectal melanoma is critical for reducing the mortality rate.

In conclusion, anorectal melanoma is a rare and aggressive disease. Because of nonspecific symptoms, it is easily mistaken for hemorrhoids. Because malignant melanoma occurs frequently in the anorectum, clinicians should suspect anorectal melanoma in cases presenting with blood in the stool. Furthermore, the prognosis depends on the staging, and it is important to detect anorectal melanoma at an early stage. Ultimately, the development of further effective adjuvant therapy may improve the survival rate.

Acknowledgment

The authors thank the patients and this paper has not been published previously.

References

[1] G. Das, S. Gupta, P. J. Shukla, and P. Jagannath, "Anorectal melanoma: a large clinicopathologic study from India," *International Surgery*, vol. 88, no. 1, pp. 21–24, 2003.

[2] A. Maqbool, R. Lintner, A. Bokhari, T. Habib, I. Rahman, and B. K. Rao, "Anorectal melanoma—3 case reports and a review of the literature," *Cutis*, vol. 73, no. 6, pp. 409–413, 2004.

[3] S. Goldman, B. Glimelius, and L. Pahlman, "Anorectal malignant melanoma in Sweden: report of 49 patients," *Diseases of the Colon and Rectum*, vol. 33, no. 10, pp. 874–877, 1990.

[4] C. Thibault, P. Sagar, S. Nivatvongs, D. M. Ilstrup, and B. G. Wolff, "Anorectal melanoma: an incurable disease?" *Diseases of the Colon and Rectum*, vol. 40, no. 6, pp. 661–668, 1997.

[5] M. S. Brady, J. P. Kavolius, and S. H. Q. Quan, "Anorectal melanoma: a 64-year experience at Memorial Sloan-Kettering Cancer Center," *Diseases of the Colon and Rectum*, vol. 38, no. 2, pp. 146–151, 1995.

[6] S. Ishizone, N. Koide, F. Karasawa et al., "Surgical treatment for anorectal malignant melanoma: report of five cases and review of 79 Japanese cases," *International Journal of Colorectal Disease*, vol. 23, no. 12, pp. 1257–1262, 2008.

[7] C. L. Slingluff and H. F. Seigler, "Anorectal melanoma: clinical characteristics and the role of abdominoperineal resection," *Annals of Plastic Surgery*, vol. 28, no. 1, pp. 85–88, 1992.

[8] A. E. Chang, L. H. Karnell, and H. R. Menck, "The National Cancer Data Base report on cutaneous and noncutaneous melanoma: a summary of 84,836 cases from the past decade. The American College of Surgeons Commission on Cancer and the American Cancer Society," *Cancer*, vol. 83, no. 8, pp. 1664–1678, 1998.

[9] J. Heyn, M. Placzek, A. Ozimek, A. K. Baumgaertner, M. Siebeck, and M. Volkenandt, "Malignant melanoma of the anal region," *Clinical and Experimental Dermatology*, vol. 32, no. 5, pp. 603–607, 2007.

[10] J. V. Klas, D. A. Rothenberger, W. D. Wong, and R. D. Madoff, "Malignant tumors of the anal canal: the spectrum of disease, treatment, and outcomes," *Cancer*, vol. 85, no. 8, pp. 1686–1693, 1999.

[11] M. M. Konstadoulakis, N. Ricaniadis, D. Walsh, and C. P. Karakousis, "Malignant melanoma of the anorectal region," *Journal of Surgical Oncology*, vol. 58, no. 2, pp. 118–120, 1995.

[12] R. M. H. Roumen, "Anorectal melanoma in the Netherlands: a report of 63 patients," *European Journal of Surgical Oncology*, vol. 22, no. 6, pp. 598–601, 1996.

[13] P. H. Cooper, S. E. Mills, and M. S. Allen, "Malignant melanoma of the anus. Report of 12 patients and analysis of 255 additional cases," *Diseases of the Colon and Rectum*, vol. 25, no. 7, pp. 693–703, 1982.

[14] R. P. Kiran, M. Rottoli, N. Pokala, and V. W. Fazio, "Long-term outcomes after local excision and radical surgery for anal melanoma: data from a population database," *Diseases of the Colon and Rectum*, vol. 53, no. 4, pp. 402–408, 2010.

[15] B. P. Whooley, P. Shaw, A. B. Astrow, I. R. Toth, and M. K. Wallack, "Long-term survival after locally aggressive anorectal melanoma," *American Surgeon*, vol. 64, no. 3, pp. 245–251, 1998.

[16] A. Malik, T. L. Hull, J. Milsom, and B. Wolff, "Long-term survivor of anorectal melanoma: report of a case," *Diseases of the Colon and Rectum*, vol. 45, no. 10, pp. 1412–1417, 2002.

[17] C. M. Balch, S. J. Soong, T. M. Murad, A. L. Ingalls, and W. A. Maddox, "A multifactorial analysis of melanoma. II. Prognostic factors in patients with stage I (localized) melanoma," *Surgery*, vol. 86, no. 2, pp. 343–351, 1979.

[18] B. C. Morson and H. Volkstädt, "Malignant melanoma of the anal canal," *Journal of Clinical Pathology*, vol. 16, no. 2, pp. 126–132, 1963.

[19] K. M. Bullard, T. M. Tuttle, D. A. Rothenberger et al., "Surgical therapy for anorectal melanoma," *Journal of the American College of Surgeons*, vol. 196, no. 2, pp. 206–211, 2003.

[20] P. Pessaux, M. Pocard, D. Elias et al., "Surgical management of primary anorectal melanoma," *British Journal of Surgery*, vol. 91, no. 9, pp. 1183–1187, 2004.

[21] J. J. Yeh, J. Shia, W. J. Hwu et al., "The role of abdominoperineal resection as surgical therapy for anorectal melanoma," *Annals of Surgery*, vol. 244, no. 6, pp. 1012–1017, 2006.

14

Jejunojejunal Intussusception Induced by a Gastrointestinal Stromal Tumor

Ali H. Zakaria and Salam Daradkeh

Istishari Hospital, The University of Jordan, P.O. Box 13261, Amman 11942, Jordan

Correspondence should be addressed to Salam Daradkeh, daradkeh@ju.edu.jo

Academic Editors: S.-i. Kosugi and M. Nikfarjam

Background. Adult intussusception is a rare entity representing less than 1% of all intestinal obstructions. Diagnosis of the condition is difficult requiring a high index of suspicion and the utilization of imaging studies, especially CT scans. Diagnostic laparoscopy and/or exploratory laparotomy can be used as a diagnostic and therapeutic intervention. In over 90% of cases, an underlying lead point is identified. In the patient described here, it was a gastrointestinal stromal tumor (GIST), a relatively rare mesenchymal tumor comprising only 0.2–1.0% of the gastrointestinal tract neoplasms and believed to originate from neoplastic transformation of the interstitial cells of Cajal. GISTs may occur anywhere along the gastrointestinal tract, but most commonly arise in the stomach and small intestine. Literature review revealed only few cases reporting GISTs as a leading point of adult's intussusception. *Case Presentation.* In this report, we are presenting a rare case of jejunojejunal intussusception in a 78-year-old female patient with a GIST located in the terminal jejunum being the leading point, demonstrating the importance of imaging studies, especially CT scan, laparoscopy, and exploratory laparotomy as diagnostic and therapeutic interventions.

1. Introduction

Intestinal invagination or intussusception is the leading cause of intestinal obstruction in children, but it is an uncommon process in adults, accounting for only 5% of all intussusceptions and 1% of all intestinal obstruction. Unlike childhood intussusception which is idiopathic in 90% of cases, 70–90% of adult cases have a demonstrable lead point, with a well-definable neoplastic abnormality being the etiology in 65% of cases [1, 2].

Adult intussusception may present with acute, subacute, or chronic nonspecific symptoms. Therefore, the initial diagnosis often is missed or delayed till the patient is in the operating room. There is a surgical consensus that adult intussusception requires surgical resection because the majority of patients have intraluminal lesions. However, there is controversy about the need for reduction of the intussusception and the extent of resection to be performed [2].

2. Case Report

A seventy-eight-year-old female patient with a previous medical history of diabetes mellitus, hypertension, ischemic heart disease, and Hypothyroidism presented with a one-week history of abdominal pain and nausea with vomiting following meals. Her symptoms progressively worsened to severe abdominal distention, anorexia and obstipation on the day of admission. She had no fever, chills, bleeding per rectum, or previous abdominal surgeries. Four weeks earlier the patient had similar symptoms. A plain abdominal X-ray and CT scan which were done at that time showed dilated small bowel loop in right lower quadrant without detected lesions or significant wall thickening, and she had been treated conservatively. After resolution of her symptoms—during the previous episode—an upper and lower GI endoscopy were done and revealed moderate erosive esophagitis, Helicobacter pylori positive gastritis and duodenitis, and an essentially normal colonic exam.

Her vital signs on admission were within normal limits. Examination showed a distended abdomen with hyperactive bowel sounds and generalized tenderness without peritoneal signs. Her laboratory investigations showed anemia with hemoglobin of 7.2 g/dL and white cell count of 9.9 × 10^3/mm^3. Abdominal X-ray revealed dilated proximal bowel loops with multiple air fluid levels. Conservative measures with bowel rest, nasogastric intubation, and intravenous fluids failed to control her symptoms. Abdominal and pelvic CT-scan showed markedly dilated fluid filled small bowel loops with one loop showing central hyperdense area, and a thick soft tissue mass around it with multiple small hypodense areas, referred to as the *target sign* [3] (Figure 1).

Diagnostic laparoscopy which revealed a distal jejunojejunal intussusception was followed by limited laparotomy and resection then anastomosis was performed (Figure 2). The leading point of the invagination was jejunal tumor (Figure 3). Histopathologic examination of the resected specimen revealed a GIST of intermediate risk, and resection was complete with viable ends.

The patient had an uneventful postoperative recovery and was discharged in a well condition. She was doing well on subsequent clinic followup.

3. Discussion

Adult intussusception is an uncommon clinical entity encountered by surgeons. The exact mechanism is unknown, and it is believed that any lesion in the bowel wall or irritant within the lumen that alters normal peristaltic activity is able to initiate invagination. It is most commonly located at the junctions between freely moving segments and retroperitoneally or adhesionally fixed segments [4].

About 90% of occurrences in adults have a well-defined pathological lead point, which may be a benign—such as benign neoplasms, inflammatory lesions, Meckel's diverticuli, appendix, and adhesions—or malignant lesion. In small intestine, malignant lesions (either primary or metastatic) account for 14–47% of cases, while malignant etiology is more prominent in large bowel representing up to 66% of the cases [2].

Most adult patients with intussusception present with chronic and nonspecific symptoms suggestive of intestinal obstruction. Abdominal pain is the most common symptom followed by nausea, vomiting, and a palpable abdominal mass [1, 2].

Preoperative imaging may help in identifying the causative lesion. Plain abdominal X-rays are typically the first diagnostic tool; with barium studies (showing "stacked coin" or "coiled spring" in upper GI series and "cup-shaped defect" in barium enema), ultrasonography (showing "target and doughnut sign" on transverse view and the "pseudokidney sign" in longitudinal view), and colonoscopy are also useful tools for evaluating intussusception [5–7].

In recent years, with a diagnostic accuracy of 58–100% in recent series, abdominal CT-scan (with the characteristic "*target sign*") has been reported to be the most useful tool for diagnosis of intestinal intussusception and is regarded superior to the above mentioned studies [3, 8, 9].

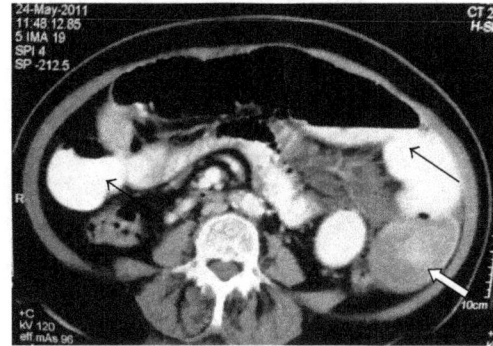

FIGURE 1: Computed tomography of abdomen showing dilated bowel loops (arrows) and the *target sign* of intussusception (white arrow).

Treatment of adult intussusception is always surgical. However, optimal management remains controversial. Most of the debate focuses on the issue of primary resection versus initial reduction followed by a more limited resection [2, 9], keeping in mind that reduction should not be attempted with any degree of suspicion of malignancy, due to possible risks of intraluminal seeding, venous embolization in regions of ulcerated mucosa, and anastomotic complications, which may potentially lead to bowel perforation [10]. Recently, there are several case reports about using laparoscopy as a minimally invasive technique for both diagnosis and treatment of adult intussusceptions.

Mesenchymal tumors constitute only 1% of primary GI cancers with GISTs being the most common. The annual incidence is between 7 and 20 cases per million per year [11]. It occurs predominantly in middle-aged and older individuals and rarely in those under the age of 40. The majority of cases are sporadic; however, several familial cases with heritable mutations in the KIT gene have been identified [12].

GISTs are thought to derive from neoplastic transformation of interstitial cells of Cajal (ICC). They may occur throughout the GI tract from the esophagus to the anus, but most commonly are found in the stomach (40–60%) and jejunum/ileum (25–30%) [12]. Duodenum (5%), colorectum (5–15%), and esophagus (≤1%) are less common sites.

Sometimes GISTs are asymptomatic and are discovered incidentally during an endoscopy or on a CT done for another purpose. More often, they are associated with nonspecific symptoms (i.e., early satiety, bloating) unless complicated with ulceration and overt GI bleeding (40% of the cases) or grow large enough to cause pain, mass or a lead point of intussusception and intestinal obstruction (20% of the cases) [12].

Contrast-enhanced CT is a preferred initial imaging study for screening and staging. However, other procedures such as ultrasound, endoscopy, intestinal capsule, and PET scan may also be used.

Surgical "en bloc" segmental resection with the goal of achieving negative resection margins is the treatment of choice for potentially resectable tumors, while initial therapy

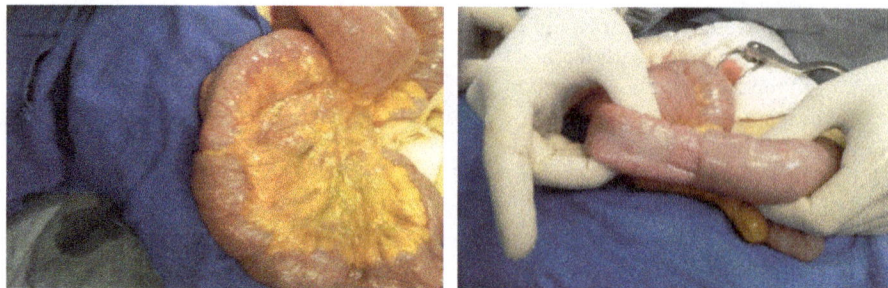

FIGURE 2: Intraoperative view showing the jejunojejunal intussusception.

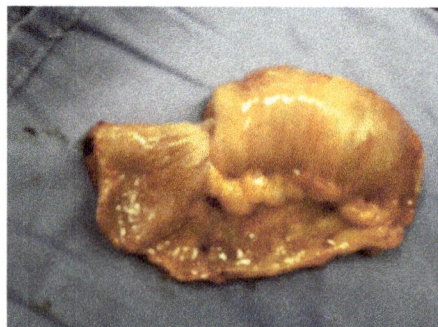

FIGURE 3: Jejunal tumor (GIST) was the leading point of intussusception.

with *imatinib* may be preferred if a tumor is borderline resectable, or if resection would necessitate extensive organ disruption.

The prognosis of small intestine GISTs depends upon the adequacy of resection, tumor size, mitotic activity, and location within the small bowel, with small intestine having a worse prognosis than stomach [13–15].

4. Conclusion

Intussusception in adults occurs relatively rarely; however, in 90% of cases a specific lead point is identified. The diagnosis may be challenging because of nonspecific symptoms, and sometimes it is impossible to reach the diagnosis of intussusception as a cause of obstruction until laparotomy is done. CT-scan is the most useful imaging modality in diagnosis. An underlying malignant lesion might be the lead point especially in large bowel. Therefore, surgeons should think of intussusception as a cause of intestinal obstruction, and they should be familiar with the various treatment options. The decision whether to undertake resection or reduction followed by resection is case specific, and it should be tailored according to the situation.

References

[1] T. Azar and D. L. Berger, "Adult intussusception," *Annals of Surgery*, vol. 226, pp. 134–138, 1997.

[2] D. G. Begos, A. Sandor, and I. M. Modlin, "The diagnosis and management of adult intussusception," *American Journal of Surgery*, vol. 173, no. 2, pp. 88–94, 1997.

[3] G. Gayer, S. Apter, C. Hofmann et al., "Intussusception in adults: CT diagnosis," *Clinical Radiology*, vol. 53, no. 1, pp. 53–57, 1998.

[4] L. T. Wang, C. C. Wu, J. C. Yu, C. W. Hsiao, C. C. Hsu, and S. W. Jao, "Clinical entity and treatment strategies for adult intussusceptions: 20 years' experience," *Diseases of the Colon and Rectum*, vol. 50, no. 11, pp. 1941–1949, 2007.

[5] L. K. Eisen, J. D. Cunningham, and A. H. Aufses Jr., "Intussusception in adults: institutional review," *Journal of the American College of Surgeons*, vol. 188, no. 4, pp. 390–395, 1999.

[6] D. L. Weissberg, W. Scheible, and G. R. Leopold, "Ultrasonographic appearance of adult intussusception," *Radiology*, vol. 124, no. 3, pp. 791–792, 1977.

[7] L. M. Hurwitz and S. L. Gertler, "Colonoscopic diagnosis of ileocolic intussusception," *Gastrointestinal Endoscopy*, vol. 32, no. 3, pp. 217–218, 1986.

[8] J. Bar-Ziv and A. Solomon, "Computed tomography in adult intussusception," *Gastrointestinal Radiology*, vol. 16, no. 3, pp. 264–266, 1991.

[9] M. Barussaud, N. Regenet, X. Briennon et al., "Clinical spectrum and surgical approach of adult intussusceptions: a multicentric study," *International Journal of Colorectal Disease*, vol. 21, no. 8, pp. 834–839, 2006.

[10] H. Yamada, T. Morita, M. Fujita, Y. Miyasaka, N. Senmaru, and T. Oshikiri, "Adult intussusception due to enteric neoplasms," *Digestive Diseases and Sciences*, vol. 52, no. 3, pp. 764–766, 2007.

[11] T. Tran, J. A. Davila, and H. B. El-Serag, "The epidemiology of malignant gastrointestinal stromal tumors: an analysis of 1,458 cases from 1992 to 2000," *American Journal of Gastroenterology*, vol. 100, no. 1, pp. 162–168, 2005.

[12] M. Miettinen and J. Lasota, "Gastrointestinal stromal tumors—definition, clinical, histological, immunohistochemical, and molecular genetic features and differential diagnosis," *Virchows Archiv*, vol. 438, no. 1, pp. 1–12, 2001.

[13] R. P. DeMatteo, J. J. Lewis, D. Leung, S. S. Mudan, J. M. Woodruff, and M. F. Brennan, "Two hundred gastrointestinal stromal tumors: recurrence patterns and prognostic factors for survival," *Annals of Surgery*, vol. 231, no. 1, pp. 51–58, 2000.

[14] W. L. Yang, J. R. Yu, Y. J. Wu et al., "Duodenal gastrointestinal stromal tumor: clinical, pathologic, immunohistochemical characteristics, and surgical prognosis," *Journal of Surgical Oncology*, vol. 100, no. 7, pp. 606–610, 2009.

[15] M. Miettinen, H. Makhlouf, L. H. Sobin, and J. Lasota, "Gastrointestinal stromal tumors of the jejunum and ileum: a clinicopathologic, immunohistochemical, and molecular genetic study of 906 cases before imatinib with long-term follow-up," *American Journal of Surgical Pathology*, vol. 30, no. 4, pp. 477–489, 2006.

15

An Unusual Case of Stercoral Perforation in a Patient with 86 cm of Small Bowel

Alfin Okullo,[1] **Ghiyath Alsnih,**[1] **and Titus Kwok**[2]

[1] *Department of Surgery, Blacktown-Mt Druitt Hospital, Blacktown Road, Blacktown, Sydney, NSW 2148, Australia*
[2] *Department of Surgery, Concord Repatriation and General Hospital, Hospital Road, Concord, Sydney, NSW 2139, Australia*

Correspondence should be addressed to Alfin Okullo; alfinokullo@gmail.com

Academic Editors: S. H. Ein, A. K. Karam, and C. Schmitz

A 77-year-old male who previously had extensive enterectomy due to ischaemic gut with loss of all but 86 cm of jejunum in addition to a right hemicolectomy presented to the emergency department (ED) with abdominal pain and constipation of 12-day duration. Abdominal imaging with X-ray and CT revealed pneumoperitoneum in addition to a grossly redundant and faecally loaded colon. At laparotomy, rectal perforation was found. In view of the patient's advanced age, comorbidities, and the absence of intraperitoneal faecal contamination, manual disimpaction followed by wedge resection and primary closure of the perforation was done. On postop day 11, a perforation in the sigmoid colon with free subdiaphragmatic gas was picked up on CT after a work up for abdominal tenderness. In the absence of peritonism and other signs of deterioration, conservative management was chosen with subsequent uneventful recovery for the patient.

1. Introduction

A patient with 86 cm of small bowel is expected to have short bowel syndrome (SBS). It is quite unusual for such a patient to present with constipation so severe that it causes stercoral perforation. We present a rare case of one such patient.

2. Case Report

A 77-year-old male presented to the (ED) with generalized abdominal pain and constipation of about 12-day duration. He was still passing wind and denied any nausea or vomiting.

His previous surgical history consisted of an extensive enterectomy 17 years ago for ischaemic gut, whereupon all but 86 cm of his jejunum was resected in addition to a right hemicolectomy. A jejunal-transverse colon anastomosis was done. Back then, his postop recovery was notable for a quick resolution of his diarrhea while on a low-fibre diet without any antimotility drugs and a return to his premorbid, chronically constipated state within about 2 months of the surgery. He thereafter required daily lactulose whose dose he had increased from 20 to 30 mls to no avail over the past 12 days. He was never on any medicines used to treat short bowel syndrome. A review of his regular medications was negative for any that would contribute to his chronic constipation prior to and after the bowel resection 17 years ago.

At this presentation, his vital signs and blood tests were all normal except for an INR of 6.6.

A chest X-ray revealed free subdiaphragmatic gas (Figure 1), while a plain erect abdominal X-ray showed gross faecal loading.

A CT abdomen and pelvis with oral and intravenous contrast demonstrated gross faecal loading in the colon up to the rectum with a very large amount of free intraabdominal gas. There was a moderate amount of gas present within a grossly redundant sigmoid colon with colonic diameter of up to 110 mm in some sections (Figure 2).

After INR reversal with prothrombinex and vitamin K, he was taken to the operating theatre.

Intraoperative findings were of gross dilatation of the sigmoid colon with massive faecal loading. A small rectal perforation approximately 1 cm in diameter was identified in the antimesenteric border. In view of the patient's advanced age, comorbidities, and the absence of intraperitoneal faecal contamination, he was manually disimpacted and the perforation wedge resected then primarily repaired.

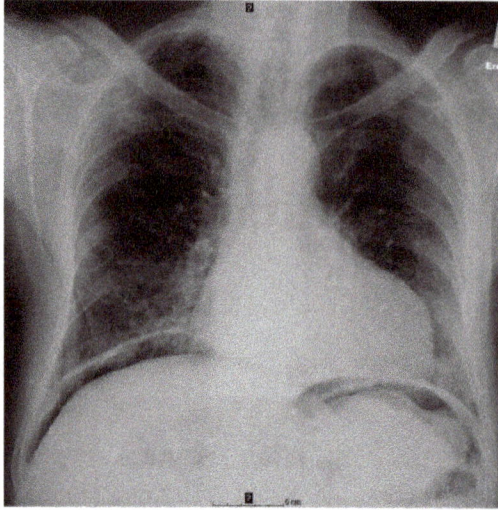

Figure 1: CXR demonstrating air under the diaphragm on presentation.

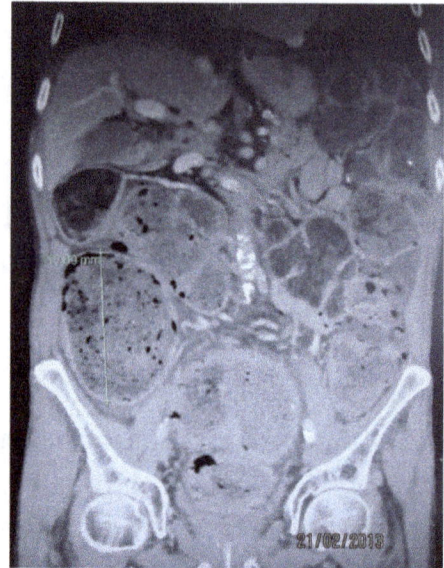

Figure 2: CT abdomen and pelvis demonstrating gross faecal loading and colonic dilatation.

The patient was subsequently admitted to the intensive care unit (ICU) for observation and ventilatory support.

His postoperative recovery was remarkable for a second perforation picked up with abdominal imaging on day 11 in ICU, after he was thought to have abdominal tenderness. However, since the patient remained nonperitonitic with no fever or signs of deterioration, he was successfully managed conservatively. The patient tolerated diet, was stepped down to the ward, and was subsequently discharged home with regular laxatives. At a follow-up visit one month after discharge, he was back to baseline with normal functioning for himself.

3. Case Discussion

Short bowel syndrome (SBS) is a complex disease that results from surgical resection, congenital defect, or disease-associated loss of absorption and is characterized by the inability to maintain protein-energy, fluid, electrolyte, or micronutrient balances when on a normal diet [1]. It is defined in adults as <200 cm of small intestine [2]. SBS presents clinically as chronic diarrhoea and severe wasting.

SBS is still a relatively rare condition with a prevalence estimated at 2 per million people in Europe. Patients often adapt clinically to the significantly reduced energy absorption associated with SBS through hyperphagia. However, the intestine adapts as well to ensure more efficient absorption per unit length. After massive enterectomy, the intestine hypertrophies and becomes more efficient in nutrient absorption; there is slight lengthening, but more importantly, diameter and villus height increase, effectively increasing the absorptive surface [2].

The patients with the greatest risk for development of SBS are those with a duodenostomy or jejunoileal anastomosis and <35 cm of residual small intestine, jejunocolic or ileocolic anastomosis, and <60 cm of residual small intestine or end jejunostomy with <115 cm of residual small intestine [3]. Patients with residual colon in continuity will have enhanced energy and fluid absorption and hence can tolerate greater loss of small intestine and retain their nutritional autonomy.

Without colon in continuity, there is a loss of inhibition on gastric emptying and intestinal transit, which is related to a significant decrease in peptide YY (PYY), glucagon-like peptide I (GLP-I), and neurotensin [4]. PYY is normally released from the L cells in the ileum and colon when stimulated by fat or bile salts. Obviously, these cells are missing in patients who had a distal ileal and colonic resection.

Stercoral perforation is defined as perforation of the bowel due to pressure necrosis from faecal masses. The latter being no more than an accumulation of stool that has hardened and has remained stationary in the bowel over a long period of time causing stagnation and colonic deformity [5].

This condition is primarily caused by chronic constipation with at least 61% of patients having a positive history and 100% of patients showing evidence of faecal impaction on the abdominal films [6].

The majority (77%) of stercoral perforations occur in the sigmoid and the rectosigmoid regions [7].

This is explained in part by the high rate of absorption of water from the stool in this part of the bowels thus making the water content in the stools the lowest in the distal colon. The narrow lumen of the distal colon also contributes by causing increased intraluminal pressure, which can become higher than the intestinal capillary perfusion pressure, causing necrosis on the antimesenteric border in the event of faecal impaction [8].

As far as we are aware, this is the first reported case of stercoral perforation in a patient with short bowel.

References

[1] S. J. D. O'Keefe, A. L. Buchman, T. M. Fishbein, K. N. Jeejeebhoy, P. B. Jeppesen, and J. Shaffer, "Short bowel syndrome and intestinal failure: consensus definitions and overview," *Clinical Gastroenterology and Hepatology*, vol. 4, no. 1, pp. 6–10, 2006.

[2] A. L. Buchman, "Etiology and initial management of short bowel syndrome," *Gastroenterology*, vol. 130, no. 2, pp. S5–S15, 2006.

[3] B. Messing, P. Crenn, P. Beau, M. C. Boutron-Ruault, J. C. Rambaud, and C. Matuchansky, "Long-term survival and parenteral nutrition dependence in adult patients with the short bowel syndrome," *Gastroenterology*, vol. 117, no. 5, pp. 1043–1050, 1999.

[4] J. M. D. Nightingale, M. A. Kamm, J. R. M. van der Sijp, M. A. Ghatei, S. R. Bloom, and J. E. Lennard-Jones, "Gastrointestinal hormones in short bowel syndrome. Peptide YY may be the "colonic brake" to gastric emptying," *Gut*, vol. 39, no. 2, pp. 267–272, 1996.

[5] A. L. Atkinson and A. Pepe, "Stercoral perforation of the colon in pregnancy," *Journal of Surgical Case Reports*, vol. 2010, 5, no. 2, 2010.

[6] J. W. Serpell and R. J. Nicholls, "Stercoral perforation of the colon," *British Journal of Surgery*, vol. 77, no. 12, pp. 1325–1329, 1990.

[7] C. Heffernan, H. L. Pachter, A. J. Megibow, and M. Macari, "Stercoral colitis leading to fatal peritonitis: CT findings," *American Journal of Roentgenology*, vol. 184, no. 4, pp. 1189–1193, 2005.

[8] A. W. Bradbury, J. Brittenden, K. McBride, and C. V. Ruckley, "Mesenteric ischaemia: a multidisciplinary approach," *British Journal of Surgery*, vol. 82, no. 11, pp. 1446–1459, 1995.

16

Gastric Glomus Tumor: A Rare Cause of Upper Gastrointestinal Bleeding

Yoshinori Handa,[1] **Mikihiro Kano,**[1] **Mayumi Kaneko,**[2] **and Naoki Hirabayashi**[1]

[1]*Department of Surgery, Hiroshima City Asa Hospital, 2-1-1 Kabeminami, Asakita-ku, Hiroshima 731-0293, Japan*
[2]*Department of Pathology, Hiroshima City Asa Hospital, 2-1-1 Kabeminami, Asakita-ku, Hiroshima 731-0293, Japan*

Correspondence should be addressed to Yoshinori Handa; qqm925e9@herb.ocn.ne.jp

Academic Editor: Fernando Turégano

A 24-year-old woman was referred to our department because of melena. These symptoms combined with severe anemia prompted us to perform an emergency upper endoscopy, which showed bleeding from an ulcerated 30 mm submucosal tumor in the gastric antrum. A computed tomography scan revealed a homogeneously enhanced mass, and endoscopic ultrasonography identified a well-demarcated mass in the third and fourth layers of the gastric wall. Because analysis of the possible medical causes remained inconclusive and the risk of rebleeding, laparoscopy-assisted gastric wedge resection was performed after administration of 10 units of red cell concentrate. Histological and immunohistological analysis revealed the tumor to be a gastric glomus tumor. Gastric submucosal tumors remain challenging to diagnose preoperatively as they show a variety of radiologic and clinicopathologic features and are associated with the risk of bleeding upon biopsy, as is indicated in the guidelines for gastric submucosal tumors. Gastric glomus tumors characteristically present with exsanguinating gastrointestinal hemorrhaging that often requires blood transfusion. Additionally, gastric submucosal tumors typically occur in elderly patients; however, this case involved a young patient who was 24 years old. Here, we describe this case in order to identify features that may aid in early differentiation of gastric submucosal tumors.

1. Introduction

Glomus tumors (GTs) are benign lesions originating from modified cells of the glomus body that are responsible for regulation of arteriolar blood flow. Although these tumors usually occur in peripheral soft tissue [1], in the gastrointestinal tract, they are most commonly found in the stomach. We encountered a case of a gastric GT that was characteristic in its clinical course, presenting with exsanguinating gastrointestinal hemorrhage and patient at the age of 24 years. Taken together with the findings in previous reports, the characteristics observed here may be useful for diagnosing gastric submucosal tumors (SMTs).

2. Case Presentation

A 24-year-old woman with no previous history of illness presented with vomiting and melena to her local primary clinic. Tachycardia was noted as a characteristic physical abnormality, and her hemoglobin level was extremely low (6.3 g/dL). The patient was transferred to our hospital and was subjected to further testing along with transfusion of 10 units of red cell concentrate. An emergency upper gastrointestinal endoscopy revealed active bleeding from an ulcer on the surface of an elevated lesion located in the lower portion of the stomach, along the greater curvature. The bleeding was successfully controlled using local sclerosis therapy.

Two days later, the patient underwent another upper gastrointestinal endoscopy, which revealed a 30 mm, well-circumscribed, soft SMT (Figure 1(a)). The gastric mucosa covering the SMT showed a small ulcer, without signs of bleeding. We did not biopsy this mass because of the probability of rebleeding. Endoscopic ultrasonography (EUS) showed a well-demarcated mass in the third and fourth layers of the gastric wall, with a hypoechoic pattern (Figure 1(b)). A computed tomography (CT) scan of the abdomen revealed a

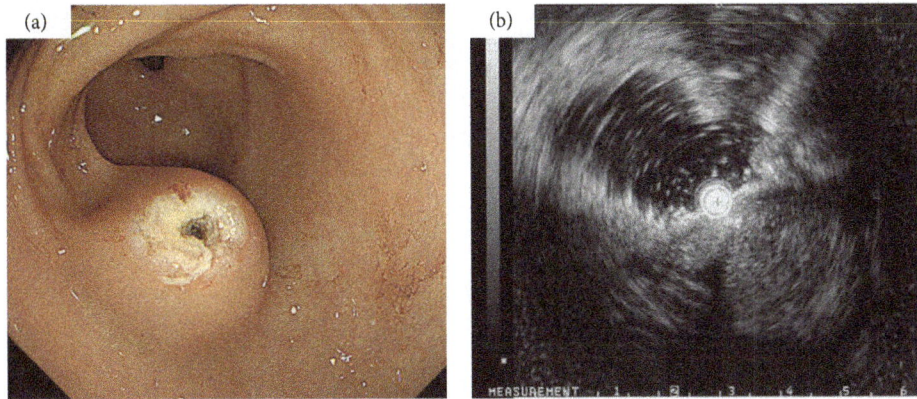

FIGURE 1: Upper gastrointestinal endoscopy and endoscopic ultrasonography findings. The image shows a well-circumscribed elevated mass, measuring 30 × 30 mm, with normal overlying mucosa in the anterior wall of the gastric antrum (a). The image shows a well-demarcated mass in the third and fourth layers of the gastric wall with a hypoechoic pattern (b).

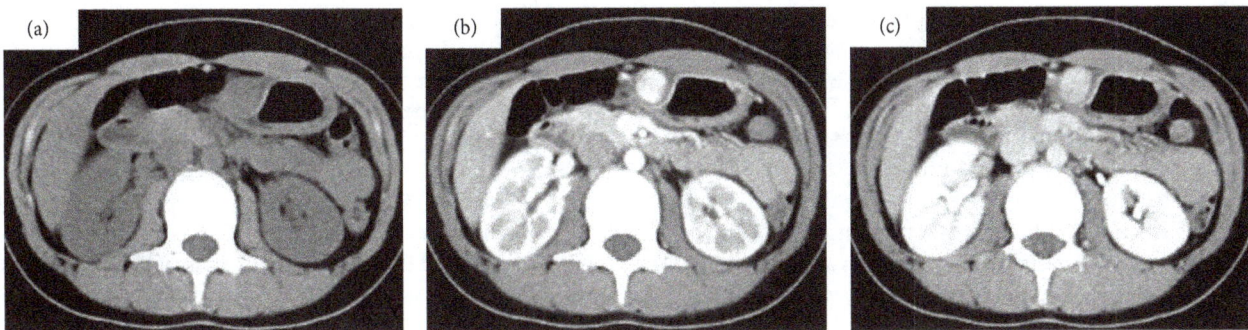

FIGURE 2: Computed tomography findings. Abdominal computed tomography revealed a well demarcated, ovoid mass at the antrum on (a) unenhanced, (b) arterial phase, and (c) delayed phase scans.

mass with dense homogeneous enhancement in the stomach wall. This scan suggested the presence of a lesion with abundant blood supply and an intact overlying mucosa using early- and delayed-phase contrast-enhanced CT, respectively (Figure 2). Because the analysis to identify the possible medical causes of the lesion remained inconclusive and because of the risk of rebleeding, the patient was referred for an elective laparoscopy-assisted surgical procedure, according to the Japanese treatment guidelines for gastric SMTs [2].

During the operation, a tumor, approximately 30 mm in diameter, was found in the antral wall of the stomach. The tumor had not invaded the adjacent organs and was successfully removed via gastric wedge resection. The patient had an uneventful postoperative course and was discharged six days after surgery.

Histologically, the tumor was composed of atypical glomus cell nests surrounding capillaries (Figure 3). Immunohistochemical staining revealed the tumor cells to be positive for vimentin, smooth muscle actin, and collagen type IV (Figure 4). Staining for CD34, synaptophysin, and chromogranin A revealed that they were not expressed in these tumor cells. Taken together, our analysis led to diagnosis of this lesion as a gastric GT.

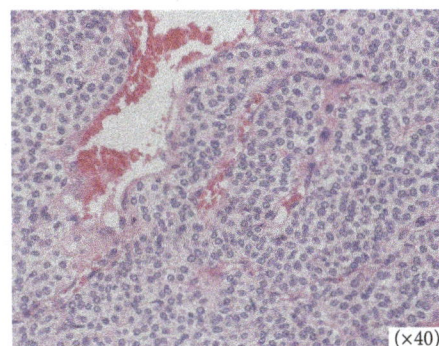

FIGURE 3: Histological findings. Microscopic examination shows numerous dilated, thin-walled vascular spaces surrounded by uniform glomus cells (hematoxylin and eosin staining; magnification, ×40).

The tumor was completely resected and was determined not to be severely malignant based on the detection of few cells undergoing mitosis and the observation of few atypical cells. We therefore chose not to provide adjuvant therapy while continuing to monitor the patient through follow-up.

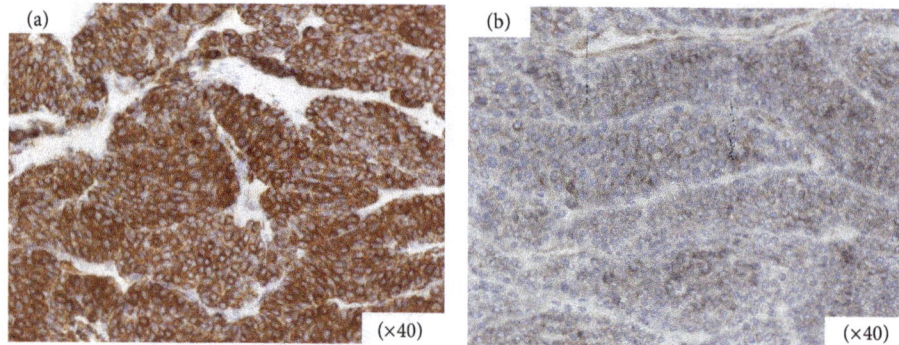

FIGURE 4: Immunohistological findings. Tumor cells are positive for smooth muscle actin (a) and collage type IV (b) (magnification, ×40).

Ten months after the operation, the postoperative course remains uneventful without signs of relapse.

3. Discussion

GTs are rare benign mesenchymal tumors arising from the glomus body. This type of tumor was first reported by De Busscher in 1948 [3], and less than 200 reports have been published in the English literature since then. Previous reports suggest that gastric GTs account for approximately 2% of all benign gastric tumors and that they are slightly more frequent in women, with a 2 : 3 male-to-female ratio [4].

Gastric SMTs vary in malignant potential from benign to highly malignant and vary in size from a small nodule to a large mass, such as gastrointestinal stromal tumors (GISTs), heterotopic pancreas, hemangiomas, carcinoid tumors, and neurilemmomas. Additionally, GTs may present as a solitary, hypervascular SMT, as in our case. Among these tumor types, GISTs are the most common ones and are often malignant, so the main diagnostic strategy when examining such a gastric SMT is to differentiate it from GISTs. An ideal course of action would be to perform a preoperative biopsy, but this is often difficult owing to the potential for rebleeding, and guidelines for gastric SMTs recommend operation without a biopsy when patients have symptoms [2]. Radiological and clinicopathologic characteristics can be used to help determine the differential diagnosis [5]. The radiological features of GISTs are diverse; namely, on examination with plain CT, GISTs exhibit low density, show strong enhancement on the arterial-phase images, and do not exhibit prolonged enhancement on delayed-phase images. On EUS, GISTs usually appear as heterogeneous tumors between the submucosal and muscularis propria layers [6]. On the other hand, GTs are reported to show different features from those described for GISTs. On examination with CT, GTs manifest as well-circumscribed submucosal masses with homogeneous density on unenhanced images and show strong enhancement on arterial-phase images as well as persistent enhancement on delayed-phase images, as was observed in our case [7]. On examination with EUS, GTs usually show well-circumscribed hypoechoic masses located in the third and/or fourth layer

of the gastric wall [8] although heterogeneous echogenicity, caused by hemorrhage or calcification, may occur.

Patients with gastric SMTs usually present with epigastric pain and distress, having been reported in over 50% of patients. Gastrointestinal bleeding and ulcer-like symptoms are occasionally observed and have been reported in 5% of patients with gastric SMTs. However, exsanguinating gastrointestinal hemorrhage from a SMT is very rare. Gastric GTs are thought to be highly vascularized because this tumor arises from cells of the arteriovenous anastomosis plexus and, in several reports, gastric GTs have led to exsanguinating gastrointestinal hemorrhaging requiring a blood transfusion [9–11].

Additionally, gastric SMTs such as GISTs generally occur in elderly patients, especially in patients above the age of 60; by comparison, this case involved a 24-year-old patient. Although the scarcity of reports may preclude a predictive conclusion, gastric GTs have been reported to occur at younger ages than GISTs, with a median age of 45 years (range, 28–79 years) [12]. Gastric GT should be included as a differential diagnosis if a solitary, hypervascular SMT is detected in the stomach, especially when it presents with exsanguinating gastrointestinal hemorrhaging and occurs in a young patient.

We confirmed that gastrointestinal GTs are histologically and immunophenotypically comparable with the GTs found in peripheral soft tissues, as previously reported [13, 14]. Histologically, the tumor was mainly located in the muscularis of the stomach and was composed of small, uniform, rounded cells surrounding capillaries with diffuse sheet distributions, but without nuclear pleomorphism or mitotic figures. The tumor was positive for α-smooth muscle actin and vimentin but negative for CD34 and KIT. These immunohistological features may help to distinguish GTs from other histologically similar tumors.

In general, gastric GTs have a good prognosis; however, several authors have reported that gastric GTs can metastasize hematogenously to the liver, lungs, and brain [15–17], and a tumor diameter of greater than 5 cm might be an indicator of risk [18]. Although gastric GTs are usually small with a median size ranging from 2 cm to 3 cm, as was observed in our case, careful follow-up is recommended.

References

[1] M. Tsuneyoshi and M. Enjoji, "Glomus tumor: a clinicopathologic and electron microscopic study," *Cancer*, vol. 50, no. 8, pp. 1601–1607, 1982.

[2] Japan Society for Cancer Therapy, Japan Gastric Cancer Association, and GIST Study Group, *Guideline 2014 for the Treatment of Gastrointestinal Stromal Tumor*, 3rd edition, 2014.

[3] G. De Busscher, "Les anatomoses arterioveineuses de l'estomac: an ultrastructural study," *Acta Neerlandica Morphologiae Normalis et Pathologicae*, vol. 6, no. 1-2, pp. 87–105, 1948.

[4] H.-W. Lee, J. J. Lee, D. H. Yang, and B. H. Lee, "A clinicopathologic study of glomus tumor of the stomach," *Journal of Clinical Gastroenterology*, vol. 40, no. 8, pp. 717–720, 2006.

[5] M. Tang, J. Hou, D. Wu, X.-Y. Han, M.-S. Zeng, and X.-Z. Yao, "Glomus tumor in the stomach: computed tomography and endoscopic ultrasound findings," *World Journal of Gastroenterology*, vol. 19, no. 8, pp. 1327–1329, 2013.

[6] C.-C. Huang, F.-J. Yu, C.-M. Jan et al., "Gastric glomus tumor: a case report and review of the literature," *The Kaohsiung Journal of Medical Sciences*, vol. 26, no. 6, pp. 321–326, 2010.

[7] V. Canzonieri and E. Bidoli, "Differential diagnosis of malignant gastric tumors. A pathological appraisal with reference to locally advanced gastric carcinoma," *I Supplementi di Tumori*, vol. 2, no. 5, p. -9, 2003.

[8] A. Imamura, M. Tochihara, K. Natsui et al., "Glomus tumor of the stomach: endoscopic ultrasonographic findings," *The American Journal of Gastroenterology*, vol. 89, no. 2, pp. 271–272, 1994.

[9] F. Ferrozzi, G. Tognini, G. Marchesi, E. Spaggiari, and P. Pavone, "Gastric tumors with fatty components. CT findings and differential diagnosis," *La Radiologia Medica*, vol. 100, pp. 343–347, 2000.

[10] E. F. R. Nascimento, F. P. Fonte, R. L. Mendonça, R. Nonose, C. A. F. de Souza, and C. A. R. Martinez, "Glomus tumor of the stomach: a rare cause of upper gastrointestinal bleeding," *Case Reports in Surgery*, vol. 2011, Article ID 371082, 5 pages, 2011.

[11] K.-C. Huang, M.-C. Tsai, and C.-C. Lin, "A rare cause of gastrointestinal bleeding in a young man," *Gastroenterology*, vol. 145, no. 4, pp. e11–e12, 2013.

[12] C. Diaz-Zorrilla, P. Grube-Pagola, J. M. Remes-Troche, and A. R.-D. la Medina, "Glomus tumour of the stomach: an unusual cause of gastrointestinal bleeding," *BMJ Case Reports*, 2012.

[13] T. Okabayashi, A. Kaneko, N. Kamioka, and I. Naoki, "Laparoscopic gastric excision of glomus tumor of stomach. A case report," *Gastric Journal of Japan Society for Endoscopic Surgery*, vol. 61, no. 8, pp. 2012–2015, 2000.

[14] M. Miettinen, V. P. Lehto, and I. Virtanen, "Glomus tumor cells: evaluation of smooth muscle and endothelial cell properties," *Virchows Archiv B*, vol. 43, no. 2, pp. 139–149, 1983.

[15] P. L. Porter, S. A. Bigler, M. McNutt, and A. M. Gown, "The immunophenotype of hemangiopericytomas and glomus tumors, with special reference to muscle protein expression: an immunohistochemical study and review of the literature," *Modern Pathology*, vol. 4, no. 1, pp. 46–52, 1991.

[16] M. Miettinen, E. Paal, J. Lasota, and L. H. Sobin, "Gastrointestinal glomus tumors: a clinicopathologic, immunohistochemical, and molecular genetic study of 32 cases," *The American Journal of Surgical Pathology*, vol. 26, no. 3, pp. 301–311, 2002.

[17] A. P. J. J. Bray, N. A. C. S. Wong, and S. Narayan, "Cutaneous metastasis from gastric glomus tumour," *Clinical and Experimental Dermatology*, vol. 34, no. 8, pp. e719–e721, 2009.

[18] S. E. Song, C. H. Lee, K. A. Kim, H. J. Lee, and C. M. Park, "Malignant glomus tumor of the stomach with multiorgan metastases: report of a case," *Surgery Today*, vol. 40, no. 7, pp. 662–667, 2010.

17

Single Incision Laparoscopic Total Gastrectomy and D2 Lymph Node Dissection for Gastric Cancer using a Four-Access Single Port: The First Experience

Metin Ertem,[1,2] **Emel Ozveri,**[1] **Hakan Gok,**[1] **and Volkan Ozben**[1]

[1] *General Surgery Clinic, Kozyatagi Acibadem Hospital, 34742 Istanbul, Turkey*
[2] *Department of General Surgery, Cerrahpasa Medical Faculty, Istanbul University, Cerrahpasa, Fatih, 34098 Istanbul, Turkey*

Correspondence should be addressed to Metin Ertem; metinertem@hotmail.com

Academic Editors: T. Çolak and S. H. Ein

Single incision laparoscopic surgery (SILS) and natural orifice transluminal endoscopic surgery (NOTES) have been developed to reduce the invasiveness of laparoscopic surgery. SILS has been frequently applied in various clinical settings, such as cholecystectomy, colectomy, and sleeve gastrectomy. So far, there have been four reports on single incision laparoscopic distal gastrectomy and one report on single incision laparoscopic total gastrectomy with D1 lymph node dissection for gastric cancer. In this report, we present our single incision laparoscopic total gastrectomy with D2 lymph node dissection technique using a four-hole single port (OctoPort) in a patient with gastric cancer.

1. Introduction

In recent years, laparoscopic gastrectomy has been increasingly performed in the surgical management of gastric cancer. In some Asian countries, especially in Japan and Korea, this procedure has become a standard therapy for early stage gastric cancer [1, 2]. Kitano et al. [1] reported excellent long-term outcomes of laparoscopic gastrectomy in a retrospective multicenter study for early gastric cancer. Experienced surgeons are trying to extend this laparoscopic approach to certain advanced gastric cancer using more aggressive techniques. Furthermore, single incision laparoscopic surgery (SILS) and natural orifice transluminal endoscopic surgery (NOTES) have been developed to reduce the invasiveness of laparoscopic surgery. SILS has been frequently applied in various clinical settings, such as cholecystectomy, colectomy, and sleeve gastrectomy [3–6]. So far, there have been four reports on single incision laparoscopic distal gastrectomy and one report on single incision laparoscopic total gastrectomy with D1 lymph node dissection for gastric cancer [7–11]. Here, we report the first experience in single incision laparoscopic total gastrectomy with D2 lymph node dissection technique in a patient with gastric cancer.

2. Case Report

A 63-year-old man presented to our clinic with the complaints of recent weight loss, indigestion, and abdominal discomfort. During diagnostic work-up, upper endoscopy and biopsy revealed adenocarcinoma located in the corpus of the stomach and endoscopic ultrasonography showed the invasion of the cancer in the submucosal layer. Abdominal CT and PET-CT demonstrated that there was no regional lymph node involvement or distant metastasis. The patient's body mass index was $22.1 \, kg/m^2$. Based on these findings, total gastrectomy was scheduled.

Operative Technique. Under general anesthesia, the patient was placed in a supine position with reverse Trendelenburg. The surgeon stood between the patient's legs. A longitudinal 3.5 cm long transumbilical skin incision was made. A four-hole single port (OctoPort, two 5 mm holes, one 10 mm, and one 12 mm hole) was placed through the umbilical incision. A carbon dioxide pneumoperitoneum was created and the pressure was maintained at 12 mmHg. There were no additional trocars used. Through the port, a rigid 30-degree 10 mm laparoscope, a liver retractor, and two dissector

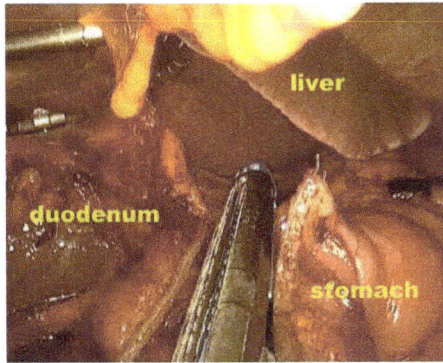

FIGURE 1: Transection of the duodenum 1-2 cm distal to the pyloric ring.

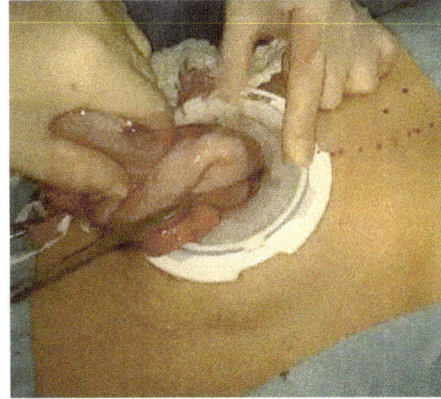

FIGURE 2: Transection of the esophagus using a linear stapler.

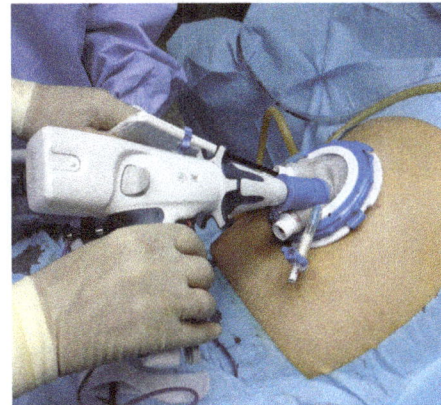

FIGURE 3: Removal of the specimen through the umbilical port.

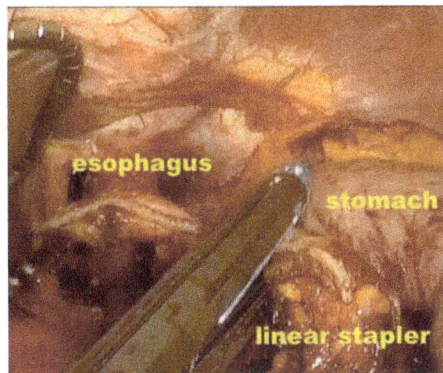

FIGURE 4: Placement of the circular stapler through the port and into the jejunal end.

forceps were introduced. The greater omentum was divided using Ligasure 5 mm (Covidien, USA). After the division and ligation of the left gastroepiploic vessels at the root, dissection around the lymph nodes was continued toward the pylorus. Then, the right gastroepiploic vessels were divided and ligated at the root. After the lesser omentum of the upper duodenum was resected, the right gastric vessels were identified from the hepatic artery and ligated. The duodenum was transected 1-2 cm distal to the pyloric ring using a laparoscopic linear stapler (Echelon Flex 60 Endopath stapler, Ethicon Endo-Surgery, Inc.) (Figure 1). The nodes along the hepatic hilus, common hepatic artery, and splenic artery were dissected. After the division and ligation of the left gastric vessels with Hem-o-lok clips (Teleflex), celiac lymph node dissection was performed. The lymph nodes around the splenic hilus were harvested and the short gastric artery was ligated. The esophagus was then transected using a linear stapler (Echelon Flex 60) and sutures were placed at the esophageal stump for the stabilization of the stump in the abdominal cavity (Figure 2). After the stomach was mobilized, the specimen was removed through the umbilical port which also served as a wound protector (Figure 3). A jejunal segment 20 cm away from the ligament of Treitz was taken outside the abdominal cavity through the port and then was transected. A side-to-side jejunojejunostomy was performed using a linear stapler extracorporeally. The port cover was removed and a circular stapler (EEA XL 25) was inserted and placed into the jejunal end (Figure 4). The main unit of the stapler with the jejunum was ligated with a silk suture. After closing the port cover, the stapler gun was inserted from port and the abdomen was reinsufflated. EEA OrVil 25 mm (Covidien) was inserted orally. A small hole was created at the closed end of the esophagus. The OrVil head and the tube were connected with two pieces of number 1 polyester yarn, which was cut to disconnect the OrVil (Figure 5). After firing the EEA XL 25 stapler, Roux-en-Y esophagojejunostomy was completed (Figure 6). The cut edge of the jejunum was closed with a linear stapler (Echelon Flex 60) (Figure 7). Methylene blue test was performed to check the anastomotic leakage. No drain was placed, and the umbilical opening was closed in layers (Figure 8).

The total operative time was 282 min. After the integrity of the esophago-intestinal tract was controlled with an oral radiopaque contrast examination on the third postoperative day, the patient was allowed to start clear fluids. The patient was discharged on the eighth day. Results of the final patho-logical analysis revealed no nodal metastasis among the 34 examined lymph nodes (pT1bN0M0). No major complica-tions including anastomotic leakage, stenosis, or bleeding

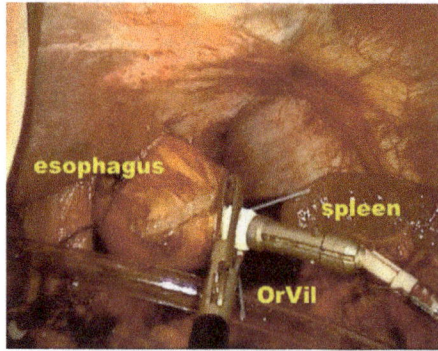

FIGURE 5: Appearance of the OrVil.

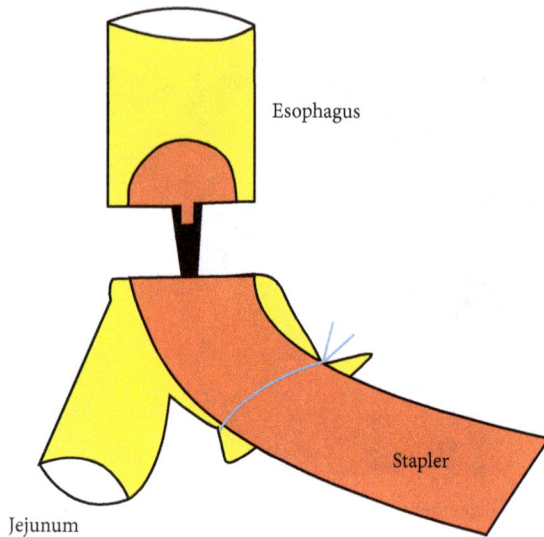

FIGURE 6: Illustration of the Roux-en-Y esophagojejunostomy.

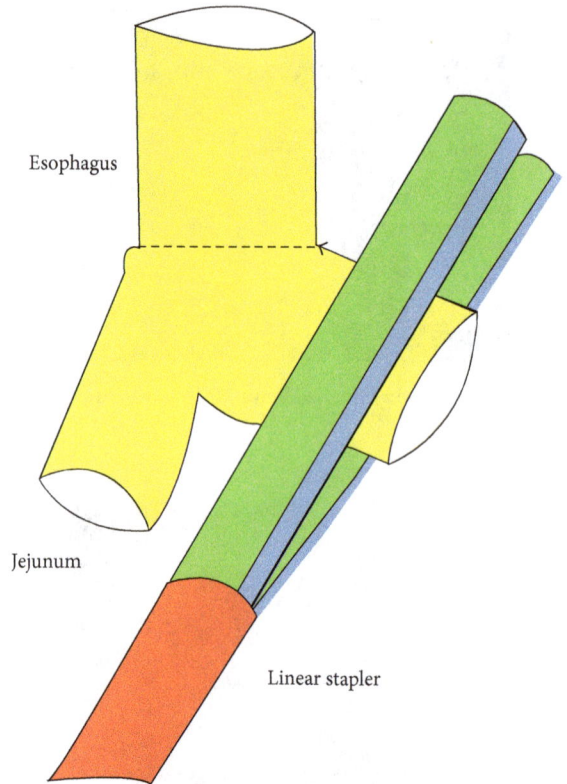

FIGURE 7: Illustration of the jejunal end closure.

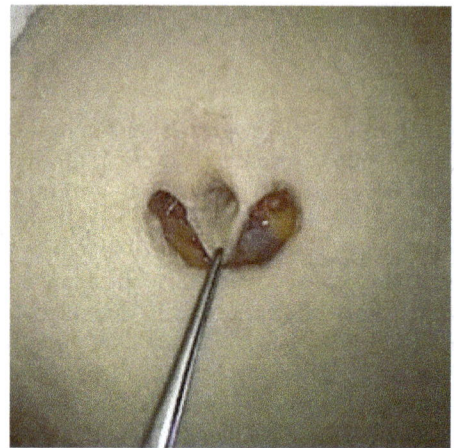

FIGURE 8: Appearance of the umbilical incision after the surgery.

were observed and no other late complications occurred during the six-month follow-up period.

3. Discussion

In recent years, laparoscopic techniques have gained worldwide clinical acceptance in the general surgery practice. Since laparoscopy-assisted distal gastrectomy for early gastric cancer was first performed in 1991 and first reported in 1994 [12], this procedure for early gastric cancer has been adapted quickly. This approach offers important advantages when compared with the open surgery such as better cosmetic results, improved quality of life, less pain, shortened hospital stay, early rehabilitation, and early return to social activity [1, 2, 13–15]. Improvements in the instruments and laparoscopic techniques have also led to widespread acceptance of this technique for other resections such as proximal, total, and functionally preserving gastrectomy [16–18].

Recently, some surgeons have been concerned with the laparoscopic surgery for advanced gastric cancer. In the case of advanced gastric cancer, it has been shown that there is no statistical difference in the number of retrieved lymph nodes with D2 lymphadenectomy in laparoscopic surgery [19, 20]. Also, several authors have shown no difference in the recurrence and survival rates following laparoscopic surgery versus open surgery for early gastric cancer. However, in the presence of an advanced gastric cancer, the results have remained controversial.

SILS was introduced to reduce the minimal invasiveness of laparoscopy to the least invasiveness possible and to achieve excellent cosmetic results. SILS has been applied in various surgical procedures with predominantly benign indications. SILS is rarely applied for gastric cancer. To our knowledge, there is very limited data on single incision laparoscopic total gastrectomy for early gastric cancer [10].

This report shows that SILS total gastrectomy with D2 lymph node dissection for gastric cancer is a feasible procedure and it can be safely performed with a proper experience in SILS and laparoscopic gastrectomy. This procedure may produce better cosmetic results. The total operative time was similar to that of conventional laparoscopic total gastrectomy.

Further experience is required to demonstrate the oncological safety of SILS for gastric cancer. We expect that all these technical advancements will finally improve the survival and quality of life of patients with gastric cancer. SILS total gastrectomy is feasible with conventional hand instruments and new laparoscopic devices (single incisional multiaccess ports, angulated linear cutter, oral inserted circular stapler, etc.). This technique can be performed safely by experienced laparoscopic surgeons and it is suitable to oncological principles.

References

[1] S. Kitano, N. Shiraishi, I. Uyama et al., "A multicenter study on oncologic outcome of laparoscopic gastrectomy for early cancer in Japan," *Annals of Surgery*, vol. 245, no. 1, pp. 68–72, 2007.

[2] M.-C. Kim, K.-H. Kim, H.-H. Kim, and G.-J. Jung, "Comparison of laparoscopy-assisted by conventional open distal gastrectomy and extraperigastric lymph node dissection in early gastric cancer," *Journal of Surgical Oncology*, vol. 91, no. 1, pp. 90–94, 2005.

[3] P. Bucher, F. Pugin, and P. Morel, "Single-port access laparoscopic radical left colectomy in humans," *Diseases of the Colon and Rectum*, vol. 52, no. 10, pp. 1797–1801, 2009.

[4] K. M. Reavis, M. W. Hinojosa, B. R. Smith, and N. T. Nguyen, "Single-laparoscopic incision transabdominal surgery sleeve gastrectomy," *Obesity Surgery*, vol. 18, no. 11, pp. 1492–1494, 2008.

[5] M. Ertem, E. Aytaç, and H. Gök, "Single port totally extraperitoneal (STEP) hernia repair: improving the benefits of one-day surgery setting," *Hernia*, vol. 16, pp. 737–738, 2012.

[6] M. Ertem, V. Özben, S. Yılmaz et al., "The use of tacker and arthroscopy cannules in SILS cholecystectomy," *Journal of Laparoendoscopic and Advanced Surgical Techniques A*, vol. 6, pp. 551–554, 2010.

[7] T. Omori, T. Oyama, H. Akamatsu, M. Tori, S. Ueshima, and T. Nishida, "Transumbilical single-incision laparoscopic distal gastrectomy for early gastric cancer," *Surgical Endoscopy and Other Interventional Techniques*, vol. 25, no. 7, pp. 2400–2404, 2011.

[8] D. J. Park, J. H. Lee, S. H. Ahn et al., "Single-port laparoscopic distal gastrectomy with D1+beta lymph node dissection for gastric cancers:report of 2 cases," *Surgical Laparoscopy Endoscopy & Percutaneous Techniques*, vol. 22, pp. e214–e216, 2012.

[9] T. Omori, K. Tanaka, M. Tori, S. Ueshima, H. Akamatsu, and T. Nishida, "Intracorporeal circular-stapled Billroth I anastomosis in single-incision laparoscopic distal gastrectomy," *Surgical Endoscopy*, vol. 26, pp. 1490–1494, 2012.

[10] S. H. Ahn, D. J. Park, S. Y. Son et al., "Single-incision laparoscopic total gastrectomy with D1+beta lymph node dissection for proximal early gastric cancer," *Gastric Cancer*, 2013.

[11] J. Kong, S. D. Wu, and Y. Su, "Translumenal single-incision laparoscopy radical gasrectomy with D2 lymph node dissection for early gastric cancer-primary experience with less invasive surgery in China," *Journal of Laparoendoscopic and Advanced Surgical Techniques A*, vol. 23, pp. 141–145, 2013.

[12] S. Kitano, Y. Iso, M. Moriyama, and K. Sugimachi, "Laparoscopy-assisted Billroth I gastrectomy," *Surgical Laparoscopy and Endoscopy*, vol. 4, no. 2, pp. 146–148, 1994.

[13] M.-C. Kim, H.-H. Kim, and G.-J. Jung, "Surgical outcome of laparoscopy-assisted gastrectomy with extraperigastric lymph node dissection for gastric cancer," *European Journal of Surgical Oncology*, vol. 31, no. 4, pp. 401–405, 2005.

[14] S. Kitano, N. Shiraishi, K. Kakisako, K. Yasuda, M. Inomata, and Y. Adachi, "Laparoscopy-assisted Billroth-I gastrectomy (LADG) for cancer: our 10 years' experience," *Surgical Laparoscopy, Endoscopy and Percutaneous Techniques*, vol. 12, no. 3, pp. 204–207, 2002.

[15] Y.-W. Kim, Y. H. Baik, Y. H. Yun et al., "Improved quality of life outcomes after laparoscopy-assisted distal gastrectomy for early gastric cancer: results of a prospective randomized clinical trial," *Annals of Surgery*, vol. 248, no. 5, pp. 721–727, 2008.

[16] I. Uyama, A. Sugioka, H. Matsui et al., "Laparoscopic side-to-side esophagogastrostomy using a linear stapler after proximal gastrectomy," *Gastric Cancer*, vol. 4, no. 2, pp. 98–102, 2001.

[17] K. O. So and J. M. Park, "Totally laparoscopic total gastrectomy using intracorporeally hand sewn-esophagojejunostomy," *Journal of Gastric Cancer*, vol. 11, pp. 206–211, 2011.

[18] N. Tanaka, H. Katai, M. Saka, S. Morita, and T. Fukagawa, "Laparoscopy-assisted pylorus-preserving gastrectomy: a matched case-control study," *Surgical Endoscopy and Other Interventional Techniques*, vol. 25, no. 1, pp. 114–118, 2011.

[19] S. I. Hwang, H. O. Kim, C. H. Yoo, J. H. Shin, and B. H. Son, "Laparoscopic-assisted distal gastrectomy versus open distal gastrectomy for advanced gastric cancer," *Surgical Endoscopy and Other Interventional Techniques*, vol. 23, no. 6, pp. 1252–1258, 2009.

[20] J. Shuang, S. Qi, J. Zheng et al., "A case control study of laparoscopy-assisted and open distal gastrectomy for advanced gastric cancer," *Journal of Gastrointestinal Surgery*, vol. 15, no. 1, pp. 57–62, 2011.

18

Management of Injury to the Common Bile Duct in a Patient with Roux-en-Y Gastric Bypass

Sheraz Yaqub,[1] Tom Mala,[2] Øystein Mathisen,[1] Bjørn Edwin,[1] Bjarte Fosby,[3] Dag Tallak Kjærsdalen Berntzen,[4] Andreas Abildgaard,[4] and Knut Jørgen Labori[1]

[1] *Department of Hepato-Pancreato-Biliary Surgery, Oslo University Hospital, Sognsvannsveien 20, 0317 Oslo, Norway*
[2] *Department of Gastrointestinal Surgery, Oslo University Hospital, Sognsvannsveien 20, 0317 Oslo, Norway*
[3] *Department of Transplantation Surgery, Oslo University Hospital, Sognsvannsveien 20, 0317 Oslo, Norway*
[4] *Department of Radiology, Oslo University Hospital, Sognsvannsveien 20, 0317 Oslo, Norway*

Correspondence should be addressed to Sheraz Yaqub; shya@ous-hf.no

Academic Editor: Boris Kirshtein

Introduction. Most surgeons prefer Roux-en-Y hepaticojejunostomy (RYHJ) for biliary reconstruction following a common bile duct (CBD) injury. However, in patients with a Roux-en-Y gastric bypass (RYGB) a RYHJ may be technically challenging and can interfere with bowel physiology induced by RYGB. The use of a hepaticoduodenostomy (HD) resolves both these issues. *Presentation of Case.* We present a case of CBD injury during laparoscopic cholecystectomy one year after laparoscopic RYGB for morbid obesity. Due to adhesions and previous surgery with RYGB, we did not want to interfere with the RYGB physiology by anastomosing the CBD to the jejunum or ileum. Succeeding a full Kocher's maneuver we performed biliary reconstruction by a tension-free end-to-side HD. The postoperative recovery was uneventful and the patient was discharged after eight days. At four-month follow-up, the patient had stable weight and normal laboratory test results. MRCP demonstrated normal intra- and extrahepatic bile ducts with status after HD. *Discussion.* We propose that HD should be considered in treatment of CBD injury in post-RYGB patients as it may reduce the risk of interfering with the post-RYGB physiology.

1. Introduction

After the introduction of laparoscopic cholecystectomy the management of bile duct injuries received increased attention [1–3]. The wave of surgery for morbid obesity (bariatric surgery) has developed a new patient cohort susceptible to gallbladder disease requiring cholecystectomy with the subsequent risk of bile duct injury. Different surgical methods are used for treatment of morbid obesity [4]. Laparoscopic Roux-en-Y gastric bypass (RYGB) is among the most common procedures. About 25–30% of the patients may develop gallbladder disease following bariatric surgery [5, 6]. An increase in laparoscopically induced bile duct injuries may be a consequence of an increasing number of cholecystectomies following RYGB. Cholecystectomy in such patients can be challenging due to the altered bowel anatomy, adhesions, and often the presence of an already constructed Roux-en-Y

loop. Repair of bile duct injuries in such patients should in addition not interfere with the weight losing effect of the previous procedure. We demonstrate herein the first case, to our knowledge, of a patient with injury of the bile duct one year after RYGB for morbid obesity.

2. Case Presentation

A 32-year-old man was referred to our hospital because of common bile duct (CBD) injury during laparoscopic cholecystectomy at a local hospital. His medical history included laparoscopic RYGB for morbid obesity with a BMI 47 kg/m². The operation was performed in East Europe and despite considerable efforts no operation record could be retrieved. One year after the operation, he presented with symptomatic cholecystolithiasis. He had no history of cholecystitis or cholangitis. During laparoscopic cholecystectomy intra-abdominal adherences were found which made the procedure more difficult and may have contributed to the transection of the CBD. As often is the case the injury was not appreciated immediately [2]. The patient developed jaundice and on postoperative day six a diagnostic laparoscopy revealed a transection of the CBD. He was immediately referred to our clinic, which is a tertiary care centre for HPB surgery.

Physical examination disclosed no abnormalities except for mild abdominal tenderness in right upper quadrant and a mild jaundice. BMI was 31 kg/m^2. Blood analyses showed CRP 9 mg/L and bilirubin 97 μmol/L; other laboratory studies were normal. Contrast-enhanced multislice computed tomography (CT) confirmed the presence of moderate water-density free fluid in the abdomen, but no free peritoneal air. Bile duct dilatation or vascular injuries were not observed. Magnetic resonance imaging (MRI) using the liver-specific contrast agent gadoxetic acid (Gd-EOB-DTPA, Primovist, Bayer-Schering, Berlin, Germany) [7] depicted transection of the CBD and pathological extrahepatic accumulation of contrast medium in the hepatobiliary phase scan (45 minutes after contrast medium injection) confirming the diagnosis of postoperative bile leakage (Figure 1).

The patient was operated with a midline laparotomy with a right-sided subcostal extension. We identified the first operation as a RYGB. The transected CBD was identified and classified as Strasberg E2 [8]. The diameter of the CBD was approximately 5 mm. As the outcome of the RYGB had been successful we did not want to interfere with the Roux-en-Y loop and decided to perform an end-to-side hepaticoduodenostomy (HD). This was done using a running 5-0 Prolene suture, after a full Kocher's maneuver to gain satisfactory mobilization to make the anastomosis tension-free. The postoperative recovery was uneventful and the patient was discharged after eight days. A four-month follow-up revealed normal physical examination. The patient had stable weight with a BMI of 31 kg/m^2 and normal lab tests. MRI showed normal intra- and extrahepatic bile ducts with a status after HD (Figure 2).

3. Discussion

Bile duct injury after elective laparoscopic cholecystectomy has been reported to range from 0.2% to 0.7% [1, 9]. The surgical approach to morbid obesity has gained wide acceptance in recent years. The risk of cholelithiasis is increased in these patients and an increased incidence of bile duct injuries would not be surprising. However, the incidence of bile duct injuries during laparoscopic cholecystectomy after previous bariatric surgery is unknown.

To avoid a second procedure due to complications from gallbladder disease, studies have looked into the benefit of concomitant cholecystectomy during the operation for morbid obesity. A recent meta-analysis recommends that prophylactic cholecystectomy during RYGB should only be performed in patients with symptomatic biliary disease [10]. However, it should be considered that a second procedure could be technically more demanding with longer operating

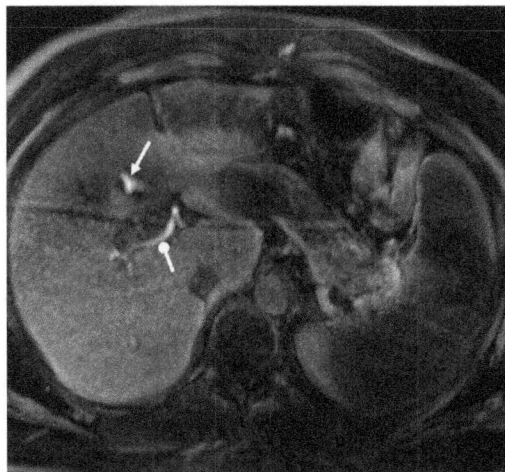

FIGURE 1: *Magnetic resonance imaging showing bile leakage.* Subvolume rendering of T1-weighted fat suppressed axial gradient echo acquisition approximately 45 minutes after intravenous administration of Gd-EOB-DTPA (Primovist; Bayer-Schering, Berlin, Germany) showing contrast-enhanced bile in central intrahepatic bile ducts (dot-head) and verifying bile leakage in gallbladder fossa (arrow).

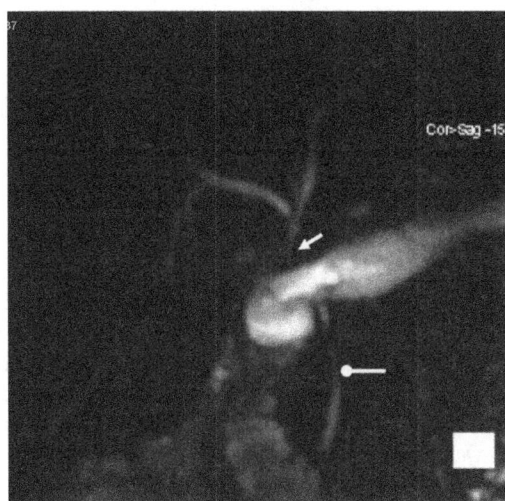

FIGURE 2: *MRCP showing hepaticoduodenostomy.* Three-dimensional rendering (right anterior oblique projection) of thin-slice MRCP (magnetic resonance cholangiopancreatography) showing normal size of intrahepatic bile ducts and a short hepatic duct with hepaticoduodenostomy (arrow). Native choledochal duct is also seen (dot-head).

time, higher conversion rate, and the risk for bile duct and vascular injuries.

Surgical repair of CBD injury can be performed using three principally different techniques: direct suture repair or bilioenteric anastomosis with either a HD or hepatico-jejunostomy Roux-en-Y (HJRY). For complete transection injuries of the bile duct most surgeons prefer HJRY as salvage therapy [2, 11, 12]. In the present case we preferred HD rather than HJRY. The reason for this was dual.

Firstly, we found it important not to interfere with the Roux-en-Y loop already constructed to treat the morbid obesity. The weight loss this patient had achieved was satisfactory and the construction of a new Roux-en-loop for HJ was not attractive since there was a possibility of jeopardizing the result of the bariatric surgery. Secondly, data from liver transplant patients and experience from our transplant center have shown that HD gives satisfactory results [13, 14]. Others have found excellent results with HD that are comparable with HJRY in a variety of indications such as benign bile duct strictures, choledochal cysts, HPB-cancer, and bile duct injuries [15–18]. A recent report advocated HD as the preferred method of biliary reconstruction and described it is as a safe and simple technique with low rates of leak, stricture, cholangitis, and bile gastritis [17]. It is however important that the anastomosis is tension-free and Kocher's maneuver should be performed if necessary.

4. Conclusions

The present case report demonstrates the management of a bile duct injury induced by laparoscopic cholecystectomy following RYGB. The treatment of such bile duct injuries may represent a new challenge for HPB-surgeons and we suggest that surgery should be planned together with bariatric surgeons to prevent interference with previous surgery. We preferred to preserve the RYGB anatomy and to perform the biliary reconstruction end-to-side HD. There were no complications and the procedure did not affect the weight loss outcome of the RYGB. However, it will be interesting and useful to collect data pointing out eventual complications.

Authors' Contribution

Dr. Sheraz Yaqub had full access to all of the data in the study and takes responsibility for the integrity of the data and the accuracy of the data analysis. Study concept and design was done by Sheraz Yaqub and Knut Jørgen Labori. Acquisition of data was done by Sheraz Yaqub, Knut Jørgen Labori, and Andreas Abildgaard. Sheraz Yaqub, Knut Jørgen Labori, and Andreas Abildgaard made analysis and interpretation of data. Sheraz Yaqub and Knut Jørgen Labori drafted the paper. Critical revision of the paper for important intellectual content was made by Sheraz Yaqub, Knut Jørgen Labori, Tom Mala, Andreas Abildgaard, Bjarte Fosby, Bjørn Edwin, Dag Tallak Kjærsdalen Berntzen, and Øystein Mathisen. Study supervision was done by Sheraz Yaqub and Knut Jørgen Labori. All authors have read and approved the final paper.

References

[1] A. Waage and M. Nilsson, "Iatrogenic bile duct injury: a population-based study of 152 776 cholecystectomies in the Swedish inpatient registry," *Archives of Surgery*, vol. 141, no. 12, pp. 1207–1213, 2006.

[2] Ø. Mathisen, O. Søreide, and A. Bergan, "Laparoscopic cholecystectomy: bile duct and vascular injuries: management and outcome," *Scandinavian Journal of Gastroenterology*, vol. 37, no. 4, pp. 476–481, 2002.

[3] S. M. Strasberg, "Avoidance of biliary injury during laparoscopic chelocystectomy," *Journal of Hepato-Biliary-Pancreatic Surgery*, vol. 9, no. 5, pp. 543–547, 2002.

[4] N. T. Nguyen, J. Root, K. Zainabadi et al., "Accelerated growth of bariatric surgery with the introduction of minimally invasive surgery," *Archives of Surgery*, vol. 140, no. 12, pp. 1198–1202, 2005.

[5] M. L. Shiffman, H. J. Sugerman, J. M. Kellum, W. H. Brewer, and E. W. Moore, "Gallstone formation after rapid weight loss: a prospective study in patients undergoing gastric bypass surgery for treatment of morbid obesity," *The American Journal of Gastroenterology*, vol. 86, no. 8, pp. 1000–1005, 1991.

[6] H. J. Sugerman, W. H. Brewer, M. L. Shiffman et al., "A multicenter, placebo-controlled, randomized, double-blind, prospective trial of prophylactic ursodiol for the prevention of gallstone formation following gastric-bypass-induced rapid weight loss," *The American Journal of Surgery*, vol. 169, no. 1, pp. 91–97, 1995.

[7] N. K. Lee, S. Kim, J. W. Lee et al., "Biliary MR imaging with Gd-EOB-DTPA and its clinical applications," *Radiographics*, vol. 29, no. 6, pp. 1707–1724, 2009.

[8] S. M. Strasberg, M. Hertl, and N. J. Soper, "An analysis of the problem of biliary injury during laparoscopic cholecystectomy," *Journal of the American College of Surgeons*, vol. 180, no. 1, pp. 101–125, 1995.

[9] D. R. Flum, A. Cheadle, C. Prela, E. P. Dellinger, and L. Chan, "Bile duct injury during cholecystectomy and survival in medicare beneficiaries," *Journal of the American Medical Association*, vol. 290, no. 16, pp. 2168–2173, 2003.

[10] R. Warschkow, I. Tarantino, K. Ukegjini et al., "Concomitant cholecystectomy during laparoscopic Roux-en-Y gastric bypass in obese patients is not justified: a meta-analysis," *Obesity Surgery*, vol. 23, no. 3, pp. 397–407, 2013.

[11] J. K. Sicklick, M. S. Camp, K. D. Lillemoe et al., "Surgical management of bile duct injuries sustained during laparoscopic cholecystectomy: perioperative results in 200 patients," *Annals of Surgery*, vol. 241, no. 5, pp. 786–795, 2005.

[12] S. Connor and O. J. Garden, "Bile duct injury in the era of laparoscopic cholecystectomy," *British Journal of Surgery*, vol. 93, no. 2, pp. 158–168, 2006.

[13] W. Bennet, M. A. Zimmerman, J. Campsen et al., "Choledochoduodenostomy is a safe alternative to roux-en-Y choledochojejunostomy for biliary reconstruction in liver transplantation," *World Journal of Surgery*, vol. 33, no. 5, pp. 1022–1025, 2009.

[14] J. Campsen, M. A. Zimmerman, M. S. Mandell et al., "Hepaticoduodenostomy is an alternative to Roux-en-Y hepaticojejunostomy for biliary reconstruction in live donor liver transplantation," *Transplantation*, vol. 87, no. 12, pp. 1842–1845, 2009.

[15] J. B. Rose, P. Bilderback, T. Raphaeli et al., "Use the duodenum, it's right there: a retrospective cohort study comparing biliary reconstruction using either the jejunum or the duodenum," *JAMA Surgery*, vol. 148, pp. 860–865, 2013.

[16] M. T. Santore, B. J. Behar, T. A. Blinman et al., "Hepaticoduodenostomy vs hepaticojejunostomy for reconstruction after resection of choledochal cyst," *Journal of Pediatric Surgery*, vol. 46, no. 1, pp. 209–213, 2011.

[17] S. K. Narayanan, Y. Chen, and K. L. Narasimhan, "Hepaticoduodenostomy versus hepaticojejunostomy after resection of choledochal cyst: a systematic review and meta-analysis," *Journal of Pediatric Surgery*, vol. 48, pp. 2336–2342, 2013.

19

Presentation and Surgical Management of Duodenal Duplication in Adults

Caroline C. Jadlowiec,[1] **Beata E. Lobel,**[1] **Namita Akolkar,**[1] **Michael D. Bourque,**[1,2] **Thomas J. Devers,**[3] **and David W. McFadden**[1,4]

[1]*University of Connecticut General Surgery Residency Program, Farmington, CT 06030, USA*
[2]*Connecticut Children's Medical Center, Department of Pediatric Surgery, Hartford, CT 06106, USA*
[3]*University of Connecticut Health Center, Division of Gastroenterology, Farmington, CT 06030, USA*
[4]*Department of Surgery, University of Connecticut Health Center, Farmington, CT 06030, USA*

Correspondence should be addressed to Caroline C. Jadlowiec; cjadlowiec@gmail.com

Academic Editor: Tahsin Colak

Duodenal duplications in adults are exceedingly rare and their diagnosis remains difficult as symptoms are largely nonspecific. Clinical presentations include pancreatitis, biliary obstruction, gastrointestinal bleeding from ectopic gastric mucosa, and malignancy. A case of duodenal duplication in a 59-year-old female is presented, and her treatment course is reviewed with description of combined surgical and endoscopic approach to repair, along with a review of historic and current recommendations for management. Traditionally, gastrointestinal duplications have been treated with surgical resection; however, for duodenal duplications, the anatomic proximity to the biliopancreatic ampulla makes surgical management challenging. Recently, advances in endoscopy have improved the clinical success of cystic intraluminal duodenal duplications. Despite these advances, surgical resection is still recommended for extraluminal tubular duplications although combined techniques may be necessary for long tubular duplications. For duodenal duplications, a combined approach of partial excision combined with mucosal stripping may offer advantage.

1. Introduction

Duodenal duplications in adults are exceedingly rare and their diagnosis remains difficult [1–3]. Treatment of duplications has traditionally involved surgical resection; however, for duodenal duplications, the anatomic proximity to the biliopancreatic ampulla makes surgical management challenging [4–6]. In our own experience, we recently encountered a symptomatic tubular duodenal duplication in an adult. Review of available literature finds that much of our knowledge of gastrointestinal duplications comes from pediatric case series [1, 7–12]. Here, we report our experience with an adult duodenal duplication and review embryology, clinical implications, and surgical management.

2. Case Discussion

A 59-year-old female was referred for evaluation secondary to several months of worsening postprandial abdominal pain, early satiety, reflux, and unplanned weight loss. The patient's laboratory values were unremarkable, and past medical and surgical history were noncontributory. Radiologic evaluation included a small bowel follow-through (Figure 1). Results of this study raised question of an abnormality involving the duodenal sweep. The duodenal C-loop was noted to be markedly dilated. At this time, two clinical diagnoses were considered. The first being that this duodenal dilation was occurring secondary to a stricture or an extrinsic compression in the fourth portion of the duodenum or at the

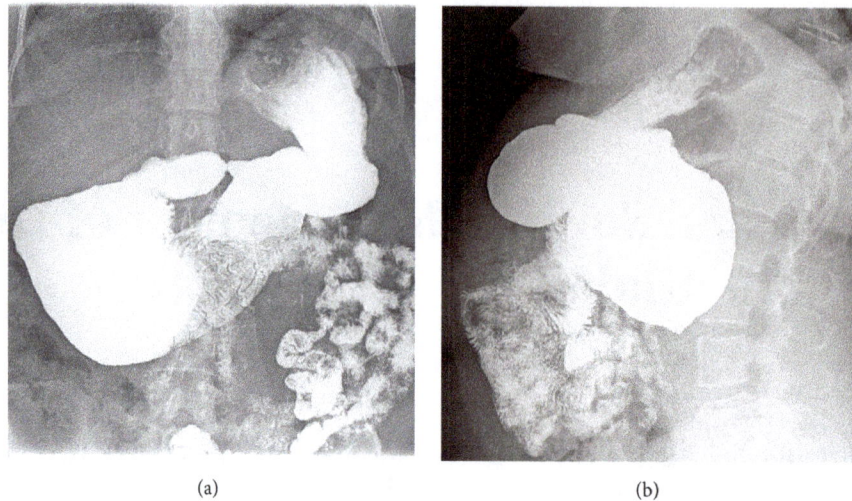

(a)   (b)

FIGURE 1: Representative images from the preoperative small bowel follow-through. There appeared to be marked abnormal dilation involving the duodenal C-loop. Of note, there was vigorous peristaltic activity involving this dilated loop although the peristaltic activity was disordered with a "to and from" movement of the barium and a marked delay in emptying into jejunum. The finding of peristaltic activity, although disordered, argued against the possibility of this being a duodenal diverticulum. (a) AP image. (b) Lateral image.

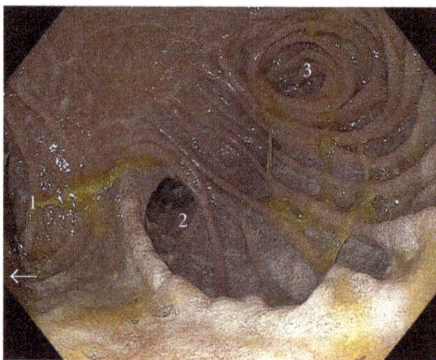

FIGURE 2: Preoperative endoscopic imaging. The second and third portions of the duodenum were noted to be markedly dilated with an accompanying finding of three downstream orifices. At this time, it was felt that the medial orifice (1) was the duplication and the lateral orifice (2) was the true lumen and that orifice (3) represented a distal common channel. White arrow denotes area of biliopancreatic ampulla which was proximal to the duplication.

duodenal-jejunal junction. The second possibility was that this finding represented some sort of enteric duplication. At this time, an upper endoscopy was performed (Figure 2). Findings from the endoscopy confirmed marked dilation to the duodenal C-loop. Bile pooling was noted to accompany this dilation. Surprisingly, three downstream orifices were found just distal to the biliopancreatic ampulla; these findings were again suggestive of a duodenal duplication. At that time, a surgical referral was obtained and the decision was made to proceed with operative exploration.

The patient underwent an open abdominal exploration. Initial inspection found the second and third portions of the duodenum to be markedly dilated as had been observed on prior imaging (Figures 3(a)-3(b)) with a normal appearing

distal jejunum. The retroperitoneal attachments of the duodenum were then taken down. The gallbladder was removed using a standard top-down approach; the cystic duct was identified and a biliary Fogarty balloon catheter was inserted into the duodenum so as to clearly delineate the location of the ampulla. Further medial mobilization of the duodenum was then performed, and at this time, it became apparent that the duplication extended superiorly, anterior to the body of the pancreas. Repeat intraoperative endoscopy was performed. Again, three orifices were confirmed to be just distal to the ampulla. A planned enterotomy was then created on the anterior surface of the duplication just distal to the ampulla; at this time it became apparent that one of these lumens was the true lumen, which connected to the distal jejunum. The other two orifices were lumens involving the duplication. Following clear delineation of anatomy, the tubular duodenal duplication was fully mobilized and resected (Figure 4(a)). A point of transection was chosen just distal to the ampulla with the distal resection line occurring at the jejunum. Accordingly, a hand-sewn end-to-side duodenojejunostomy was then fashioned (Figure 4(b)). In combining preoperative imaging and intraoperative findings, the final defined anatomy was consistent with that of a tubular duodenal duplication of the third and fourth portions of the duodenum.

3. Embryology

Duplications of the gastrointestinal (GI) tract are rare congenital anomalies that occur in either cystic or tubular form. Because of their relative infrequency, they tend to be clinically challenging with regard to diagnosis and treatment. Features common to all enteric duplications include their intimate attachment to the GI tract, epithelial mucosal lining, and a well-developed smooth muscle layer [7]. Duplications may or may not share a common communication with the native GI tract, and they may likewise be multiple. To date, the

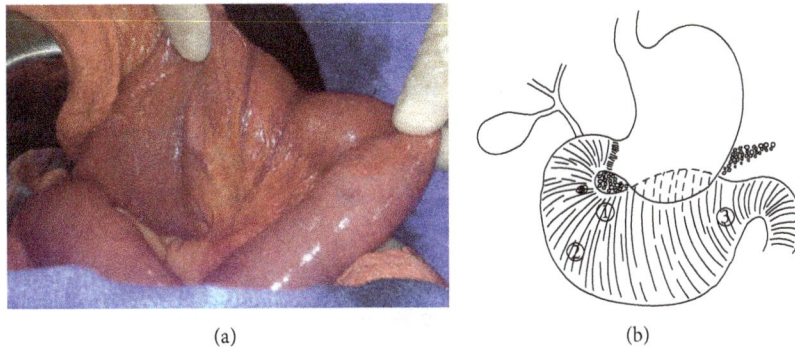

FIGURE 3: (a) Intraoperative photograph showing the duodenal duplication. (b) Schematic representation of intraoperative findings; included numbers correlate with endoscopic findings shown in Figure 2.

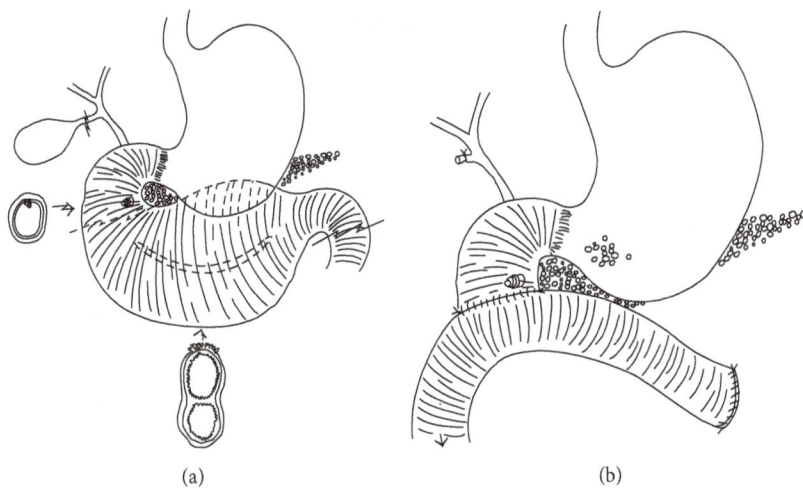

FIGURE 4: (a) Schematic of operative proceedings. The cystic duct was identified and a biliary Fogarty catheter was inserted into the duodenum. A duodenotomy was created and point of transection was chosen just distal to the ampulla so as to fully resect the duplication. The distal resection line occurring at the jejunum just beyond the ligament of Treitz. (b) Schematic of end-to-side duodenojejunostomy used for operative reconstruction.

cause of GI duplications remains debated. The split notochord theory is commonly used to explain thoracic duplications where it is believed that there is incomplete separation of the notochord from the GI endoderm [7]. Alternatively, enteric duplications are hypothesized to arise as a result of recanalization errors involving the neonatal solid GI tract [2, 7, 8, 13]. Enteric duplications as a whole are believed to occur with an incidence of 1 per 4000–5000 live births [1, 3]. In comparison to other alimentary tract duplications, duodenal duplications are comparatively rare. In order of descending approximated frequency, jejunoileal duplications occur most commonly (52%), followed by esophageal (17%), colonic (14%), gastric (8%), duodenal (6%), and rectal (6%) duplications (Table 1 and Figure 5) [4, 9–12, 14–30].

4. Clinical Findings

Most enteric duplications are identified by the age of two years, with less than thirty percent being diagnosed in adults [3]. The large majority of duodenal duplications are cystic and intraluminal [31]. They most commonly arise from

the mesenteric border of the second and third portions of the native duodenum, and accordingly, there is a tendency for them to be closely associated with both the pancreatic and biliary ducts. By comparison, extraluminal tubular duodenal duplications are rare [31, 32]. Cystic duodenal duplications are typically fluid-filled and however may, on occasion, contain gallstones, bile, or pancreatic fluid [32, 33]. Both computer tomography (CT) and ultrasound are useful imaging modalities [26, 28]. Ultrasound of cystic duplications should reveal an anechoic fluid-filled double-walled cyst composed of an inner hyperechoic rim of mucosa-submucosa and an outer hypoechoic layer of smooth muscle consistent with the muscularis propria; in contrast, although frequently difficult to capture, a classically identifying feature of tubular duplications is peristalsis [34]. For CT imaging, oral contrast used with CT imaging can be helpful as it will not fill a cystic duplication because of lack of communication with the gastrointestinal tract but rather may delineate it by demonstrating compression effect on adjacent structures whereas a tubular duplication would be expected to fill [29].

TABLE 1: Alimentary tract duplications.

Ref.	Pub. yr.	Number of patients	Location								
			Oral	Esophageal	Thoracoabdominal	Gastric	Duodenal	Jejunal and ileal	Colonic	Rectal	Other
[7]	1935	90	—	10	—	6	8	59	3	3	1
[8]	1953	67	1	13	3	2	4	32	9	4	—
[9]	1956	25	—	5	—	4	2	16	5	—	—
[10]	1960	28	1	7	—	1	3	16	4	2	—
[11]	1961	38	—	6	2	1	—	18	6	4	—
[12]	1966	8	—	1	1	—	—	6	—	—	—
[13]	1970	23	3	4	2	1	4	9	7	—	—
[14]	1971	37	—	4	—	3	6	20	4	2	—
[1]	1978	64	—	15	1	6	1	34	12	5	2
[15]	1981	53	—	8	2	8	2	32	4	1	—
[16]	1988	11	—	1	—	1	—	4	2	—	—
[17]	1988	17	—	6	—	1	2	5	8	5	—
[18]	1989	96	1	20	3	8	1	47	15	1	—
[19]	1994	14	—	8	1	—	3	1	3	6	—
[20]	1995	72	2	15	6	10	1	21	10	6	4
[21]	1995	27	2	—	—	3	—	9	8	—	—
[22]	1996	17	—	2	—	1	3	14	3	2	—
[23]	2000	38	1	7	2	1	1	17	9	1	—
[24]	2000	12	—	—	—	3	—	8	—	—	—
[25]	2003	73	—	—	—	6	7	51	5	4	—
Total		810	11 (1.4%)	132 (16.3%)	23 (2.8%)	66 (8.1%)	48 (5.9%)	419 (51.7%)	117 (14.4%)	46 (5.7%)	7 (0.9%)

Thoracoabdominal, intrathoracic duplication originating from below the diaphragm.

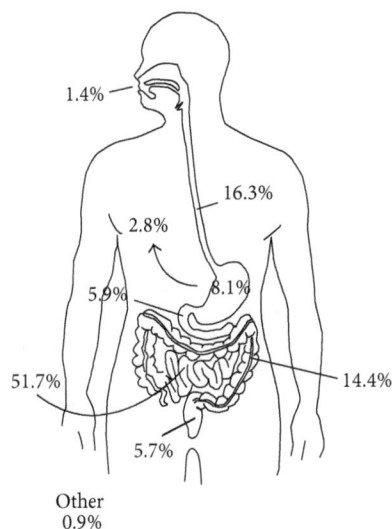

1.4%

16.3%

2.8%

5.9%

8.1%

51.7%

14.4%

5.7%

Other
0.9%

FIGURE 5: Alimentary tract duplications.

In adults, duodenal duplications remain difficult to diagnose, as presenting symptoms tend to be nonspecific [2]. With regard to duodenal duplications, commonly reported presenting symptoms include abdominal pain with weight loss, nausea, vomiting, and reflux. Accompanying clinical presentations include pancreatitis, biliary obstruction, gastrointestinal bleeding from ectopic gastric mucosa, and malignancy, and of these, pancreatitis appears to be the most frequent [32–38].

5. Treatment Options

Review of earlier literature highlights the complexity and surgical difficulty in treating enteric duplications. It is important to note that management of cystic intraluminal and tubular extraluminal duodenal duplications typically varies. Cystic intraluminal duplications are increasingly more amendable to drainage alone whereas extraluminal tubular duplications typically necessitate formal surgical resection.

Historically, prior attempts to create a drainage limb while leaving an intraluminal cystic duplication intact via a surgical cystjejunostomy resulted in incomplete long-term success primarily because of retained heterotrophic gastric tissue and long-term risk of peptic ulceration, bleeding, or malignancy [4, 5, 39]. Recent advances in endoscopy have expanded on this idea with successful drainage accomplished via endoscopic marsupialization [39]. Review of the literature finds that there are eight children who underwent endoscopic management and remained asymptomatic after mean follow-up of over seven years, thus suggesting that this may be a safe and effective technique [40, 41]. Concerns regarding malignancy or bleeding from peptic ulceration still exist in this setting, as endoscopic therapy does not always result in complete ablation of the cyst mucosa; this risk, however, appears to be low.

In contrast, current surgical understanding and practice still largely recommends resection for tubular extraluminal duplications. Complete resection for short segmental duplications may be possible whereas combined techniques may be necessary for longer segmental duplications. Duodenal duplications, in particular, pose a unique challenge as their anatomic proximity to the ampulla makes surgical management more complex. Of note, duodenal duplications typically arise just distal to the biliopancreatic ampulla in comparison to choledochoceles which are typically found proximal [41]. A combined approach of partial excision combined with mucosal stripping offers one such solution [5, 6, 22]. From the pediatric literature, mucosal stripping is a practical surgical option as it removes the secretory mucosa and also reduces the future risk of peptic ulceration and malignancy. Of note, during this process, the shared blood supply between the duplication and the native bowel must be protected and preserved so as to avoid the need for resection [3].

6. Conclusion

Despite a large historic experience, duodenal duplications in adults continue to be rare and their diagnosis remains difficult. Clinical symptoms in adults are nonspecific and potential risks, if untreated, including risk of peptic ulceration and malignant transformation. The treatment of duplications has traditionally involved surgical resection; however, for duodenal duplications, the anatomic proximity to the ampulla makes surgical management more challenging. For intraluminal cystic duodenal duplications, advances in endoscopy have changed current practice; however management of extraluminal tubular duplications remains challenging. In this setting, a combined approach of partial excision combined with mucosal stripping may offer advantage.

References

[1] M. Lima, F. Molinaro, G. Ruggeri, T. Gargano, and B. Randi, "Role of mini-invasive surgery in the treatment of enteric duplications in paediatric age: a survey of 15 years," *La Pediatria Medica e Chirurgica*, vol. 34, no. 5, pp. 217–222, 2012.

[2] J. L. Bremer, "Diverticula and duplications of the intestinal tract," *Archives of Pathology*, vol. 38, pp. 132–140, 1944.

[3] M. P. Arias, F. G. Lorenzo, M. M. Sánchez, and R. M. Vellibre, "Enteric duplication cyst resembling umbilical cord cyst," *Journal of Perinatology*, vol. 26, no. 6, pp. 368–370, 2006.

[4] C. P. Iyer and G. H. Mahour, "Duplications of the alimentary tract in infants and children," *Journal of Pediatric Surgery*, vol. 30, no. 9, pp. 1267–1270, 1995.

[5] E. L. Wrenn Jr., "Tubular duplication of the small intestine," *Surgery*, vol. 52, no. 3, pp. 494–498, 1962.

[6] T. W. Adams, "Obstructing enterogenous cyst of the duodenum treated by cystojejunostomy," *Annals of Surgery*, vol. 144, no. 5, pp. 902–906, 1956.

[7] R. J. Bower, W. K. Sieber, and W. B. Kiesewetter, "Alimentary tract duplications in children," *Annals of Surgery*, vol. 188, no. 5, pp. 669–674, 1978.

[8] P. Laje, A. W. Flake, and N. S. Adzick, "Prenatal diagnosis and postnatal resection of intraabdominal enteric duplications," *Journal of Pediatric Surgery*, vol. 45, no. 7, pp. 1554–1558, 2010.

[9] H. E. Houston and H. B. Lynn, "Duplications of the small intestine in children: mayo clinic experience and review of the literature," *Mayo Clinic Proceedings*, vol. 41, no. 4, pp. 246–256, 1966.

[10] J. L. Grosfeld, J. A. O'Neill Jr., and H. W. Clatworthy Jr., "Enteric duplications in infancy and childhood: an 18-year review," *Annals of Surgery*, vol. 172, no. 1, pp. 83–90, 1970.

[11] J. J. Bissler and R. L. Klein, "Alimentary tract duplications in children: case and literature review," *Clinical Pediatrics*, vol. 27, no. 3, pp. 152–157, 1988.

[12] I. Kamak, T. Öcal, M. E. Şenocak, F. C. Tanyel, and N. Büyükpamukçu, "Alimentary tract duplications in children: report of 26 years' experience," *Turkish Journal of Pediatrics*, vol. 42, no. 2, pp. 118–125, 2000.

[13] P. Menon, K. L. N. Rao, B. R. Thapa et al., "Duplicated gall bladder with duodenal duplication cyst," *Journal of Pediatric Surgery*, vol. 48, no. 4, pp. E25–E28, 2013.

[14] H. W. Hudson Jr., "Giant diverticula or reduplications of the intestinal tract—report of three cases," *The New England Journal of Medicine*, vol. 213, no. 23, pp. 1123–1131, 1935.

[15] R. E. Gross and W. E. Ladd, *The Surgery of Infancy and Childhood: Its Principles and Techniques*, WB Saunders, 1953.

[16] W. K. Sieber, "Alimentary tract duplications," *AMA Archives of Surgery*, vol. 73, no. 3, pp. 383–392, 1956.

[17] R. Basu, I. Forshall, and P. P. Rickham, "Duplications of the alimentary tract," *The British Journal of Surgery*, vol. 47, pp. 477–484, 1960.

[18] R. W. Mellish and C. E. Koop, "Clinical manifestations of duplication of the bowel," *Pediatrics*, vol. 27, pp. 397–407, 1961.

[19] B. E. Favara, R. A. Franciosi, and D. R. Akers, "Enteric duplications. Thirty-seven cases: a vascular theory of pathogenesis," *American Journal of Diseases of Children*, vol. 122, no. 6, pp. 501–506, 1971.

[20] M. Hocking and D. G. Young, "Duplications of the alimentary tract," *British Journal of Surgery*, vol. 68, no. 2, pp. 92–96, 1981.

[21] S. T. Ildstad, D. J. Tollerud, R. G. Weiss, D. P. Ryan, M. A. McGowan, and L. W. Martin, "Duplications of the alimentary tract. Clinical characteristics, preferred treatment, and associated malformations," *Annals of Surgery*, vol. 208, no. 2, pp. 184–189, 1988.

[22] G. W. Holcomb, A. Gheissari, J. A. O'Neill Jr., N. A. Shorter, and H. C. Bishop, "Surgical management of alimentary tract duplications," *Annals of Surgery*, vol. 209, no. 2, pp. 167–174, 1989.

[23] M. Bajpai and M. Mathur, "Duplications of the alimentary tract: clues to the missing links," *Journal of Pediatric Surgery*, vol. 29, no. 10, pp. 1361–1365, 1994.

[24] M. D. Stringer, L. Spitz, R. Abel et al., "Management of alimentary tract duplication in children," *British Journal of Surgery*, vol. 82, no. 1, pp. 74–78, 1995.

[25] M.-C. Yang, Y.-C. Duh, H.-S. Lai, W.-J. Chen, C.-C. Chen, and W.-T. Hung, "Alimentary tract duplications," *Journal of the Formosan Medical Association*, vol. 95, no. 5, pp. 406–409, 1996.

[26] J. Schalamon, J. Schleef, and M. E. Höllwarth, "Experience with gastro-intestinal duplications in childhood," *Langenbeck's Archives of Surgery*, vol. 385, no. 6, pp. 402–405, 2000.

[27] P. S. Puligandla, L. T. Nguyen, D. St-Vil et al., "Gastrointestinal duplications," *Journal of Pediatric Surgery*, vol. 38, no. 5, pp. 740–744, 2003.

[28] S. J. Keckler and G. W. Holcomb III, "Alimentary tract duplications," in *Ashcraft's Pediatric Surgery*, G. W. Holcomb III and J. P. Murphy, Eds., pp. 517–525, Saunders, Philadelphia, Pa, USA, 5th edition, 2010.

[29] D. P. Lund, "Alimentary tract duplications," in *Pediatric Surgery*, A. G. Coran, Ed., pp. 1155–1163, Saunders, Philadelphia, Pa, USA, 7th edition, 2012.

[30] J. J. Aiken, "Intestinal duplications," in *Principles and Practice of Pediatric Surgery*, K. T. Oldham, P. M. Colombani, R. P. Foglia, and M. A. Skinner, Eds., pp. 1329–1345, Lippincott Williams & Wilkins, Philadelphia, Pa, USA, 2nd edition, 2004.

[31] T. Merrot, R. Anastasescu, T. Pankevych et al., "Duodenal duplications. Clinical characteristics, embryological hypotheses, histological findings, treatment," *European Journal of Pediatric Surgery*, vol. 16, no. 1, pp. 18–23, 2006.

[32] S. Y. Ko, S. H. Ko, S. Ha, M. S. Kim, H. M. Shin, and M. K. Baeg, "A case of a duodenal duplication cyst presenting as melena," *World Journal of Gastroenterology*, vol. 19, no. 38, pp. 6490–6493, 2013.

[33] R. J. Lad, P. Fitzgerald, and K. Jacobson, "An unusual cause of recurrent pancreatitis: duodenal duplication cyst," *Canadian Journal of Gastroenterology*, vol. 14, no. 4, pp. 341–345, 2000.

[34] G. Cheng, D. Soboleski, A. Daneman, D. Poenaru, and D. Hurlbut, "Sonographic pitfalls in the diagnosis of enteric duplication cysts," *American Journal of Roentgenology*, vol. 184, no. 2, pp. 521–525, 2005.

[35] T. Stelling, W. J. J. von Rooij, and T. L. Tio, "Pancreatitis associated with congenital duodenal duplication cyst in an adult," *Endoscopy*, vol. 19, no. 4, pp. 171–173, 1987.

[36] O. Sezgin, E. Altiparmak, U. Yilmaz, Ü. Sarita, and B. Ahin, "Endoscopic management of a duodenal duplication cyst associated with biliary obstruction in an adult," *Journal of Clinical Gastroenterology*, vol. 32, no. 4, pp. 353–355, 2001.

[37] G. L. Falk, C. J. Young, and J. Parer, "Adenocarcinoma arising in a duodenal duplication cyst: a case report," *Australian and New Zealand Journal of Surgery*, vol. 61, no. 7, pp. 551–553, 1991.

[38] C. D. Knight Jr., M. J. Allen, D. M. Nagorney, L. E. Wold, and E. P. DiMagno, "Duodenal duplication cyst causing massive bleeding in an adult: an unusual complication of a duplication cyst of the digestive tract," *Mayo Clinic Proceedings*, vol. 60, no. 11, pp. 772–775, 1985.

[39] W. Y. Inouye, C. Farrell, W. T. Fitts Jr., and T. A. Tristan, "Duodenal duplication: case report and literature review," *Annals of Surgery*, vol. 162, no. 5, pp. 910–916, 1965.

[40] F. Antaki, A. Tringali, P. Deprez et al., "A case series of symptomatic intraluminal duodenal duplication cysts: presentation, endoscopic therapy, and long-term outcome (with video)," *Gastrointestinal Endoscopy*, vol. 67, no. 1, pp. 163–168, 2008.

[41] R. Liu and D. G. Adler, "Duplication cysts: diagnosis, management, and the role of endoscopic ultrasound," *Endoscopic Ultrasound*, vol. 3, no. 3, pp. 152–160, 2014.

20

Gastrotracheal Fistula as a Result of Transhiatal Esophagectomy for Esophageal Cancer: An Unusual Complication

Heshmatollah Salahi,[1] Mehdi Tahamtan,[2] Bijan Ziaian,[3] Mansoor Masjedi,[4] Zahra Saadati,[5] Nazanin Hoseini,[5] and Elahe Torabi[6]

[1] *Transplant Research Center, Shiraz University of Medical Sciences, Shiraz, Iran*
[2] *Colorectal Research Center, Shiraz University of Medical Sciences, Shiraz, Iran*
[3] *Department of Thoracic Surgery, Shiraz University of Medical Sciences, Shiraz, Iran*
[4] *Department of Anesthesiology, Shiraz University of Medical Sciences, Shiraz, Iran*
[5] *Shiraz University of Medical Sciences, Shiraz, Iran*
[6] *Department of Internal Medicine, Shiraz University of Medical Sciences, Shiraz, Iran*

Correspondence should be addressed to Mehdi Tahamtan; mehditahamtan@yahoo.com

Academic Editor: Kevin Reavis

Gastrotracheal fistula following open transhiatal esophagectomy (Orringer's technique) for esophageal cancer is an unusual but lethal complication. Surgical intervention with resection of the fistula tract and primary interrupted suturing of gastric and tracheal orifices using a muscle flap interposition has proved to be a successful method. We report the case of a 73-year-old male with an adenocarcinoma of the distal part of the esophagus, who underwent open transhiatal esophagectomy (Orringer's technique) with gastric tube reconstruction and cervical anastomosis. The patient did not receive induction chemoradiotherapy before the esophagectomy. Two attempts of surgical repair of fistula failed and the patient died. Being aware of warning signs such as dyspnea and respiratory distress accompanied by bilious content in the tracheal tube is helpful in the early detection and treatment of this type of fistula.

1. Introduction

The development of gastrotracheal fistula after esophagectomy is a rare but life-threatening condition. Despite close anatomical relationship between the trachea and the stomach after esophagectomy, literature about gastrotracheal fistula is limited mainly to case reports. Diagnosis is based on both radiologic and endoscopic studies. The confirmation is often made by direct visualization of the fistula orifice by means of bronchoscopic or esophagoscopic modalities. Treatment options are conservative, endoscopic, and surgical, but the treatment of choice remains controversial.

2. Case Presentation

A 73-year-old male patient, who we knew to have had COPD and CABG, came to our clinic with uT3. No poorly differentiated adenocarcinoma at distal part of the esophagus was found. Endoscopy showed a 3.5 cm segment of narrowing in the lower third of the esophagus. He did not receive induction chemoradiotherapy before surgery.

The patient underwent an open transhiatal esophagectomy and reconstruction by gastric pull-up according to Orringer's technique.

Postoperative outcome was acceptable at first days and the patient was extubated successfully. On the 8th postoperative day, however, our patient developed dyspnea, cough, and respiratory distress. Intubation was therefore performed again. The patient underwent conservative management with supportive care and on the 30th postoperative day the patient was extubated successfully. During the next 6 days the patient developed respiratory distress with metabolic acidosis. Chest X-ray revealed bilateral basal consolidation with diffuse patchy infiltration. Consequently, the patient underwent

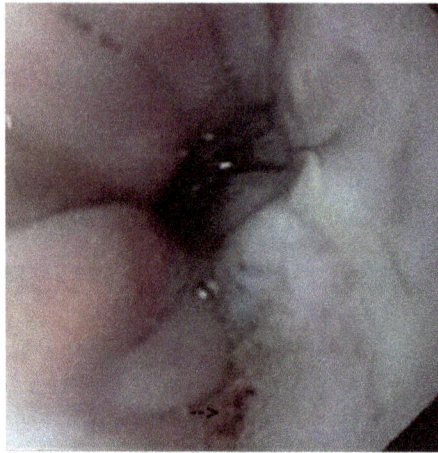

FIGURE 1: Gastrotracheal fistula just above the level of anastomosis.

intubation again. When the patient was reintubated, plenty large amount of bilious fluid was extracted from the endotracheal tube. Fiberoptic bronchoscopy was performed in the ICU and a fistula was detected 6 cm above the carina, just adjacent to the site of esophagogastric anastomosis. On the basis of bronchoscopic finding and clinical evidences, the diagnosis of gastrotracheal fistula was confirmed.

Because of the patient's bad general condition, conservative management and endoscopic approach for insertion of a stent in the trachea were not allowed. After a multidisciplinary team consultation, the patient was scheduled for operative intervention.

At the 1st operation, we carried out the left side neck exploration through the previous incision site. It showed severe inflammation and adhesion. A partial sternotomy was done to allow better access and exposure to the high retrotracheal portion of the esophagus [1]. After insertion of a nasogastric tube above the level of esophagogastric anastomosis, methylene blue was injected via NG tube to clarify the site of leakage. No leakage of dye appeared in the operating field. Then the gastric tube and cervical esophagus were mobilized and freed from fibrosis and adhesions. A fistula tract was identified in the posterior aspect of the anastomosis adjacent to the trachea. It was transected and repaired with interrupted primary sutures. Because the location of fistula was in the neck adjacent to the esophagogastric anastomosis, we could not interpose an intercostal muscle bundle, pericardial, pleural, or omental flap to protect the suture lines. Besides, the presence of severe inflammation and adhesions made interposition of strap muscle flap or sternocleidomastoid muscle (SCM) impossible. The patient was then transferred to the ICU.

After this operation, secretions of the endotracheal tube reduced dramatically but increased again at the 3rd postoperative day. Unfortunately, the subsequent endoscopy showed the persistence of the fistula about 16 cm from incisors, just above the level of anastomosis (Figure 1). The decision for the next neck exploration through the previous incision site was implemented 1 day later.

After exploration of the neck via previous incision, rigid esophagoscopy with transillumination of the esophagus was performed to detect the fistula orifice by one surgeon and at the same time gastrotracheal fistula and anastomosic leak was sutured by another surgeon. Besides, tracheostomy was done for the patient to eliminate the endotracheal tube cuff pressure on suture lines. As mentioned previously, interposing a muscle bundle was impossible.

The patient was then transferred to the ICU. In the ICU, the patient condition worsened and bilious secretions from the endotracheal tube continued. A new chest X-ray showed whitish lung which was in favor of chemical pneumonitis. Blood pressure and O_2 saturation dropped and finally, the patient expired the next day after the second neck exploration.

3. Discussion

Literature on gastrotracheal fistula following esophagectomy for cancer consists mainly of case reports. This entity is rare (0.3–0.5%) but potentially lethal [1].

Several parameters contribute to selecting the best remedy such as general condition and severity of the disease and location and size of the fistula. In a patient with a good general condition, localized small fistula orifice, and no sign of necrosis, an endoscopic modality is the best option. In this method, abrasion-coagulation is followed by fibrin glue injection and, finally, approximation of the orifice with endoscopic clips [2]. As mentioned previously, if conservative management fails or if the patient's general condition worsens, a surgical intervention is imperative [3].

Surgical intervention consists of dissection of the fistula tract and repair of the esophageal and tracheal defects [4]. Additionally, the use of tissues with a rich blood supply (pleural, pericardial, myocutaneous, and muscle flaps) in the dead space between suture lines may protect the tracheal and gastroesophageal suture lines and prevent recurrent fistulization [5].

Symptoms vary widely from coughing to severe pneumonia, chemical pneumonitis, and mediastinitis [6]. There are various identified predisposing factors, the most important of which are previous chemoradiotherapy and en bloc resection with extensive lymphadenectomy [7].

But, what is the pathophysiology of fistula?

(1) Leakage of the anastomosis causing mediastinal abscess formation and, in turn, secondary fistulization to the trachea [7].

(2) Tracheal ischemia secondary to extensive dissection.

(3) Iatrogenic tracheal injuries.

(4) Cuff-induced tracheal ischemia secondary to prolonged intubation.

(5) Tracheal injuries by gastric staplers.

(6) Erosion of the stomach by tracheostomy tube.

(7) Tumor recurrence.

(8) Radiation.

(9) Gastric ulcer [6].

One of the most important factors in preventing complications such as fistula is meticulous dissection of the tumors and careful esophagogastric anastomosis. Technical errors that must be avoided are tension on anastomosis, impairment of gastric or esophageal blood supply, mucosal defect of anastomosis, and overdistended gastric tube [5].

Gastrotracheal fistula after esophagectomy for cancers is a rare but life-threatening and challenging complication. It seems that the best choice in treating such kinds of fistula is surgical intervention, along with transposed pedicled pericardial, omental, pleural, or muscle flap. Even in a previously irradiated field, closure of the fistula with muscle bundle interposition such as SCM and pectoralis major myocutaneous (PMM) flap has showed excellent outcomes [8].

The SCM muscle flap for repair of an esophageal fistula and perforation is a well-known technique [9]. But in some reports there was a high rate of flap necrosis due to poor blood supply. So the pectoralis major muscle flap is the preferred method to repair the esophageal anastomotic leakage after gastric pull-up [10, 11]. However, the PMM flap is less flexible and requires a longer and difficult surgical procedure. In addition, cosmetic and functional complications at the donor site are more than those of the SCM flap [9]. PMM flap was not a good choice for our debilitated and asthenic patient. Most of the time, these two approaches are safe and feasible, especially when conservative management proves unsuccessful [3].

4. Conclusion

We report a case of gastrotracheal fistula after transhiatal esophagectomy (Orringer's technique) without a history of induction chemoradiotherapy. In our case, two attempts of gastrotracheal fistula repair with interrupted primary sutures without transposed flap were unsuccessful. If feasible, SCM muscle could help our patient. However, we refrained from SCM muscle flap because of the risk of flap necrosis and inability to interpose it in the appropriate place which had severely inflamed and adhesive tissue. We could not find an appropriate treatment for situations in which flap interposition is impossible. Being aware of warning signs such as dyspnea and respiratory distress accompanied by bilious content in the tracheal tube is helpful in the early detection and treatment of this type of fistula [12].

References

[1] C. J. Buskens, J. B. F. Hulscher, P. Fockens, H. Obertop, and J. J. B. Van Lanschot, "Benign tracheo-neo-esophageal fistulas after subtotal esophagectomy," Annals of Thoracic Surgery, vol. 72, no. 1, pp. 221–224, 2001.

[2] C. Gutiérrez San Román, J. E. Barrios, J. Lluna et al., "Long-term assessment of the treatment of recurrent tracheoesophageal fistula with fibrin glue associated with diathermy," Journal of Pediatric Surgery, vol. 41, no. 11, pp. 1870–1873, 2006.

[3] J. P. Freire, S. M. Feijó, L. Miranda, F. Santos, and H. B. Castelo, "Tracheo-esophageal fistula: combined surgical and endoscopic approach," Diseases of the Esophagus, vol. 19, no. 1, pp. 36–39, 2006.

[4] A. Baisi, L. Bonavina, S. Narne, and A. Peracchia, "Benign tracheoesophageal fistula, results of surgical therapy," Diseases of the Esophagus, vol. 12, no. 3, pp. 209–211, 1999.

[5] S.-W. Song, H.-S. Lee, M. S. Kim, J. M. Lee, J. H. Kim, and J. I. Zo, "Repair of gastrotracheal fistula with a pedicled pericardial flap after Ivor Lewis esophagogastrectomy for esophageal cancer," Journal of Thoracic and Cardiovascular Surgery, vol. 132, no. 3, pp. 716–717, 2006.

[6] C. J. Buskens, J. B. F. Hulscher, P. Fockens, H. Obertop, and J. J. B. Van Lanschot, "Benign tracheo-neo-esophageal fistulas after subtotal esophagectomy," Annals of Thoracic Surgery, vol. 72, no. 1, pp. 221–224, 2001.

[7] H. E. Bartels, H. J. Stein, and J. R. Siewert, "Tracheobronchial lesions following oesophagectomy: prevalence, predisposing factors and outcome," British Journal of Surgery, vol. 85, no. 3, pp. 403–406, 1998.

[8] I. Ökten, A. K. Cangir, N. Özdemlr, Ş. Kavukçu, H. Akay, and Ş. Yavuzer, "Management of esophageal perforation," Surgery Today, vol. 31, no. 1, pp. 36–39, 2001.

[9] C.-H. Lin, C.-H. Lin, C.-W. Wu, and C.-T. Liao, "Sternocleidomastoid muscle flap: an option to seal off the esophageal leakage after free jejunal flap transfer—a case report," Chang Gung Medical Journal, vol. 32, no. 2, pp. 224–229, 2009.

[10] M. Hirao, S. Yoshitatsu, T. Tsujinaka et al., "Pectoralis myocutaneous flap with T-tube drainage for cervical anastomotic leakage after salvage operation," Esophagus, vol. 3, no. 1, pp. 33–36, 2006.

[11] K. R. Shen, W. G. Austen Jr., and D. J. Mathisen, "Use of a prefabricated pectoralis major muscle flap and pedicled jejunal interposition graft for salvage esophageal reconstruction after failed gastric pull-up and colon interposition," Journal of Thoracic and Cardiovascular Surgery, vol. 135, no. 5, pp. 1186–1187, 2008.

[12] C.-H. Marty-Ané, M. Prudhome, J.-M. Fabre, J. Domergue, M. Balmes, and H. Mary, "Tacheoesophagogastric anastomosis fistula: a rare complication of esophagectomy," The Annals of Thoracic Surgery, vol. 60, no. 3, pp. 690–693, 1995.

21

Esophagojejunal Anastomosis Fistula, Distal Esophageal Stenosis, and Metalic Stent Migration after Total Gastrectomy

Nadim Al Hajjar,[1,2] **Calin Popa,**[1,3] **Tareg Al-Momani,**[3,4] **Simona Margarit,**[5,6] **Florin Graur,**[1,2] **and Marcel Tantau**[7,8]

[1]*Department of Surgery, Regional Institute of Gastroenterology and Hepatology "Prof. Dr. Octavian Fodor", Croitorilor Street, No. 19-21, 400162 Cluj-Napoca, Romania*

[2]*3rd Surgical Clinic, Iuliu Hatieganu University of Medicine and Pharmacy, Croitorilor Street, No. 19-21, 400162 Cluj-Napoca, Romania*

[3]*Training and Research Center "Prof. Dr. Sergiu Duca", Petre Ispirescu Street, No. 1, 400090 Cluj-Napoca, Romania*

[4]*Department of Oncological Surgery, The Oncology Institute "Prof. Dr. Ion Chiricuță" Republicii Street, No. 34-36, 400015 Cluj-Napoca, Romania*

[5]*Department of Intensive Care Unit, Regional Institute of Gastroenterology and Hepatology "Prof. Dr. Octavian Fodor", Croitorilor Street, No. 19-21, 400162 Cluj-Napoca, Romania*

[6]*1st Anesthesiology and Critical Care Clinic, Iuliu Hatieganu University of Medicine and Pharmacy, Croitorilor Street, No. 19-21, 400162 Cluj-Napoca, Romania*

[7]*Department of Gastroenterology, Regional Institute of Gastroenterology and Hepatology "Prof. Dr. Octavian Fodor", Croitorilor Street, No. 19-21, 400162 Cluj-Napoca, Romania*

[8]*3rd Medical Clinic, Iuliu Hatieganu University of Medicine and Pharmacy, Croitorilor Street, No. 19-21, 400162 Cluj-Napoca, Romania*

Correspondence should be addressed to Calin Popa; calinp2003@yahoo.com

Academic Editor: Shin-ichi Kosugi

Esophagojejunal anastomosis fistula is the main complication after a total gastrectomy. To avoid a complex procedure on friable inflamed perianastomotic tissues, a coated self-expandable stent is mounted at the site of the anastomotic leak. A complication of stenting procedure is that it might lead to distal esophageal stenosis. However, another frequently encountered complication of stenting is stent migration, which is treated nonsurgically. When the migrated stent creates life threatening complications, surgical removal is indicated. We present a case of a 67-year-old male patient who was treated at our facility for a gastric adenocarcinoma which developed, postoperatively, an esophagojejunostomy fistula, a distal esophageal stenosis, and a metallic coated self-expandable stent migration. To our knowledge, this is the first reported case of an esophagojejunostomy fistula combined with a distal esophageal stenosis as well as with a metallic coated self-expandable stent migration.

1. Introduction

With every year passing, the incidence of complications following a total gastrectomy is decreasing; literature review shows it occurs in approximately 7–27% of cases [1–4]. Esophagojejunal anastomosis fistula is the main complication of this procedure, with a high mortality rate of around 20%, which represents 30–65% of global postgastrectomy mortality [4–8].

Surgeons tried since the beginning to treat these postoperative leaks and fistulae with drainage and repair, complete parenteral nutrition with no oral intake, and combining these with antibiotics. Nonetheless, this approach had a significant morbidity and mortality rates of up to 60% [9, 10].

Interventional endoscopy comes to the rescue by placing coated self-expandable stents in patients with esophagojejunostomies at the site of the anastomotic leakage. This

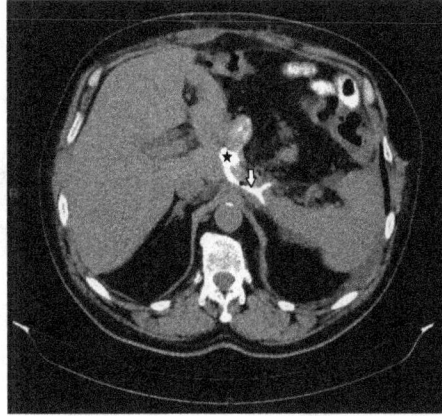

FIGURE 1: Axial contrast-enhanced abdominal computer tomography (CT): esophageal lumen (star); esophagojejunal anastomotic fistula (arrow).

helps to avoid a complex procedure on friable inflamed perianastomotic tissues [1, 11–13].

The most encountered complication of coated self-expandable stents is stent migration; this according to published literature occurs in up to 28% of cases [14–16]. Management of this condition usually is nonsurgical, being either repositioned endoscopically, waiting for the stent to be eliminated spontaneously through the rectum, or it might even remain in the body if it does not create complications [17, 18]. When the migrated stents create complications, surgical removal is indicated [19].

2. Case Report

We present the case of a 67-year-old male patient who was diagnosed with gastric adenocarcinoma intestinal type T2N0M0 (Stage I B), mild microcytic hypochromic anemia, gall bladder lithiasis, essential hypertension grade I, and obesity grade I.

A total gastrectomy with D2 lymphadenectomy with End-to-Side esophagojejunostomy in a transmesocolic Roux-en-Y anastomosis, cholecystectomy, and a feeding jejunostomy were performed.

Postoperative outcome was favorable initially after which his status suddenly worsened, with fever of 38.2°C, loss of appetite, and leukocytosis with neutrophilia. An oral contrast-enhanced CT was performed which showed an esophagojejunal anastomotic fistula (Figure 1).

A 28 mm diameter metallic coated self-expandable stent (CSES) was mounted endoscopically on the anastomotic site after which the patient showed a favorable outcome (no reflux complaints) (Figure 2).

48 hours before discharging the patient and 39 days postoperatively, a barium swallow upper GI radiography was performed which showed good esophageal transit with no contrast material leakage at the anastomotic site (Figure 3).

Histopathological examination of the surgical specimen revealed a gastric adenocarcinoma pT3N0MxL0V0R0 (37 lymph nodes were examined). This puts the patient in the IIA stage of the disease.

The metallic CSES was removed one month after placement, after which the patient started having dysphagia episodes three weeks later. Initially the cause of dysphagia was thought to be a stenosis of the esophagojejunal anastomosis; however, it was further investigated where results showed that the stenosis was situated proximal to the anastomosis, which we interpreted as scar tissue after prolonged local pressure on the esophageal wall due to the presence of the proximal stent tulip.

In the following three-month period he received chemotherapy (FU-FOL protocol) and continued having recurrent dysphagia episodes, for which he was being treated repeatedly by interventional endoscopy with balloon and plug dilation (Figure 4).

To avoid recurrent balloon and plug dilatations, a second (22 mm diameter) CSES was placed two months after the removal of the first one on the distal esophageal stenosis, which was removed one month after placement. A third (22 mm diameter) CSES was placed due to the persisting dysphagia (Figure 5) two months after the removal of the second stent.

One month after the placement of the third stent, the patient presented to the emergency department complaining of diffuse abdominal pain and mixed dysphagia. On physical examination the patient was pale with altered general status and dehydration, and a mass could be palpated in the left paraumbilical region. A fluoroscopy of the abdomen was done, which revealed that the metallic stent has migrated into the jejunum.

Correlating the migration of the stent with the increasing intensity of the abdominal pain, a decision of exploratory laparotomy was made, where exploration revealed that the esophageal stenosis was proximal to the esophagojejunal anastomosis, and a migrated metallic stent located just distally to the anastomotic site of the blind loop of the Roux-en-Y procedure performed initially (Figure 6).

A distal esophagectomy with a new End-to-Side esophagojejunostomy using a 25 mm circular stapler and an *en bloc* segmentary enterectomy at the site of the stent (Figure 7), with an End-to-End anastomosis, were performed.

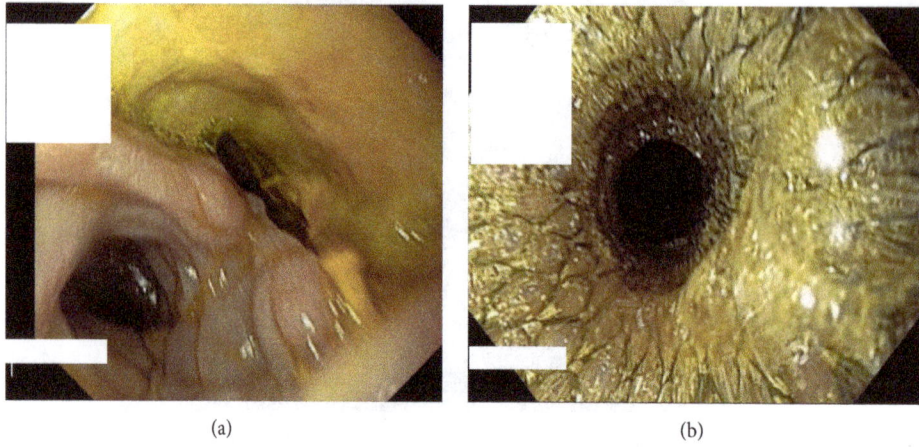

FIGURE 2: Esophagoscopy: esophagojejunal anastomotic fistula before (a) and after (b) stent placement.

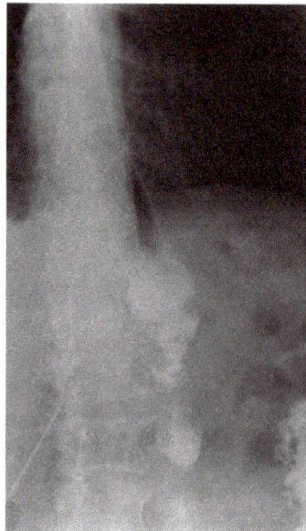

FIGURE 3: Barium swallow: without extraluminal contrast leakage.

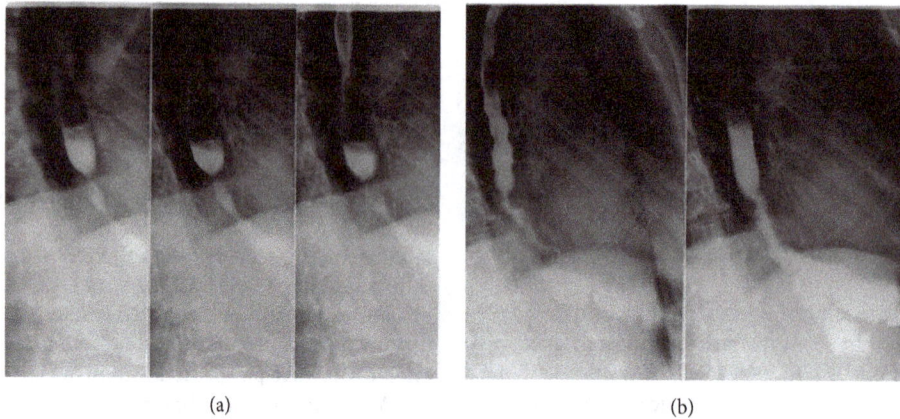

FIGURE 4: Abdominal X-ray: before (a) and after (b) balloon dilatation.

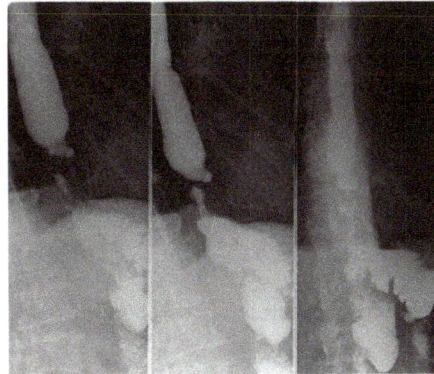

FIGURE 5: Moderate distal esophageal stenosis before the third stent placement.

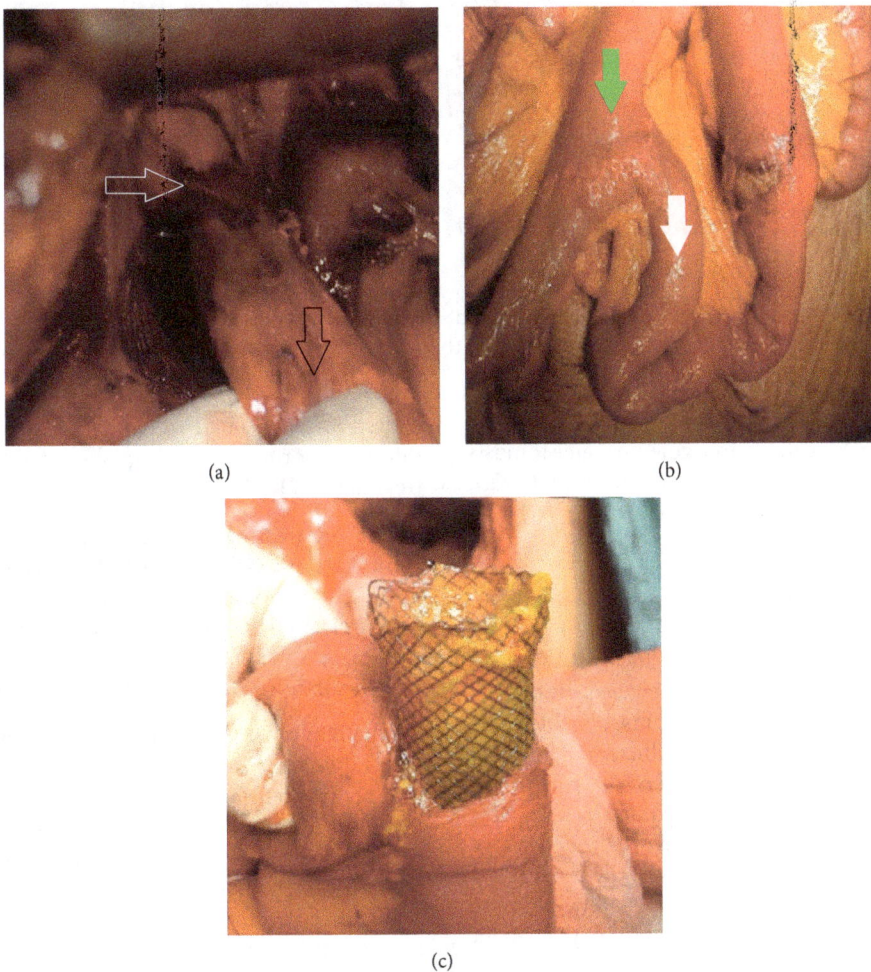

(a)

(b)

(c)

FIGURE 6: Intraoperative aspects: (a) circumferential distal esophageal stenosis (white arrow), site of esophagojejunal anastomosis (black arrow); (b) migrated stent: direction of migration (white arrow), end-loop proximal small bowel (green arrow); (c) metallic stent into the jejunal lumen.

Postoperative evolution was favorable, with nutrition per os reestablished after CT evaluation 2 weeks after the last operation, and the patient was discharged a week later.

Histopathological examination of the specimens showed that the esophageal stenosis was of benign nature (Figure 8).

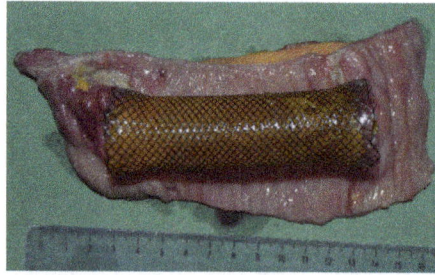

FIGURE 7: Segmentary enterectomy: postresection specimen and metallic stent.

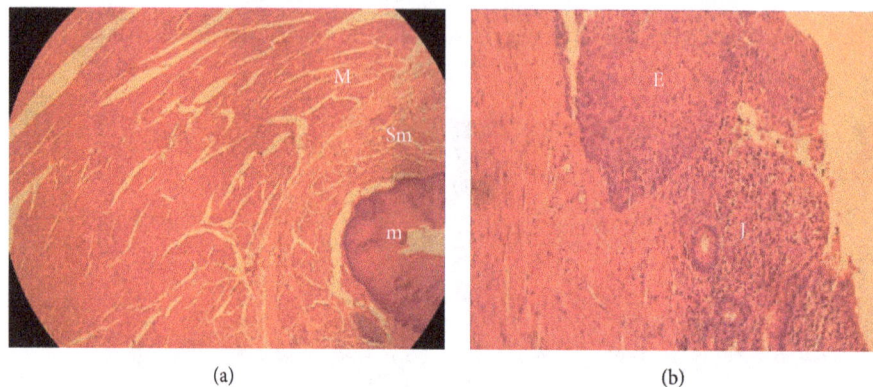

(a)

(b)

FIGURE 8: Histopathological findings (H&E ×4) revealing benign distal esophageal stenosis: (a) cross section above anastomotic site (m: mucosa, Sm: submucosa, and M: hypertrophic muscularis propria); (b) esojejunal anastomosis (E: esophageal mucosa, J: jejunal mucosa).

The patient was followed up after 6 months after the second intervention, where the esophagojejunal anastomosis was patent with good oral nutrition and gain in weight (6 Kg).

3. Discussion

Anastomotic fistula is a complication that is encountered in some patients who underwent gastric surgeries and might lead to poor outcome, poor quality of life, and even life threatening complications. The current management of such cases concentrates on relieving the symptoms, possible complications of the leakage, and providing efficient nutritional support for the patients. This management consists of the drainage of the leaked collections accompanied by long term parenteral nutrition. In more severe cases when the leakage is associated with peritonitis or paralytic ileus, surgical intervention is indicated, despite the possibility of more severe complications due to poor general status of the patient and the high invasiveness of the procedure [20, 21].

In cases of minimal leakage, management consists of discontinuing oral intake and feeding through a jejunal feeding tube or parenterally. Literature shows minimally invasive treatments for esophageal anastomotic leaks like fibrin glue application and endoscopic clipping which showed satisfactory results in some cases, but when the anastomotic leak is large, repeated complex interventions are required to seal these fistulas [22, 23]. Meanwhile endoscopic stenting as a treatment for such fistulas is showing advantages to the patient over immediate surgical reintervention, such as earlier resumption of oral intake, shorter hospitalization, minimal morbidity, better quality of life, and less costs of treatments [21, 24].

As any treatment modality, endoscopic stenting has its complications such as hemorrhage, stent migration, strictures, and perforations. Most migrated stents are removed nonsurgically [19]. However, we believe that in such cases surgical intervention is absolutely necessary if life threatening complications (obstruction, perforation) are imminent.

Benign refractory strictures of the esophagus are the ones where dilation to an appropriate diameter fails and strictures that recur after short periods of time as well as the ones that need continuous dilation [25]. These strictures lower the patient's quality of life due to their possible complications like malnutrition, pain, or perforation [26]. Many techniques are available for treating such strictures, out of which is temporary stenting. Stenting is an appealing approach as the placed stent is performing the dilation function for the complete period of placement, and it can be removed when needed. Nonetheless, temporary stenting must be used in carefully chosen patients as it has a high rate of complications. These temporary stents are useful tools in restoring the lumen of the esophagus until the patient's status or treatment plan allows surgical intervention [27].

Reintervention in our patient had a particularity that it had two purposes: to resolve the imminent complication of stent migration and the distal esophageal stenosis.

The multidisciplinary treatment, interventional endoscopy, and surgery were complementary approaches as interventional endoscopy managed the surgical complication being an esophagojejunal fistula, and later surgery for managing the endoscopic stenting complication being the distal esophageal stenosis and stent migration.

For this case, endoscopic stenting seemed to be the most appropriate immediate management for the esophagojejunostomy fistula. Operative management for the distal esophageal stenosis would have delayed chemotherapy, whereas stenting enabled chemotherapy administration as early as possible and offered the patient a better quality of life during this phase of treatment as well as avoiding repeated balloon and plug dilatation sessions. Taking into account that the stenosis before the third stent mounting was moderate, it might have contributed to the migration of the stent. When the patient's symptoms indicate an upcoming complication of a migrated stent, we consider the operative removal an essential step for a better prognosis.

References

[1] J. Hoeppner, B. Kulemann, G. Seifert et al., "Covered self-expanding stent treatment for anastomotic leakage: outcomes in esophagogastric and esophagojejunal anastomoses," *Surgical Endoscopy and Other Interventional Techniques*, vol. 28, no. 5, pp. 1703–1711, 2014.

[2] A. Fernández Villaverde, J. J. Vila, S. Vázquez et al., "Self-expanding plastic stents for the treatment of post-operative esophago-jejuno anastomosis leak. A case series study," *Revista Espanola de Enfermedades Digestivas*, vol. 102, no. 12, pp. 704–710, 2010.

[3] H. Lang, P. Piso, C. Stukenborg, R. Raab, and J. Jähne, "Management and results of proximal anastomotic leak in a series of 1114 total gastrectomies for gastric carcinoma," *European Journal of Surgical Oncology*, vol. 26, no. 2, pp. 168–171, 2000.

[4] P. Nowakowski, K. Ziaja, T. Ludyga et al., "Self-expandable metallic stents in the treatment of post-esophagogastrostomy/post-esophagoenterostomy fistula," *Diseases of the Esophagus*, vol. 20, no. 4, pp. 358–360, 2007.

[5] H. J. Fahn, L. S. Wang, M.-S. Huang, B.-S. Huang, W.-H. Hsu, and M.-H. Huang, "Leakage of intrathoracic oesophagovisceral anastomoses in adenocarcinoma of the gastric cardia: changes in serial APACHE II scores and their prognostic significance," *European Journal of Surgery*, vol. 163, no. 5, pp. 345–350, 1997.

[6] T. Aparicio, M. Yacoub, P. Karila-Cohen, and E. René, "Adénocarcinome gastrique: notions fondamentales, diagnostic et traitement," *Encyclopédie Médico-Chirurgicale—Chirurgie*, vol. 1, no. 1, pp. 47–66, 2004.

[7] A. Sauvanet, L. Berthoux, B. Gayet, J. F. Fléjou, J. Belghiti, and F. Fekete, "Adénocarcinome du cardia: l'étendue de l'éxérèse gastrique et du curage ganglionnaire influence t elle la survie?" *Gastroentérologie Clinique et Biologique*, vol. 19, pp. 244–251, 1995.

[8] K. Alanezi and J. D. Urschel, "Mortality secondary to esophageal anastomotic leak," *Annals of Thoracic and Cardiovascular Surgery*, vol. 10, no. 2, pp. 71–75, 2004.

[9] R. C. Karl, R. Schreiber, D. Boulware, S. Baker, and D. Coppola, "Factors affecting morbidity, mortality, and survival in patients undergoing ivor lewis esophagogastrectomy," *Annals of Surgery*, vol. 231, no. 5, pp. 635–643, 2000.

[10] N. Kumar and C. C. Thompson, "Endoscopic therapy for postoperative leaks and fistulae," *Gastrointestinal Endoscopy Clinics of North America*, vol. 23, no. 1, pp. 123–136, 2013.

[11] R. Kochar and N. Shah, "Enteral stents: from esophagus to colon," *Gastrointestinal Endoscopy*, vol. 78, no. 6, pp. 913–918, 2013.

[12] I. I. El Hajj, T. F. Imperiale, D. K. Rex et al., "Treatment of esophageal leaks, fistulae, and perforations with temporary stents: evaluation of efficacy, adverse events, and factors associated with successful outcomes," *Gastrointestinal Endoscopy*, vol. 79, no. 4, pp. 589–598, 2014.

[13] R. Babor, M. Talbot, and A. Tyndal, "Treatment of upper gastrointestinal leaks with a removable, covered, self-expanding metallic stent," *Surgical Laparoscopy, Endoscopy and Percutaneous Techniques*, vol. 19, no. 1, pp. 1–4, 2009.

[14] N. Vakil, A. I. Morris, N. Marcon et al., "A prospective, randomized, controlled trial of covered expandable metal stents in the palliation of malignant esophageal obstruction at the gastroesophageal junction," *The American Journal of Gastroenterology*, vol. 96, pp. 1791–1796, 2001.

[15] N. A. Christie, P. O. Buenaventura, H. C. Fernando et al., "Results of expandable metal stents for malignant esophageal obstruction in 100 patients: short-term and long-term follow-up," *Annals of Thoracic Surgery*, vol. 71, no. 6, pp. 1797–1802, 2001.

[16] M. Y. V. Homs, E. W. Steyerberg, E. J. Kuipers et al., "Causes and treatment of recurrent dysphagia after self-expanding metal stent placement for palliation of esophageal carcinoma," *Endoscopy*, vol. 36, no. 10, pp. 880–886, 2004.

[17] S. R. Puli, I. S. Spofford, and C. C. Thompson, "Use of self-expandable stents in the treatment of bariatric surgery leaks: a systematic review and meta-analysis," *Gastrointestinal Endoscopy*, vol. 75, no. 2, pp. 287–293, 2012.

[18] Y. S. Oh and M. L. Kochman, "Polyflex esophageal stent migration with elimination per rectum," *Gastrointestinal Endoscopy*, vol. 66, no. 3, p. 633, 2007.

[19] O. Karatepe, E. Acet, M. Altiok, M. Battal, G. Adas, and S. Karahan, "Esophageal stent migration can lead to intestinal obstruction," *North American Journal of Medical Sciences*, vol. 1, no. 2, pp. 63–65, 2009.

[20] R. Morgan and A. Adam, "Use of metallic stents and balloons in the esophagus and gastrointestinal tract," *Journal of Vascular and Interventional Radiology*, vol. 12, no. 3, pp. 283–297, 2001.

[21] Y. P. Cho, D. H. Lee, H. J. Jang et al., "Leakage of jejunal end of Roux limb after total gastrectomy: management with a placement of a covered metallic stent. Case report," *Journal of Korean Medical Science*, vol. 18, no. 3, pp. 437–440, 2003.

[22] G. Curcio, F. Mocciaro, I. Tarantino et al., "Self-expandable metal stent for closure of a large leak after total gastrectomy," *Case Reports in Gastroenterology*, vol. 4, no. 2, pp. 293–297, 2010.

[23] L. Cipolletta, M. A. Bianco, G. Rotondano, R. Marmo, R. Piscopo, and C. Meucci, "Endoscopic clipping of perforation following pneumatic dilation of esophagojejunal anastomotic strictures," *Endoscopy*, vol. 32, no. 9, pp. 720–722, 2000.

[24] M. A. Mauro, R. E. Koehler, and T. H. Baron, "Advances in gastrointestenal intervention: The treatment of gastroduodenal and colorectal obstructions with metallic stents," *Radiology*, vol. 215, no. 3, pp. 659–669, 2000.

[25] P. D. Siersema and M. M. C. Hirdes, "What is the optimal duration of stent placement for refractory, benign esophageal strictures?" *Nature Clinical Practice Gastroenterology and Hepatology*, vol. 6, no. 3, pp. 146–147, 2009.

[26] J. H. Kim, H.-Y. Song, E. K. Choi, K. R. Kim, J. H. Shin, and J.-O. Lim, "Temporary metallic stent placement in the treatment of refractory benign esophageal strictures: results and factors associated with outcome in 55 patients," *European Radiology*, vol. 19, no. 2, pp. 384–390, 2009.

[27] J. H. Kim, J. H. Shin, and H.-Y. Song, "Benign strictures of the Esophagus and Gastric outlet: interventional management," *Korean Journal of Radiology*, vol. 11, no. 5, pp. 497–506, 2010.

22

Concomitant Gastrointestinal Stromal Tumor of the Stomach and Gastric Adenocarcinoma in a Patient with Billroth 2 Resection

Federico Sista, Valentina Abruzzese, Mario Schietroma, and Gianfranco Amicucci

Dipartimento di Scienze Cliniche Applicate e Biotecnologie, Università degli Studi di L'Aquila, 67100 Coppito, Italy

Correspondence should be addressed to Federico Sista; silversista@gmail.com

Academic Editors: M. Ganau, A. Protopapas, M. L. Quek, and B. Tokar

Background. With this study we focus on the etiopathogenesis and on the therapy of the simultaneous occurrence of Gastric gastrointestinal stromal tumor (gGIST) and adenocarcinoma of the stomach in a patient with Billroth II gastric resection (BIIGR). We report the first case of this event and a review of the literature. *Methods.* A 70-year-old man with a BIIGR, affected by adenocarcinoma of the stomach, was successfully treated with total gastrectomy. The histological examination showed a gastric adenocarcinoma with a synchronous GIST sized 2 cm and S-100, CD117, and CD34 positive. The mutation of PDGFR gene was detected. *Discussion.* This tumor is a rare mesenchymal neoplasm of the gastrointestinal tract. Few cases of synchronous gastric adenocarcinoma and GIST are observed in the literature and no case in patients with BIIGR. Various hypotheses have been proposed to explain this occurrence. It is frequently attributed to Metallothioneins genes mutations or embryological abnormalities, but this has not been proven yet. We suggest a hypothesis about the etiopathogenesis of this event in a BIIGR patient. *Conclusion.* GIST may occur synchronously with gastric adenocarcinoma. This simultaneous occurrence needs more studies to be proven. The study of Cajal cells' proliferation signalling is crucial to demonstrate our hypotesis.

1. Introduction

gGISTs are rare; they represent 0.2% of all gastrointestinal tumors [1]. They are also the most common mesenchymal tumors of the gastrointestinal tract. Inappropriately classified in the past as Leiomyomas, Leiomyoblastomas, and Schwannomas, in the late 1990s they were classified as a single neoplastic entity, when immunohistochemistry had identified the gene KIT (CD117) [2]. They derive from Cajal cells arising from cells of the smooth muscle of the viscera [3, 4]. 50–60% of GIST are localized in the stomach, 30–40% in the small intestine, and 5–10% in the colon and rectum. GISTs represent 1% of gastric malignant tumors; they are symptomatic in 60% of cases although the diagnosis is often incidental [4, 5]. Unlike gastric carcinomas, that are often associated with other cancers such as lymphomas, GISTs are rarely synchronous to other gastric neoplasms. Here we report a rare case of gGIST synchronous to adenocarcinoma in a patient with a previous Billroth II gastric resection (BIIGR).

2. Case Report

A 70-year-old man suffered from dyspepsia, chronic anemia, and epigastric pain for about six months, and he also had a weight loss of 15 kg and melena. The patient underwent BIIGR for a gastric ulcer 35 years before. A gastroscopy was performed, and it showed a "polypoid neoformation that occupies one third of the anastomosis and extends along the greater curvature of the gastric stump for about 3 cm." Biopsies were performed, and they showed "adenocarcinoma infiltrating the stroma and focally the smooth muscle." Bioumoral findings (CEA, GICA, AFP, and NSE) were negative. The abdominal computed tomography (CT), executed for the staging of the neoplasia, showed parietal thickening of the gastric stump without secondary repetitions (Figure 1). The patient then underwent a total gastrectomy with a Roux-en-Y reconstruction and D2 lymphadenectomy. The histological examination of the surgical specimen showed a "moderately differentiated tubulo-papillary adenocarcinoma infiltrating deep into the muscle layer" (Figure 2). A 3 cm GIST of

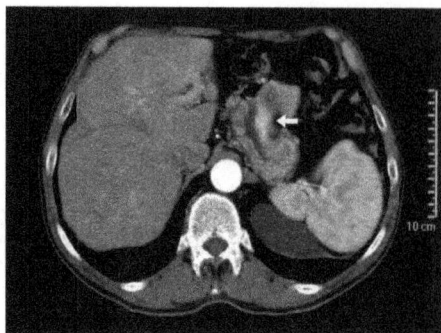

FIGURE 1: Computer tomography with intravenous contrast of the abdomen showing a thickening of gastric stump (white arrow).

the gastric corpus muscle layer coexists. It is composed by proliferating spindle-shaped cells with nuclear palisading (Figure 3). Its cellularity is low, its mitotic index (number of mitoses per 50 high-power fields) is 1/50 HPF, and scattered hyalinization and calcification are observed. There was positivity for KIT/CD117 (Figure 4) and negativity for SMA (smooth muscle actin) and S-100 (Figure 5). The molecular analysis of this tumor showed a PDGFR gene mutation; this error makes the tumor sensitive to the oral treatment with Imatinib Mesylate (Glivec @). The final staging was T3 N2 M0. The postoperative was normal without complications. The patient was discharged in the IXth postoperative day and entrusted to an oncologist consultant.

3. Discussion

GIST is a rare cancer that originates from Cajal cells, interstitial pacemaker cells [1, 3, 4]; it shows positivity to tumor markers that can be found also in normal Cajal cells [1, 3]. The immunohistochemical examination highlights the over expression of KIT or CD34 gene in 90% of cases. Therefore, the positivity for the KIT gene is enough to make anatomopathological diagnosis of GIST [2, 3, 6]. Other histological features are the negativity to S-100 and SMA (smooth muscle actin), over expressed in nerve cells and muscular cells (Figure 5), respectively; in this way it is possible to make differential diagnosis with gastric Schwannoma and Sarcoma. Genetic analysis of the PDGFRA is necessary to evaluate an eventual postoperative therapy with Imatinib Mesylate. Over expression of PGFRA is not associated with its mutation; it occurs in up to 85% of cases, while the mutation occurs in up to 5–7% [6–8].

Just few cases in the literature report GISTs synchronous to gastric adenocarcinomas [9–14]. In our case there was a low grade GIST (according to the Bucher Grading System [15]), associated with an infiltrating adenocarcinoma. The percentage of loco regional lymph node repetitions is estimated from 1 to 3,4% [16–18] for GISTs (in our case it was 0%: the repetitions found derived from the adenocarcinoma). Disease progression and patients' outcome depend on tumor's size and on mitosis number [15]. Patients with malignant gGIST have usually a better survival if compared to those with an intestinal localization. In fact, patients

with malignant gGIST who undergo a complete resection have a recurrence rate of about 50%, a median time to recurrence of 18–24 months, and a 5-year survival of 50% [8]. Liver and peritoneum are the main organs involved in case of relapse [8, 19]. Liver is involved in more than 60% of cases, representing the only repetition site in 44% of cases [8], while extra-abdominal repetitions are found just in the advanced phases of the disease. Novitsky et al. [20] reported a 92% of 5-year disease-free survival for 4, 4 cm tumors. Other authors reported similar results for gGISTs up to 5 cm [21]. Chaudhry and DeMatteo [8] highlighted that the responsivity to the biological treatment with Imatinib determines a better survival, which is 100% in the first 2 year, with a disease progression just in 61% of cases. The refractoriness to this biological treatment results in a 2-years survival of 36%, with a disease progression in 100% of cases. In our case, the disease-free survival was 18 months for the metastatic progression of gastric adenocarcinoma, without the biological therapy.

GIST in combination with other synchronous malignant disease is a rare event. The studies reported in the literature about this tumor are still few. Some authors [14, 22, 23] report that about 20% of patients with GIST develop another type of tumor, but they do not suggest a common etiology. Liu et al. [14] carried out a study of 54 GISTs synchronous to other digestive tract malignant neoplasia; they showed that the highest incidence of synchrony occurs with esophagus squamous cell carcinoma, with gastric adenocarcinoma and with pancreatic cancer, in a percentage of 1.13%, 0.53% and 0.38% respectively. They also found a higher prevalence in females. In all cases the most frequent location was the gastric corpus. Some other authors noted a higher prevalence of synchrony between GIST and female genital neoplastic pathology. Li et al. reported: "As the full spectra of ovarian epithelial neoplasm may develop in the endometrium and other anatomic components of the female upper genital tract, an "extended or secondary Müllerian system" has been proposed to describe the similarity of the female upper genital tract in common undergoing metaplastic changes giving rise to synchronous neoplasm" [23]. In this respect they hypothesized an embryological origin of these neoplasm. Kawanowa et al. [24] analyzed 100 cases of gastric cancer; they found a high incidence of microscopic GIST (35%), suggesting that other genetic changes (in addition to the gene kit) may be necessary for the evolution in malignant form. These alterations are probably involved even in the genesis of gastric carcinomas. Finally some authors suggested that the coexistence of these neoplasms can be attributed to mutations in Metallothioneins genes; their lack could reduce the cellular oncosuppression necessary to block the onset and progression of GISTs, as well as other epithelial tumors [25, 26].

However, no study highlights if there is a higher GIST preponderance in gastrectomized subjects. In patients with BIIGR in fact, biles' role in the genesis of gastric adenocarcinoma on the anastomotic mucosa is known; there is no evidence so far for an analogous effect for GIST. A common metabolic pathway may be shown through the study of the proliferation signal. It is known that Cajal cell proliferation

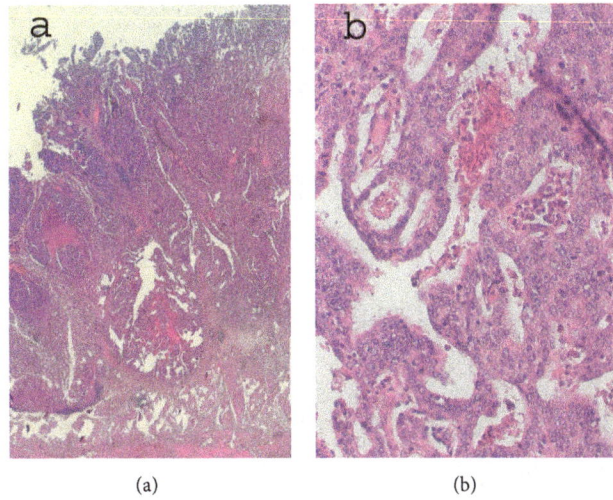

FIGURE 2: Gastric adenocarcinoma: (a) adenocarcinoma infiltrating depth muscular wall—10x and (b) moderately differentiated tubulo-papillary adenocarcinoma—20x.

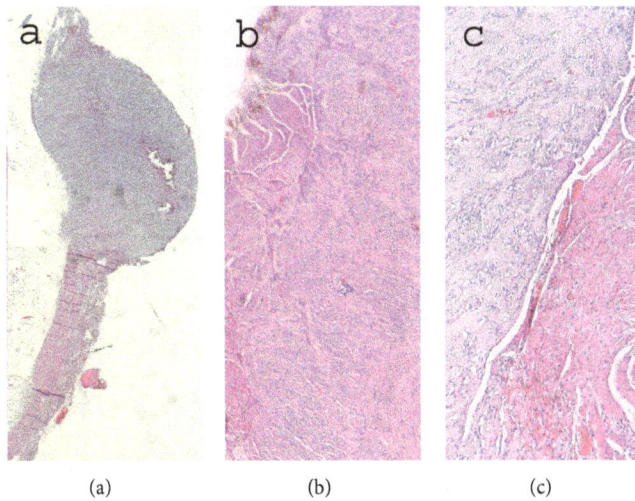

FIGURE 3: coexistent GIST EE: (a) GIST of the muscle wall of the gastric corpus—2x, (b) fusiform low grade GIST cells composed of spindle cells with ovoid nuclei arranged in short fascicles (nuclear palisading) —4x and (c) interface between GIST and gastric muscle wall—10x.

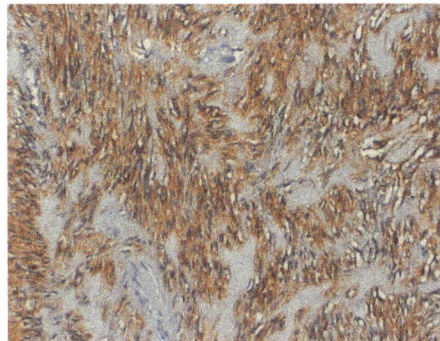

FIGURE 4: Immunohistochemical features of GIST: c-KIT/CD117 (tyrosine kinase growth factor receptor) positivity—20x.

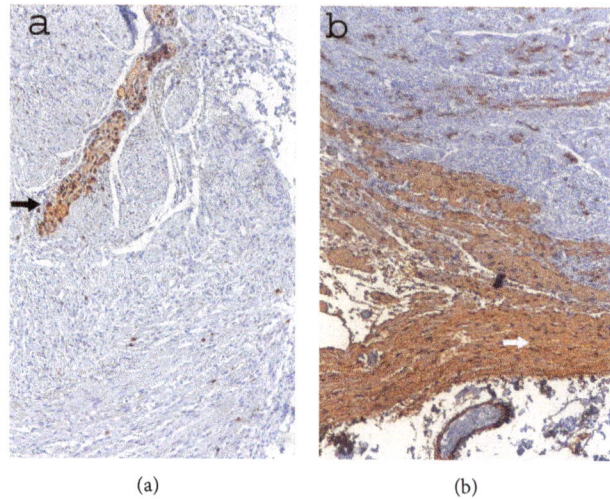

(a)   (b)

FIGURE 5: Immunohistochemical features of GIST: (a) S-100 negativity. Instead overexpressed in nerve cells (black arrow) —10x (b) SMA (smooth muscle actin) negativity. Instead overexpressed in muscular gastric wall cells (white arrow) —10x.

persists throughout the postnatal period. KIT and Ki-67 signal are observed in the proliferation and development of this kind of cell [27]. Ki-67 protein is associated with cellular proliferation and it can be detected in the cell nucleus during the active phases of the cell cycle [28]. Ki-67 is thus a useful marker to determine the growth fraction of normal or neoplastic cell population. The *Ki-67 labeling index* assesses the fraction of Ki-67-positive tumor cells and is often correlated with the clinical course of cancer [29].

We propose that the genesis of these neoplasms can be the overstimulation of the enteric sympathetic plexus as a result of increased gastric clearance. The absence of a parasympathetic stimulus due to vagotomy can lead to the hypertrophy and hyperplasia of Cajal cells, pacemakers of the enteric sympathetic plexus. The study of Cajal cells' proliferation signal in GISTs and in healthy muscular tunica of resected stomachs could demonstrate the etiopathogenesis of these tumors, justifying the synchronism with adenocarcinomas in gastrectomized subjects. This kind of research could provide useful information on the origins of these tumors, but also they could be the starting point for new therapies. Anyway, because of the GIST's low malignant potential, its probability of recurrence is considerably lower than synchronous gastric adenocarcinoma's one. For this reason, incidental GISTs should not be over treated, in order not to invalidate the outcome of surgical and oncological treatment of the primary disease.

4. Conclusion

gGIST in combination with other synchronous malignant diseases is a rare event. GIST's malignancy is considerably lower than gastric adenocarcinoma's one; in this respect, the surgeon has to pay attention to a possible primary GIST, synchronous to other primary malignancies. The coexistence of these neoplasms is an intriguing oncologic model. There is not a unique interpretation of the biochemical mechanisms

behind this synchronism, and further studies are needed. Our hypothesis is that in gastrectomized patients there is an overstimulation on Cajal cells, because an increased clearance is necessary. PGFRA mutation affects the treatment of GIST and therefore its prognosis. The GIST overtreatment in terms of survival however could not be effective in case of synchronous neoplasm, because of the worse prognosis of the other tumor. Further studies on the molecular biology of these neoplasms are necessary to detect their biochemical mechanisms; if we could understand the genesis of these synchronisms we also could be able to produce new therapies, such as the biological one.

Authors' Contribution

Federico Sista has made substantial contributions to conception and design of the study. Valentina Abruzzese has made analysis and interpretation of the literature data. Mario Schietroma and Gianfranco Amicucci have given final approval of the version to be published.

References

[1] R. P. DeMatteo, J. J. Lewis, D. Leung, S. S. Mudan, J. M. Woodruff, and M. F. Brennan, "Two hundred gastrointestinal stromal tumors: recurrence patterns and prognostic factors for survival," *Annals of Surgery*, vol. 231, no. 1, pp. 51–58, 2000.

[2] S. Hirota, K. Isozaki, Y. Moriyama et al., "Gain-of-function mutations of c-kit in human gastrointestinal stromal tumors," *Science*, vol. 279, no. 5350, pp. 577–580, 1998.

[3] M. Koelz, N. Wick, T. Winkler, F. Längle, and F. Wrba, "The impact of c-kit mutations on histomorphological risk assessment of gastrointestinal stromal tumors," *European Surgery*, vol. 39, no. 1, pp. 45–53, 2007.

[4] M. Miettinen and J. Lasota, "Gastrointestinal stromal tumors—definition, clinical, histological, immunohistochemical, and molecular genetic features and differential diagnosis," *Virchows Archiv*, vol. 438, no. 1, pp. 1–12, 2001.

[5] B. Nilsson, P. Bümming, J. M. Meis-Kindblom et al., "Gastrointestinal stromal tumors: the incidence, prevalence, clinical course, and prognostication in the preimatinib mesylate era—a population-based study in western Sweden," *Cancer*, vol. 103, no. 4, pp. 821–829, 2005.

[6] T. Terada, "Gastrointestinal stromal tumor of the digestive organs: a histopathologic study of 31 cases in a single Japanese institute," *International Journal of Clinical and Experimental Pathology*, vol. 3, no. 2, pp. 162–168, 2009.

[7] B. Liegl-Atzwanger, J. A. Fletcher, and C. D. M. Fletcher, "Gastrointestinal stromal tumors," *Virchows Archiv*, vol. 456, no. 2, pp. 111–127, 2010.

[8] U. I. Chaudhry and R. P. DeMatteo, "Management of resectable gastrointestinal stromal tumor," *Hematology/Oncology Clinics of North America*, vol. 23, no. 1, pp. 79–96, 2009.

[9] A. Maiorana, R. Fante, A. M. Cesinaro, and R. A. Fano, "Synchronous occurrence of epithelial and stromal tumors in the stomach: a report of 6 cases," *Archives of Pathology and Laboratory Medicine*, vol. 124, no. 5, pp. 682–686, 2000.

[10] S. Bircan, Ö. Candir, Ş. Aydin et al., "Synchronous primary adenocarcinoma and gastrointestinal stromal tumor in the stomach: a report of two cases," *Turkish Journal of Gastroenterology*, vol. 15, no. 3, pp. 187–191, 2004.

[11] F. Rauf, Z. Ahmad, S. Muzzafar, and A. S. Hussaini, "Synchronous occurrence of gastrointestinal stromal tumor and gastric adenocarcinoma: a case report," *Journal of the Pakistan Medical Association*, vol. 56, no. 4, pp. 184–186, 2006.

[12] S. Uchiyama, M. Nagano, N. Takahashi et al., "Synchronous adenocarcinoma and gastrointestinal stromal tumors of the stomach treated laparoscopically," *International Journal of Clinical Oncology*, vol. 12, no. 6, pp. 478–481, 2007.

[13] I. E. Katsoulis, M. Bossi, P. I. Richman, and J. I. Livingstone, "Collision of adenocarcinoma and gastrointestinal stromal tumour (GIST) in the stomach: report of a case," *International Seminars in Surgical Oncology*, vol. 4, article 2, 2007.

[14] Y.-J. Liu, Z. Yang, L.-S. Hao, L. Xia, Q.-B. Jia, and X.-T. Wu, "Synchronous incidental gastrointestinal stromal and epithelial malignant tumors," *World Journal of Gastroenterology*, vol. 15, no. 16, pp. 2027–2031, 2009.

[15] P. Bucher, J.-F. Egger, P. Gervaz et al., "An audit of surgical management of gastrointestinal stromal tumours (GIST)," *European Journal of Surgical Oncology*, vol. 32, no. 3, pp. 310–314, 2006.

[16] D. A. Arber, R. Tamayo, and L. M. Weiss, "Paraffin section detection of the c-kit gene product (cd117) in human tissues: value in the diagnosis of mast cell disorders," *Human Pathology*, vol. 29, no. 5, pp. 498–504, 1998.

[17] T. Aparicio, V. Boige, J.-C. Sabourin et al., "Prognostic factors after surgery of primary resectable gastrointestinal stromal tumours," *European Journal of Surgical Oncology*, vol. 30, no. 10, pp. 1098–1103, 2004.

[18] T. Tashiro, T. Hasegawa, M. Omatsu, S. Sekine, T. Shimoda, and H. Katai, "Gastrointestinal stromal tumour of the stomach showing lymph node metastases," *Histopathology*, vol. 47, no. 4, pp. 438–439, 2005.

[19] R. P. DeMatteo, J. J. Lewis, D. Leung, S. S. Mudan, J. M. Woodruff, and M. F. Brennan, "Two hundred gastrointestinal stromal tumors: recurrence patterns and prognostic factors for survival," *Annals of Surgery*, vol. 231, no. 1, pp. 51–58, 2000.

[20] Y. W. Novitsky, K. W. Kercher, R. F. Sing, and B. T. Heniford, "Long-term outcomes of laparoscopic resection of gastric gastrointestinal stromal tumors," *Annals of Surgery*, vol. 243, no. 6, pp. 738–745, 2006.

[21] Y. Otani, T. Furukawa, M. Yoshida et al., "Operative indications for relatively small (2-5 cm) gastrointestinal stromal tumor of the stomach based on analysis of 60 operated cases," *Surgery*, vol. 139, no. 4, pp. 484–492, 2006.

[22] R. K. Pandurengan, A. G. Dumont, D. M. Araujo et al., "Survival of patients with multiple primary malignancies: a study of 783 patients with gastrointestinal stromal tumor," *Annals of Oncology*, vol. 21, no. 10, pp. 2107–2111, 2010.

[23] W. Li, X. Wu, N. Wang, D. Yin, and S.-L. Zhang, "Gastrointestinal stromal tumor with synchronous isolated parenchymal splenic metastasis of ovarian cancer," *Chinese Medical Journal*, vol. 124, no. 24, pp. 4372–4375, 2011.

[24] K. Kawanowa, Y. Sakuma, S. Sakurai et al., "High incidence of microscopic gastrointestinal stromal tumors in the stomach," *Human Pathology*, vol. 37, no. 12, pp. 1527–1535, 2006.

[25] M. Ø. Pedersen, A. Larsen, M. Stoltenberg, and M. Penkowa, "The role of metallothionein in oncogenesis and cancer prognosis," *Progress in Histochemistry and Cytochemistry*, vol. 44, no. 1, pp. 29–64, 2009.

[26] E. T.-L. Soo, C.-T. NG, G. W.-C. Yip et al., "Differential expression of metallothionein in gastrointestinal stromal tumors and gastric carcinomas," *Anatomical Record*, vol. 294, no. 2, pp. 267–272, 2011.

[27] X. He, W.-C. Yang, X.-Y. Wen et al., "Late embryonic and postnatal development of interstitial cells of cajal in mouse esophagus: distribution, proliferation and kit dependence," *Cells Tissues Organs*, vol. 196, no. 2, pp. 175–188, 2012.

[28] J. Bullwinkel, B. Baron-Lühr, A. Lüdemann, C. Wohlenberg, J. Gerdes, and T. Scholzen, "Ki-67 protein is associated with ribosomal RNA transcription in quiescent and proliferating cells," *Journal of Cellular Physiology*, vol. 206, no. 3, pp. 624–635, 2006.

[29] T. Scholzen and J. Gerdes, "The Ki-67 protein: from the known and the unknown," *Journal of Cellular Physiology*, vol. 182, no. 3, pp. 311–322, 2000.

23

Superior Mesenteric Venous Thrombosis after Laparoscopic Exploration for Small Bowel Obstruction

Hideki Katagiri,[1] **Shozo Kunizaki,**[1] **Mayu Shimaguchi,**[1] **Yasuo Yoshinaga,**[1]
Yukihiro Kanda,[1] **Alan T. Lefor,**[2] **and Ken Mizokami**[1]

[1] *Department of Surgery, Tokyo Bay Urayasu Ichikawa Medical Center (Noguchi Hideyo Memorial International Hospital),*
3-4-34 Todaijima, Urayasu, Chiba 279-0001, Japan
[2] *Department of Surgery, Jichi Medical University, 1-3311 Yakushiji, Shimotsuke, Tochigi 329-0498, Japan*

Correspondence should be addressed to Hideki Katagiri; x62h20k38@yahoo.co.jp

Academic Editors: S. Bhatt, M. Güvener, and S. Landen

Mesenteric venous thrombosis is a rare cause of intestinal ischemia which is potentially life-threatening because it can lead to intestinal infarction. Mesenteric venous thrombosis rarely develops after abdominal surgery and is usually associated with coagulation disorders. Associated symptoms are generally subtle or nonspecific, often resulting in delayed diagnosis. A 68-year-old woman underwent laparoscopic exploration for small bowel obstruction, secondary to adhesions. During the procedure, an intestinal perforation was identified and repaired. Postoperatively, the abdominal pain persisted and repeat exploration was undertaken. At repeat exploration, a perforation was identified in the small bowel with a surrounding abscess. After the second operation, the abdominal pain improved but anorexia persisted. Contrast enhanced abdominal computed tomography was performed which revealed superior mesenteric venous thrombosis. Anticoagulation therapy with heparin was started immediately and the thrombus resolved over the next 6 days. Although rare, this complication must be considered in patients after abdominal surgery with unexplained abdominal symptoms.

1. Introduction

Mesenteric venous thrombosis is an unusual cause of intestinal ischemia and potentially life-threatening because it can result in intestinal infarction. Mesenteric venous thrombosis accounts for 5 to 15% of all mesenteric ischemic events and usually involves the superior mesenteric vein [1–4]. Several cases of mesenteric venous thrombosis after abdominal surgery have been reported; however, mesenteric venous thrombosis after surgery for abdominal sepsis is especially uncommon. We report a case of superior mesenteric venous thrombosis after abdominal abscess with small intestinal perforation, successfully treated by systemic anticoagulation therapy.

2. Case Presentation

A 68-year-old woman with a history of previous abdominal surgery presented with abdominal pain and vomiting. One day prior to admission, she noted the gradual onset of abdominal pain. She had one bowel movement but the abdominal pain persisted. The pain was intermittent and gradually worsened. She vomited several times. She underwent a hernia repair 15 years previously and had a lower midline incision, although the details of that procedure were unavailable. On physical examination, her lower abdomen was slightly distended with mild tenderness to palpation. Dilated intestine was palpable, but there were no signs of peritonitis. Nasogastric suction was initiated but inadequate and the abdominal pain persisted. Abdominal CT scan revealed dilated loops of small intestine with a small amount of ascites.

The diagnosis of small bowel obstruction was established and exploration undertaken. This was begun laparoscopically which demonstrated multiple areas of adherent loops of small bowel. The adhesions were lysed sharply and further exploration revealed a small bowel perforation, which was repaired in a conventional manner after conversion to open laparotomy.

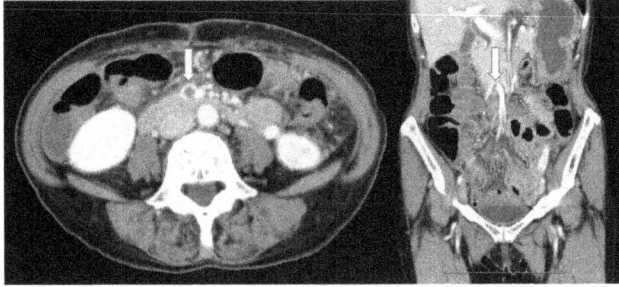

FIGURE 1: Contrast enhanced computed tomographic scan (axial and coronal views) of the abdomen demonstrated a filling defect in the superior mesenteric vein (arrow), suggesting thrombus.

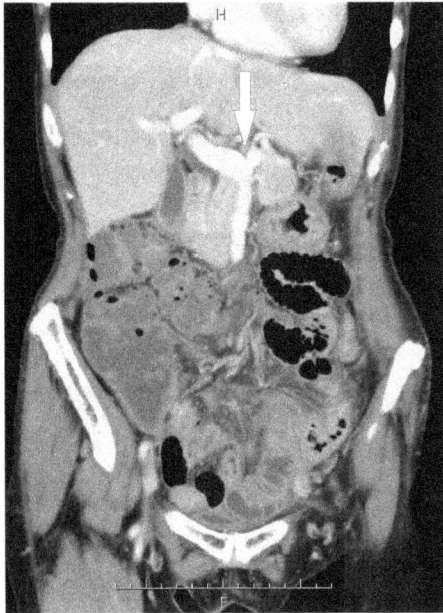

FIGURE 2: Contrast enhanced computed tomographic scan of the abdomen (coronal view) six days after starting anticoagulation therapy. The superior mesenteric vein is patent (arrow) and the thrombus has resolved.

On postoperative day (POD) 1, her temperature increased to 39°C; however, it resolved over five days without specific treatment. The abdominal pain persisted and became more intense on POD 6. Abdominal CT scan was performed on POD 7, which showed a small fluid collection with some air. Due to persistence and increasing severity of the abdominal pain, repeat operative exploration was undertaken on POD 8. Exploration revealed abscesses in the abdominal wall and between loops of small bowel, as well as a site of perforation, which was resected and repaired with a primary anastomosis.

The postoperative course was uneventful except for persistent anorexia. Ten days after the second exploration, CT scan was obtained due to the persistent anorexia. The CT scan revealed edematous small intestine and dilatation of the mesenteric veins. The scan also revealed a filling defect in the superior mesenteric vein (Figure 1) suggestive of a thrombus. She had no evidence of intestinal gangrene or peritonitis, and

systemic heparin was begun followed by warfarin therapy. Laboratory data were not consistent with protein C, protein S, or antithrombin III deficiencies. She had no past history or family history of deep venous thrombosis or other coagulation disorders. Over the next six days, the thrombus resolved on repeat imaging studies (Figure 2), and her appetite recovered. She was discharged without further complications, continuing oral anticoagulation with warfarin.

3. Discussion

Mesenteric venous thrombosis is a rare cause of intestinal ischemia which rarely occurs after abdominal surgery. Its frequency remains obscure but Kim et al. reported that 0.3% of patients after laparoscopic bariatric surgery develop portomesenteric venous thrombosis [4]. James et al. reviewed 18 cases of portomesenteric venous thrombosis after laparoscopic procedures including Roux-en-Y gastric bypass, Nissen fundoplication, partial colectomy, cholecystectomy, and appendectomy [3]. To the best of our knowledge, this is the first reported case of superior mesenteric venous thrombosis after surgery for abdominal sepsis. Intra-abdominal inflammation such as acute pancreatitis can lead to mesenteric venous thrombosis [1, 3, 5, 6]. In the present patient, we believe that inflammation due to intestinal perforation led to superior mesenteric venous thrombosis. While the exact etiology of this complication is unclear, the use of the laparoscope in the first operation may also have contributed to this complication.

The etiologic factors associated with mesenteric venous thrombosis are varied, most commonly associated with coagulation disorders such as Factor V Leiden, protein C and protein S deficiencies, and antithrombin III deficiency [1–3, 5, 6]. In young women, oral-contraceptive use can lead to mesenteric venous thrombosis [1, 2, 6]. Other etiologic factors include inflammatory conditions such as pancreatitis, intra-abdominal sepsis, cirrhosis, portal hypertension, neoplasms, and blunt abdominal trauma [1, 2, 5, 6].

The diagnosis of mesenteric venous thrombosis is often delayed because the associated symptoms are usually subtle or nonspecific. The most common symptom is unexplained abdominal pain. Abdominal distension, anorexia, diarrhea, and vomiting have also been associated with mesenteric venous thrombosis [1–3, 5]. Severe abdominal pain, fever, and peritoneal signs suggest intestinal infarction or perforation. In the present patient, she had only unexplained anorexia which resolved after treatment. CT scan is considered to be the best way to establish the diagnosis of mesenteric venous thrombosis, with a sensitivity as high as 90% [1, 2]. In patients with mesenteric venous thrombosis, a central lucency in the mesenteric vein may be seen on CT scan. Other CT findings include enlargement of the superior mesenteric vein, a sharply defined vein wall with a rim of increased density, and intestinal edema [1].

The treatment of mesenteric venous thrombosis includes systemic anticoagulation. Surgical intervention is sometimes required. When the diagnosis of mesenteric venous thrombosis is made, systemic anticoagulation with heparin should be started immediately [1, 2]. Brunaud et al. reported that, in patients without bowel necrosis or perforation, the morbidity, mortality, and survival rate are similar to both surgical and nonoperative management [2]. However, in patients with intestinal infarction, peritonitis, or bowel stricture due to ischemia, surgery is essential. Warfarin should be started in the absence of intestinal ischemia [1]. Nasogastric suction, fluid resuscitation, and bowel rest are included as supportive care [1, 4].

This rare complication must be considered when evaluating patients after abdominal surgery with unexplained abdominal symptoms. Nonoperative management is feasible when indicated.

References

[1] S. Kumar, M. G. Sarr, and P. S. Kamath, "Mesenteric venous thrombosis," *The New England Journal of Medicine*, vol. 345, no. 23, pp. 1683–1688, 2001.

[2] L. Brunaud, L. Antunes, S. Collinet-Adler et al., "Acute mesenteric venous thrombosis: case for nonoperative management," *Journal of Vascular Surgery*, vol. 34, no. 4, pp. 673–679, 2001.

[3] A. W. James, C. Rabl, A. C. Westphalen, P. F. Fogarty, A. M. Posselt, and G. M. Campos, "Portomesenteric venous thrombosis after laparoscopic surgery: a systematic literature review," *Archives of Surgery*, vol. 144, no. 6, pp. 520–526, 2009.

[4] H. K. Kim, J. M. Chun, and S. Huh, "Anticoagulation and delayed bowel resection in the management of mesenteric venous thrombosis," *World Journal of Gastroenterology*, vol. 19, no. 30, pp. 5025–5028, 2013.

[5] D. Goitein, I. Matter, A. Raziel et al., "Portomesenteric thrombosis following laparoscopic bariatric surgery: incidence, patterns of clinical presentation, and etiology in a bariatric patient population," *JAMA Surgery*, vol. 148, no. 4, pp. 340–346, 2013.

[6] S. Acosta, A. Alhadad, P. Svensson, and O. Ekberg, "Epidemiology, risk and prognostic factors in mesenteric venous thrombosis," *British Journal of Surgery*, vol. 95, no. 10, pp. 1245–1251, 2008.

24

Duplication Cyst in the Third Part of the Duodenum Presenting with Gastric Outlet Obstruction and Severe Weight Loss

Osama Shaheen,[1] **Samer Sara,**[1] **Mhd Firas Safadi,**[1] **and Bayan Alsaid**[1,2]

[1]Department of Surgery, Almouwasat University Hospital, Damascus, Syria
[2]Laboratory of Anatomy, Faculty of Medicine, University of Damascus, Damascus, Syria

Correspondence should be addressed to Mhd Firas Safadi; doctor.safadi@gmail.com

Academic Editor: Boris Kirshtein

Duodenal duplication is a rare developmental abnormality which is usually diagnosed in infancy and childhood, but less frequently in adulthood. We report a case of a 16-year-old female with a duplication cyst in the third part of the duodenum. The patient presented with symptoms of gastric outlet obstruction, including severe anorexia and weight loss. The diagnosis was made preoperatively by CT scan and upper endoscopy. The cyst was successfully treated by marsupialization on the duodenum using a GIA stapler. Duodenal duplication presents with a wide variety of symptoms. Although illusive, many cases can be properly diagnosed preoperatively by using the appropriate imaging modalities. Treatment choices are tailored according to the size and location of the cyst, in addition to its relation to adjacent structures. The outcomes are favorable in the majority of patients.

1. Introduction

Duplications of the alimentary tract are rare developmental abnormalities. The overall incidence of this condition is 1 : 25,000, and duodenal duplication constitutes 5–12% of all cases [1]. Most cases of duodenal duplication are seen at the medial border of the first and second portions of the duodenum. Duplication of the third portion is even less frequent [2, 3].

Here, we report a rare case of a duplication cyst that compresses the third part of the duodenum. The cyst presented with gastric outlet obstruction and severe anorexia. To our knowledge, this is the first reported case that presents with severe weight loss and malnutrition in adolescence.

2. Case Presentation

A 16-year-old female presented to the emergency department of our hospital complaining of recurrent abdominal pain in the epigastrium especially after meals, with occasional radiation to the left shoulder. She reported a recent history of persistent nausea and vomiting in addition to severe anorexia and weight loss.

The patient looked anxious, dehydrated, and debilitated. She had tachycardia and her BMI was only 15.8 kg/m². Abdominal examination revealed mild tenderness in the epigastrium without rigidity or palpable masses. Laboratory findings showed anemia (hemoglobin 8.2 g/dL), hypokalemia (potassium 3.1 mEq/L), and hypoalbuminemia (albumin 2.2 g/dL). Gastric aspiration yielded about one liter of non-bloody aspirate.

Abdominal ultrasonography (US) showed severe gastric distension with a big cystic mass in the upper abdomen. Abdominal computed tomography (CT) showed a cystic lesion measuring 8 × 4 × 7 cm, which extends along the third part of the duodenum in the retroperitoneum. The lumen of the third part of the duodenum was completely obscured. The cyst was suspicious for duodenal duplication (Figure 1). Upper endoscopy showed a copious amount of fluids in the stomach with severe gastric dilatation. The third part of the duodenum was nearly occluded, supposedly due to external compression.

Upon laparotomy, a cystic structure was found behind the transverse mesocolon. An extended Kocher maneuver was performed, and exploration revealed a big cyst along the third part of the duodenum with close relation to the head

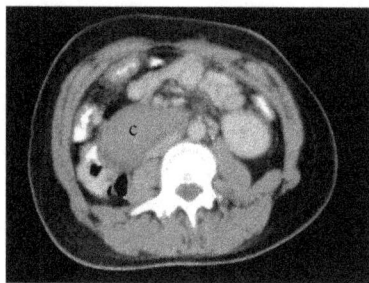

FIGURE 1: Oral and intravenous contrast-enhanced CT scan of the abdomen. The noncommunicating cyst extends along the third portion of the duodenum (c: cyst).

of the pancreas (Figure 2(a)). The duodenum was opened on the lower lateral wall, and duodenotomy revealed the cyst which was protruding inside the lumen of the third duodenal portion (Figure 2(b)).

The cyst was opened widely through the common wall, and blood clots were extracted from the cyst. No abnormal pathology was noted inside the cyst. Part of the common wall was resected, and the cyst was marsupialized on the duodenum with the aid of a GIA stapler. Finally, a side-to-side anastomosis was performed between the duodenotomy site and a jejunal loop about 30 cm after the ligament of Treitz (Figure 2(c)).

Histopathologic examination confirmed the diagnosis by identifying a duodenal mucosa that lines a smooth muscle coat within the wall of the cyst (Figure 3). The patient was well and free from symptoms after 12 months of follow-up. She regained her nutritional state and her BMI was 20.5 kg/m^2.

3. Discussion

Duplication cysts of gastrointestinal tract were first documented in the mid-19th century by Reginald Fitz [4]. Three criteria are required for the diagnosis of a duplication cyst: an intimate relation to the gastrointestinal tract, the presence of a smooth muscular coat, and the presence of an alimentary mucosal lining [4].

Duodenal duplications represent a low percentage of all duplications. They can be cystic or tubular, and they may communicate with the duodenal lumen, the pancreatic duct, or rarely the biliary system [4]. These cysts often contain mucosal secretions from the epithelial lining, but many authors reported the presence of purulent content or bile [5, 6].

The abnormality is usually diagnosed in infancy and childhood [1]. However, many patients can remain asymptomatic until adulthood, and about one third of patients present after 20 years of age [7].

The clinical features of duodenal duplication cysts vary from asymptomatic cases to nonspecific symptoms such as abdominal pain, abdominal distention, and vomiting [5, 7]. Some patients develop symptoms of gastric outlet obstruction or small bowel obstruction. Ulceration or perforation due to

the presence of an ectopic mucosa may cause duodenal bleeding or peritonitis, respectively [8]. Duodenal duplication cysts may also cause recurrent episodes of acute pancreatitis because of the direct pressure applied against the pancreatic duct. Stone formation was reported in some cases due to stasis inside the cyst. Jaundice and intussusceptions have also been reported [6]. Hemorrhagic ascites is a very rare complication of duplication cysts [9].

Most cysts are 2–5 cm in size. The largest diameter of the cyst in our case was 8 cm, which is relatively large. Only few cases in the literature were larger than 5 cm [6]. This was responsible for the severe compressive symptoms which included anorexia, vomiting, malnutrition, and weight loss. The BMI of our patient was 15.8 kg/m^2 with severe laboratory derangement, and this was not previously reported in any case of duodenal cysts.

The preoperative diagnosis of intestinal duplications is rarely accurate. The differential diagnosis encompasses all cystic lesions in this region, which include choledochoceles, pancreatic pseudocysts, cystic tumors of the pancreas, mesenteric cysts, and duodenal diverticulums [6].

Endoscopic US could differentiate the duplication cyst by the "gut signature" or "the double-layer wall" sign of its wall. CT is valuable in identifying the type, location, and the size of the duplication cyst, and the technetium scan can aid in the detection of heterotopic gastric mucosa in cases complicated with bleeding [10]. Magnetic resonance imaging (MRI) and gastroduodenoscopy are other modalities that can be used for diagnosis. Magnetic resonance cholangiopancreatography (MRCP) is a valuable noninvasive tool for the identification of cysts that communicate with the biliary tree. Endoscopic retrograde cholangiopancreatography (ERCP) was also recommended to visualize the pancreaticobiliary tract and to determine its relationship with the cyst, but ERCP-related complications limit its role [9, 11].

The appropriate surgical procedure for a duodenal duplication cyst depends on its type and location. Consequently, several operative choices are feasible [12]. Total excision is indicated when the cyst is small and not related to the pancreaticobiliary tree or the head of the pancreas, or when the cyst is complicated with an ulcer, either in the cystic mucosa or in the adjacent mucosa. Excision is considered the procedure of choice to avoid possible malignant transformation, which was reported in three cases in the literature [7, 13]. Pancreaticoduodenectomy is rarely required, but it may be the only choice in complicated cysts which are intimately related to the head of the pancreas or the pancreaticobiliary tree [11].

Partial resection of the common wall with internal marsupialization on the duodenum is a good management option to avoid injury to the pancreas, pancreatic and bile ducts, or any related structure as we did in our case. Other possibilities include cystojejunostomy by a jejunal loop or Roux-en-Y anastomosis [8].

The surgeon should judge the best treatment that relieves the symptoms without causing serious complications. Total excision was not possible in our case due to the close relation of the cyst to the head of the pancreas, and marsupialization

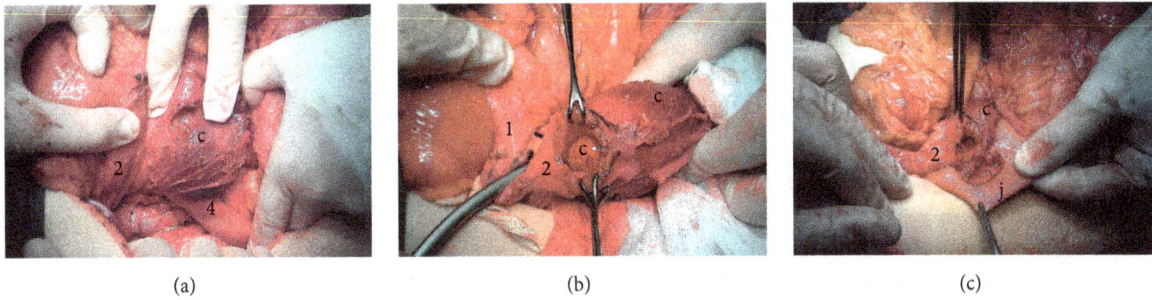

(a)   (b)   (c)

FIGURE 2: Operative views of the cyst illustrating management steps. (a) Extended Kocher maneuver revealed a big cyst compressing the third part of the duodenum, with close relation to the head of the pancreas. (b) The duodenum was opened through the lateral wall of the second part, which showed the internal common wall between the cyst and the third part of the duodenum. The lumen of the of the third part of the duodenum was completely occluded. The common wall was opened using a GIA-stapler (not shown). (c) The cyst collapsed after marsupialization and duodenojejunal anastomosis was performed (c: cyst, j: jejunum, numbers: corresponding parts of the duodenum).

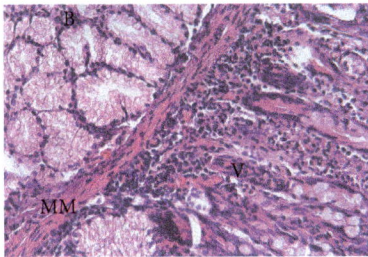

FIGURE 3: Histological view of the cyst wall showing typical structure of duodenal mucosa (hematoxylin and eosin, ×100) (B: Brunner's glands, MM: mucosa muscularis, V: duodenal villi).

was a safer option for draining the cyst and relieving the compressive symptoms.

Advances in therapeutic endoscopy, such as endoscopic mucosal resection, were recently used in the management of some duodenal cysts [5]. More recently, many cases of duodenal duplication were managed laparoscopically, including resection or anastomosis, with favorable outcomes [14].

Although duodenal cysts are considered a rare entity, we believe that further research is needed to design a specific classification system and management criteria for these lesions. Such diagnostic and therapeutic criteria would spare many patients the sequelae of laparotomy by taking advantage of the recent advances in minimally invasive and endoscopic techniques. This would only be possible through accumulation of more cases. Therefore, we encourage surgeons to report any lesion of this type with enough details about location and appropriate treatment options.

4. Conclusion

Duodenal duplication should be considered in the differential diagnosis of vague upper abdominal symptoms, especially when a cystic structure neighboring the duodenum is demonstrated on radiology. Ideal treatment is total excision when feasible. Otherwise the cyst may be treated with subtotal excision and/or internal anastomosis. When treated properly, these lesions usually have favorable outcomes.

Acknowledgments

The authors would like to thank Dr. Hadeel Shamma for her help with histopathologic considerations and Dr. Anas Shawa for his help with reference material.

References

[1] R. W. Browning, "Duodenal duplications," *Review of Surgery*, vol. 20, pp. 226–229, 1963.

[2] W. Y. Inouye, C. Farrell, W. T. Fitts, and T. A. Tristan, "Duodenal duplication: case report and literature review," *Annals of Surgery*, vol. 162, no. 5, pp. 910–916, 1965.

[3] H. Hata, N. Hiraoka, H. Ojima, K. Shimada, T. Kosuge, and T. Shimoda, "Carcinoid tumor arising in a duplication cyst of the duodenum," *Pathology International*, vol. 56, no. 5, pp. 272–278, 2006.

[4] R. E. Gross, G. W. Holcomb Jr., and S. Farber, "Duplications of the alimentary tract," *Pediatrics*, vol. 9, no. 4, pp. 448–468, 1952.

[5] H. S. You, S. B. Park, J. H. Kim et al., "A case of duodenal duplication cyst manifested by duodenal polyp," *Clinical Endoscopy*, vol. 45, no. 4, pp. 425–427, 2012.

[6] J.-J. Chen, H.-C. Lee, C.-Y. Yeung, W.-T. Chan, C.-B. Jiang, and J.-C. Sheu, "Meta-analysis: the clinical features of the duodenal duplication cyst," *Journal of Pediatric Surgery*, vol. 45, no. 8, pp. 1598–1606, 2010.

[7] B. Seeliger, T. Piardi, E. Marzano, D. Mutter, J. Marescaux, and P. Pessaux, "Duodenal duplication cyst: a potentially malignant disease," *Annals of Surgical Oncology*, vol. 19, no. 12, pp. 3753–3754, 2012.

[8] B. K. Rai, S. Zaman, B. Mirza, G. Hanif, and A. Sheikh, "Duodenal duplication cyst having ectopic gastric and pancreatic tissues," *APSP Journal of Case Reports*, vol. 3, no. 2, article 15, 2012.

[9] E. Redondo-Cerezo, J. Pleguezuelo-Diaz, M. L. de Hierro et al., "Duodenal duplication cyst and pancreas divisum causing acute pancreatitis in an adult male," *World Journal of Gastrointestinal Endoscopy*, vol. 2, no. 9, pp. 318–320, 2010.

[10] N. S. Salemis, C. Liatsos, M. Kolios, and S. Gourgiotis, "Recurrent acute pancreatitis secondary to a duodenal duplication cyst in an adult. A case report and literature review," *Canadian Journal of Gastroenterology*, vol. 23, no. 11, pp. 749–752, 2009.

[11] Y. C. Jo, K. R. Joo, D. H. Kim et al., "Duodenal duplicated cyst manifested by acute pancreatitis and obstructive jaundice in an elderly man," *Journal of Korean Medical Science*, vol. 19, no. 4, pp. 604–607, 2004.

[12] T. Merrot, R. Anastasescu, T. Pankevych et al., "Duodenal duplications: clinical characteristics, embryological hypotheses, histological findings, treatment," *European Journal of Pediatric Surgery*, vol. 16, no. 1, pp. 18–23, 2006.

[13] M. M. Orr and A. J. Edwards, "Neoplastic change in duplications of the alimentary tract," *British Journal of Surgery*, vol. 62, no. 4, pp. 269–274, 1975.

[14] U. K. Ballehaninna, T. Nguyen, and S. C. Burjonrappa, "Laparoscopic resection of antenataly identified duodenal duplication cyst," *Journal of the Society of Laparoendoscopic Surgeons*, vol. 17, no. 3, pp. 454–458, 2013.

25

Esophageal Gastrointestinal Stromal Tumor: Diagnostic Complexity and Management Pitfalls

Charalampos G. Markakis,[1] Eleftherios D. Spartalis,[1] Emmanouil Liarmakopoulos,[1] Evangelia G. Kavoura,[2] and Periklis Tomos[1]

[1] *Second Department of Propedeutic Surgery, University of Athens, Medical School, "Laiko" General Hospital,*
  Agiou Thoma 17, 11527 Athens, Greece
[2] *First Department of Pathology, University of Athens, Medical School, 11527 Athens, Greece*

Correspondence should be addressed to Eleftherios D. Spartalis; eleftherios.spartalis@gmail.com

Academic Editors: J. J. Andreasen and D. E. Jaroszewski

Introduction. Gastrointestinal stromal tumors of the esophagus are rare. *Case Presentation.* This is a case of a 50-year-old male patient who was referred to our department complaining of atypical chest pain. A chest computed tomographic scan and endoscopic ultrasound revealed a submucosal esophageal tumor measuring 5 cm in its largest diameter. Suspecting a leiomyoma, we performed enucleation via right thoracotomy. The pathology report yielded a diagnosis of an esophageal gastrointestinal stromal tumor. The patient has shown no evidence of recurrence one year postoperatively. *Conclusions.* This report illustrates the complexity and dilemmas inherent in diagnosing and treating esophageal GISTs.

1. Introduction

Gastrointestinal stromal tumors (GISTs) are the most common mesenchymal neoplasms of the gastrointestinal tract [1]. After the discovery of c-kit mutations, their accurate diagnosis and differentiation from other mesenchymal tumors became possible and the use of imatinib mesylate provided new therapeutic options. Consequently, there was interest in these tumors and their management and prognosis has been extensively investigated and standardized.

Esophageal GISTs, in contrast, are rare, amounting to 12.7–28% of mesenchymal esophageal tumors or 2% of all GISTs [1–3] and their diagnosis and management are still challenging, as illustrated in the following case.

2. Case Presentation

A 50 year old Caucasian male was referred to the thoracic surgery department for evaluation of an intramural esophageal mass. The patient complained of atypical chest pain of gradual onset over the previous 6 months. He denied weight loss, dysphagia, upper GI bleeding, reflux, or other symptoms. The patient's medical history included hypertension and a 30-pack-year smoking history. After a chest radiograph failed to show any pathology, a computed tomography (CT) scan was ordered which revealed showed a 5 cm mass on the midesophagus at the junction of the azygos vein with the superior vena cava (Figure 1). Endoscopy showed a normal esophageal mucosa and endoscopic ultrasound a smooth, submucosal mass. A CT scan of the abdomen did not show any evidence of distant metastases.

The mass was approached via a right posterolateral thoracotomy (Figure 1). The subcarinal lymph nodes were found to be enlarged and were sent for frozen section, which was negative for malignancy. The mass was enucleated from the esophageal wall by gently detaching it from the mucosa. No adhesions with the mucosa or muscularis were noted, and the mass was excised with its capsule intact. A frozen section of the mass indicated the mesenchymal origin, with a possible diagnosis of leiomyoma. The muscular layer of the

(a)

(b)

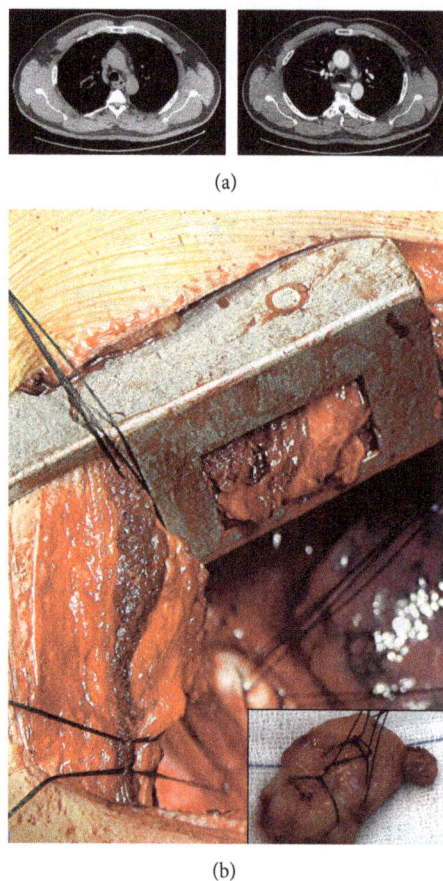

FIGURE 1: (a) CT scan of the chest, showing a well-circumscribed 5 cm submucosal esophageal mass. (b) Intraoperative view of the tumor (inset: macroscopic view of the resected specimen).

esophagus was repaired with vicryl 4-0 interrupted sutures and covered with parietal pleura. Integrity of the esophageal mucosa was established by intraoperative endoscopy. An upper gastrointestinal series on postoperative day 1 showed no evidence of a leak, and the patient was uneventfully discharged on the 6th postoperative day.

On macroscopic examination, the mass was $5.5 \times 3.5 \times 1.5$ cm in size and grayish in color with a fasciated texture (Figure 1). Histologically the mass corresponded to an encapsulated mesenchymatous neoplasm, consisting of fibrous and muscle fascicles with sparse round and spindle cells (Figure 2(a)). No neoplastic cells were found to infiltrate the margins of the capsule. There was no evidence of necrosis and <2 mitoses per 50 high-power fields. Less than 1% of cells stained positive for Ki67. The diagnosis of a GIST was established by immunohistochemistry, which revealed a positive immunoreaction to c-kit and CD34 (Figures 2(b) and 2(c)). There was also an unusual positive reaction to smooth muscle actin (SMA) (Figure 2(d)) [3, 4]. All excised lymph nodes were negative.

After a multidisciplinary meeting the patient received adjuvant therapy (imatinib mesylate 400 mg/d for 1 year). He is closely followedup with endoscopy and CT scans every 3 months and is currently free of disease one year after surgery.

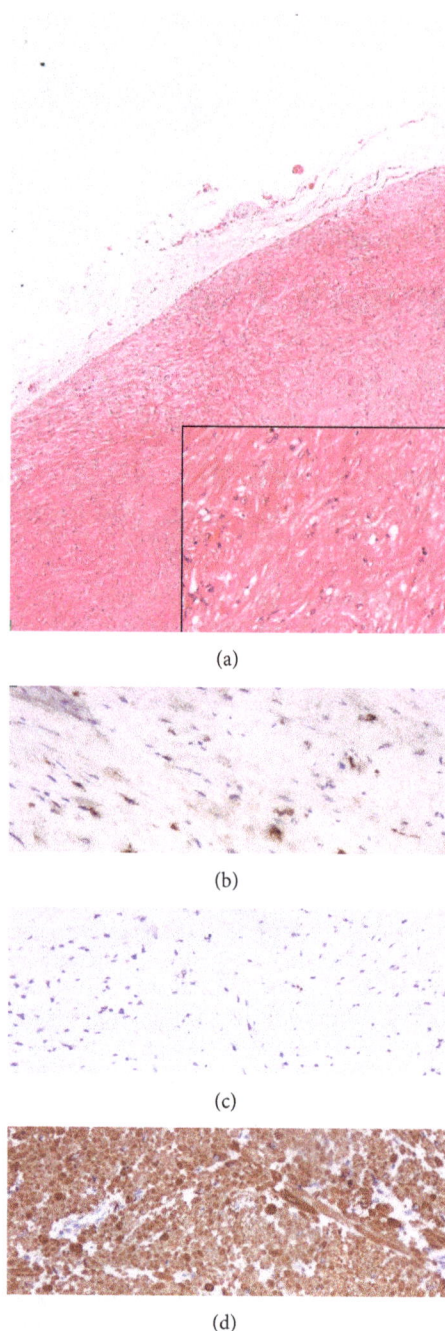

(a)

(b)

(c)

(d)

FIGURE 2: Microscopic view of the tumor. (a) H/E ×40 (inset H/E X200), (b) c-kit ×200, (c) Ki-67 ×200, and (d) SMA (a smooth muscle actin) ×200.

3. Discussion

Esophageal GISTs are difficult to diagnose preoperatively since there are no specific findings to differentiate them from far more common leiomyomas when their clinical presentation, endoscopy, endoscopic ultrasound, or CT scan is reviewed [1, 4, 5]. Both GISTs and leiomyomas are hypoechoic lesions originating from the muscularis propria or muscularis mucosa on endoscopic ultrasound, while lipomas are hyperechoic and can be easily differentiated [6]. Definitive diagnosis can be made by fine-needle aspiration but is not usually performed for esophageal submucosal lesions. This is due to the concern that it may spread malignant disease or induce scarring that might make safe enucleation impossible [1, 3]. Blum et al. recommended biopsy for tumors larger than 2 cm, enlarging tumors, or tumors positive on PET scan. In their series they encountered adhesions to the mucosa or muscularis in all GISTs (but not in 2 leiomyomas) after biopsy, in contrast to other reports [1, 2, 5]. A selective approach to biopsy based on tumor size (>5 cm) and suspicious radiological appearance is warranted until the risks of biopsy compared to the benefit of accurate preoperative diagnosis and planning are determined. As stated above, we did not perform a preoperative biopsy in our patient, while a PET scan might have been appropriate, but it was not possible to obtain it with the patient's insurance in our institution. Immunohistochemical staining can differentiate GISTs, which have c-kit mutations and are positive for CD117 and CD34 from leiomyomas, which are CD34 and CD117 negative, with no c-kit mutations. Leiomyomas are also positive for desmin and smooth muscle actin, while GISTs are usually (but not always) negative [4].

Another contentious point is the type of surgery indicated for esophageal GISTs. While the recommendation for GISTs found in other locations is a wide local excision, the increased morbidity of esophageal resection has to be taken into account. Conflicting data exist in the literature; while some authors report poor results with mortality of up to 59% [3, 4], it is difficult to attribute these to the extent of resection, as other studies such as that of Lee et al. reporting no recurrences in 5 GISTs treated by enucleation [1]. With no strong evidence available, the recommendations from the small existing case series are contradictory to suggested approaches ranging from esophagectomy to endoscopic enucleation [1, 2, 4]. The National Institute of Health (NIH) risk stratification criteria as well as other risk factors described subsequently can be used [7, 8]. There appears to be a poor prognosis in patients with tumors >9 cm and the opposite is true for tumors <5 cm [3, 4]. Our patient had several favorable prognostic factors, namely, low mitotic count, no necrosis, low percentage of Ki-67 positive cells, and negative lymph nodes. Furthermore, the tumor had a clearly defined capsule which was not breached and the tumor margins were clear. On the other hand, the size of the patient's tumor and its localization in the esophagus are reasons to consider enucleation a possibly risky strategy. We felt that we had to offer this patient, who was of low surgical risk, formal resection of the tumor site, which he refused. Concern over a possibly inadequate resection led us to administer adjuvant therapy, which has been shown to result in increased recurrence-free survival in large tumors at high risk of recurrence in the ACOSOG Z9001 trial [9].

4. Conclusions

This case illustrates the complexity and dilemmas in diagnosing and treating esophageal GISTs. To accumulate high-level evidence sufficient to support specific guidelines, a multi-institutional study or even an international registry

of such lesions is needed. Until then, each patient should be evaluated individually by surgical risk, tumor size and biology and should actively participate in the management decision process.

Authors' Contribution

C. G. Markakis and E. D. Spartalis analyzed and interpreted patient's files, assisted at the operation and wrote the paper; E. Liarmakopoulos contributed to the writing; E. G. Kavoura is the pathologist who performed the histological examination; P. Tomos is the supervising professor, who planned and performed the operation; All authors read and approved the final version of the paper.

References

[1] H. J. Lee, S. I. Park, D. K. Kim, and Y. H. Kim, "Surgical resection of esophageal gastrointestinal stromal tumors," *The Annals of Thoracic Surgery*, vol. 87, no. 5, pp. 1569–1571, 2009.

[2] B. H. A. Von Rahden, H. J. Stein, H. Feussner, and J. R. Siewert, "Enucleation of submucosal tumors of the esophagus: minimally invasive versus open approach," *Surgical Endoscopy and Other Interventional Techniques*, vol. 18, no. 6, pp. 924–930, 2004.

[3] P. Jiang, Z. Jiao, B. Han et al., "Clinical characteristics and surgical treatment of oesophageal gastrointestinal stromal tumours," *European Journal of Cardio-thoracic Surgery*, vol. 38, no. 2, pp. 223–227, 2010.

[4] M. Miettinen, M. Sarlomo-Rikala, L. H. Sobin, and J. Lasota, "Esophageal stromal tumors: a clinicopathologic, immunohistochemical, and molecular genetic study of 17 cases and comparison with esophageal leiomyomas and leiomyosarcomas," *The American Journal of Surgical Pathology*, vol. 24, no. 2, pp. 211–222, 2000.

[5] M. G. Blum, K. Y. Bilimoria, J. D. Wayne, A. L. de Hoyos, M. S. Talamonti, and B. Adley, "Surgical considerations for the management and resection of esophageal gastrointestinal stromal tumors," *The Annals of Thoracic Surgery*, vol. 84, no. 5, pp. 1717–1723, 2007.

[6] V. Bhatia, M. Tajika, and A. Rastogi, "Upper gastrointestinal submucosal lesions—clinical and endosonographic evaluation and management," *Tropical gastroenterology*, vol. 31, no. 1, pp. 5–29, 2010.

[7] C. D. M. Fletcher, J. J. Berman, C. Corless et al., "Diagnosis of gastrointestinal stromal tumors: a consensus approach," *Human Pathology*, vol. 33, no. 5, pp. 459–465, 2002.

[8] P. Rutkowski, Z. I. Nowecki, W. Michej et al., "Risk criteria and prognostic factors for predicting recurrences after resection of primary gastrointestinal stromal tumor," *The Annals of Surgical Oncology*, vol. 14, no. 7, pp. 2018–2027, 2007.

[9] R. P. Dematteo, K. V. Ballman, C. R. Antonescu et al., "Adjuvant imatinib mesylate after resection of localised, primary gastrointestinal stromal tumour: a randomised, double-blind, placebo-controlled trial," *The Lancet*, vol. 373, no. 9669, pp. 1097–1104, 2009.

26

Portomesenteric Vein Thrombosis, Bowel Gangrene, and Bilateral Pulmonary Artery Embolism Two Weeks after Laparoscopic Sleeve Gastrectomy

David G. Darcy, Ali H. Charafeddine, Jenny Choi, and Diego Camacho

Department of Surgery, Montefiore Medical Center, New York, NY 10467, USA

Correspondence should be addressed to David G. Darcy; ddarcy@montefiore.org

Academic Editor: Dimitrios Mantas

Sleeve gastrectomy and gastric bypass surgery are popular and effective options for weight loss surgery. Portomesenteric vein thrombosis (PMVT) is a documented but rare complication of bariatric surgery. Proper surgical technique, careful postoperative prophylaxis, and early mobilization are essential to prevent this event. The diagnosis of PMVT in the postoperative period requires a high index of suspicion and early directed intervention to prevent a possibly fatal outcome. We present a case of PMVT complicated by small bowel ischemia resulting in gangrene that necessitated resection.

1. Introduction

Sleeve gastrectomy has recently become a very popular weight loss surgery [1] and portomesenteric vein thrombosis (PMVT) is a rare but documented complication after this operation [2]. The diagnosis can be challenging, and early intervention is key in the management of these patients. The case we are reporting is a PMVT complicated by small bowel gangrene that necessitated resection and primary anastomosis. Further workup for hypercoagulable state was negative; a high index of suspicion for venous thrombosis in the surgical bariatric patient must be maintained at all times, including several weeks after operation.

2. Case Presentation

Our patient is a 55-year-old female with a body mass index (BMI) of 41.1, with multiple medical problems including coronary artery disease, diabetes mellitus, hypertension, and hyperlipidemia. She failed nonsurgical attempts at weight loss with diet and exercise and elected to undergo a laparoscopic sleeve gastrectomy (LSG).

The patient is placed on the operating room table in supine position with sequential compression devices (SCD) on both lower extremities. Subcutaneous heparin is given preoperatively as well as 2 grams of cefoxitin thirty minutes before incision time. The surgeon stands on the right side of the patient and the assistant on the left. The abdomen is insufflated with CO2 to achieve pneumoperitoneum at 15 mm Hg. A LigaSure device (Covidien, Dublin, Ireland) is used to dissect the greater curvature of the stomach starting 5 cm from the pylorus. A 34F bougie was introduced and placed along the lesser curvature. Gastric resection is performed with Tri-Staple (Covidien, Dublin, Ireland) devices using black and purple loads, directed towards the angle of His. The resected stomach is finally extracted by extending a 12 mm trocar incision in the supraumbilical midline by 2-3 cm. Operative time was 53 minutes.

In the postoperative period, the patient remained on subcutaneous heparin as chemical prophylaxis against deep vein thrombosis, and her SCD were on for the entire hospital stay. She tolerated a clear liquid diet on her first postoperative day and was ambulating with minimal pain. She was sent home on post-operative day (POD) #2. She was seen in the clinic a week after discharge and was doing well, free of pain, and tolerating her diet.

On POD #14 the patient presented to the ED with acute onset abdominal pain, nausea, and vomiting (nonbloody, nonbilious). Her vital signs were within normal limits, and

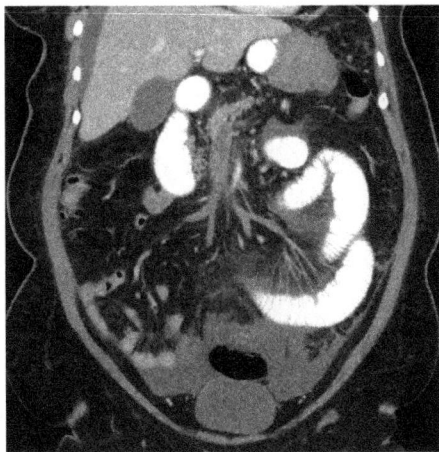

FIGURE 1: Coronal view with PO and IV contrast showing large portal venous thrombosis and dilated loops of small bowel in the left lower quadrant.

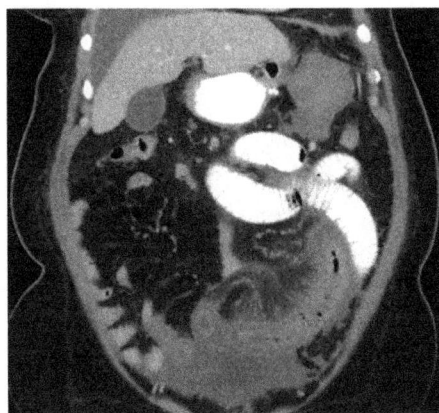

FIGURE 2: Coronal view with PO and IV contrast showing dilated loops of small bowel with wall thickening and pneumatosis denoting ischemia.

physical exam was significant for a soft abdomen, which was nondistended, with tenderness in the right upper quadrant. An abdominal ultrasound showed thickened small bowel loops. Her labs were significant for leukocytosis and acidosis, and her heart rate increased as she was in the emergency department. A decision was made to obtain a CT of the abdomen and pelvis with PO and IV contrast for further assessment. The CT showed extensive superior mesenteric vein thrombosis (Figure 1), nonocclusive thrombi within the splenic vein, right common iliac vein, and its external and internal iliac branches. Additionally, there were concerns for ischemia/necrosis over a long segment of small bowel (Figure 2).

A heparin drip was started immediately to treat the PMVT and the patient consented to an emergent exploratory laparotomy. On exploratory laparotomy, gangrenous bowel in the mid-jejunum was found and resected (43 cm) and bowel continuity was achieved with primary stapled anastomosis.

The sleeve gastrectomy staple line was examined and was intact.

The patient tolerated the surgery well; however she went into respiratory failure requiring intubation on POD #2. Despite being on a heparin drip at a therapeutic level, she developed bilateral pulmonary artery emboli. She improved clinically, and an IVC filter was placed on POD #5; she was extubated on POD #6, was started on the bariatric diet on POD #8 and warfarin on POD #9, and was eventually discharged home in good condition on warfarin. Her factor V Leiden and thrombophilia tests all came back negative. The patient returned to clinic 1 week after discharge; she was doing well, tolerating a bariatric diet without pain. She has been seen in hematology clinic at 1, 3, and 6 months after the readmission, doing well on warfarin. Hematology has suggested that she remain on lifelong anticoagulation for persistent portal thrombosis.

3. Discussion

The incidence of PMVT after LSG is reported at 1% [3], and following Roux-en-Y gastric bypass, the incidence is even lower [4]. The etiology of PMVT after LSG is still not clear. The classic Virchow triad explains that endothelial damage, stasis of venous blood, and a hypercoagulable state are the reasons behind formation of a thrombus. It has been suggested that induction of pneumoperitoneum is associated with decreased splanchnic circulation contributing to the formation of a clot; however, this operation does not require a higher pressure than others [5]. Morbid obesity and those patients with metabolic syndrome are at increased risk for clot formation, and morbidly obese patients are thought to have a baseline inflammatory state, further contributing to the formation of blood clots [6, 7]. It is our practice to send patients with BMI >60 home on prophylactic enoxaparin for two weeks, and they are seen in clinic at that time.

Although placement of IVC filter was considered early on, the patient was managed with heparin drip after her bowel resection and PMVT, given that filters themselves are thrombogenic. Deep venous thrombosis alone is not an indication for IVC filter placement when therapeutic heparin drip can be employed. The development of bilateral pulmonary embolism on treatment with therapeutic heparin prompted IVC filter placement.

Patients with PMVT after surgery present with a wide variety of symptoms [8]. Our patient had tenderness in the right upper quadrant and symptoms that could have been mistaken for acute cholecystitis, but her overall clinical picture was more consistent with bowel ischemia. As in our case, PMVT can lead to catastrophic outcomes including necrotic bowel, septic shock, and death. Although arterial insufficiency is a more common cause of bowel ischemia, the gangrene that developed in this patient was due to impaired venous outflow. Therefore, early diagnosis and intervention (anticoagulation and prompt surgical exploration if needed) are critical in saving this subset of patients with a highly morbid and possibly fatal complication.

References

[1] S. M. Han, W. W. Kim, and J. H. Oh, "Results of laparoscopic sleeve gastrectomy (LSG) at 1 year in morbidly obese Korean patients," *Obesity Surgery*, vol. 15, no. 10, pp. 1469–1475, 2005.

[2] P. Singh, M. Sharma, K. Gandhi, J. Nelson, and A. Kaul, "Acute mesenteric vein thrombosis after laparoscopic gastric sleeve surgery for morbid obesity," *Surgery for Obesity and Related Diseases*, vol. 6, no. 1, pp. 107–108, 2010.

[3] J. Salinas, D. Barros, N. Salgado et al., "Portomesenteric vein thrombosis after laparoscopic sleeve gastrectomy," *Surgical Endoscopy*, vol. 28, no. 4, pp. 1083–1089, 2014.

[4] D. E. Swartz and E. L. Felix, "Acute mesenteric venous thrombosis following laparoscopic Roux-en-Y gastric bypass," *Journal of the Society of Laparoendoscopic Surgeons*, vol. 8, no. 2, pp. 165–169, 2004.

[5] J. Jakimowicz, G. Stultiëns, and F. Smulders, "Laparoscopic insufflation of the abdomen reduces portal venous flow," *Surgical Endoscopy*, vol. 12, no. 2, pp. 129–132, 1998.

[6] A. W. James, C. Rabl, A. C. Westphalen, P. F. Fogarty, A. M. Posselt, and G. M. Campos, "Portomesenteric venous thrombosis after laparoscopic surgery: a systematic literature review," *Archives of Surgery*, vol. 144, no. 6, pp. 520–526, 2009.

[7] A. T. Rocha, Â. G. de Vasconcellos, E. R. da Luz Neto, D. M. A. Araújo, E. S. Alves, and A. A. Lopes, "Risk of venous thromboembolism and efficacy of thromboprophylaxis in hospitalized obese medical patients and in obese patients undergoing bariatric surgery," *Obesity Surgery*, vol. 16, no. 12, pp. 1645–1655, 2006.

[8] M. D. Morasch, J. L. Ebaugh, A. C. Chiou, J. S. Matsumura, W. H. Pearce, and J. S. T. Yao, "Mesenteric venous thrombosis: a changing clinical entity," *Journal of Vascular Surgery*, vol. 34, no. 4, pp. 680–684, 2001.

27

Carcinoma of the Colon in an Adult with Intestinal Malrotation

Michael Donaire, James Mariadason, Daniel Stephens,
Sitaram Pillarisetty, and Marc K. Wallack

Department of Surgery, Metropolitan Hospital, New York Medical College, USA

Correspondence should be addressed to Michael Donaire; m_donaire@hotmail.com

Academic Editors: T. Çolak, S.-i. Kosugi, and M. Picchio

Colon cancer is the third most common cancer in the USA. Intestinal malrotation diagnosed in adulthood was, until recently, a very rare phenomenon. While patients may present with intestinal obstruction or abdominal pain, the diagnosis is now often made as an incidental finding by computed tomography (CT). Surprisingly we found only seven case reports of carcinoma of the colon in patients with malrotation; CT failed to make the preoperative diagnosis in a majority. Laparoscopic colon surgery is rapidly becoming standard of care for colon cancer. We present a case of carcinoma of the colon in an adult that thwarted attempts at laparoscopic resection due to failure to recognize malrotation preoperatively. The literature is reviewed, and the implications of malrotation in patients with colon cancer are examined.

1. Introduction

Intestinal malrotation is a congenital anomaly that generally presents in the first month of life. Until a spate of recent reports, adult malrotation was considered extremely rare. Carcinoma of the colon, on the other hand, is the second most common cancer. Surprisingly reports of carcinoma of the colon in adults with malrotation are so rare that we found only 7 case reports in the literature. We present our case and discuss the implications.

2. Case Report

A 52-year-old male was admitted to an outside institution with lethargy, weight loss of 30 kg, and severe unexplained anemia (hemoglobin 4.5 g/dL; hematocrit 15%). The patient felt better after transfusion of 4 units of packed red blood cells, and gastroscopy performed at the time revealed a healed duodenal ulcer and erosive gastritis.

When he lost his medical insurance, he was discharged and advised to have further workup performed elsewhere. During a difficult colonoscopy at a charity clinic, a large tumor was found in his right colon that precluded passage of the scope to the cecum (see Figure 1). Biopsy confirmed an infiltrating adenocarcinoma. Polyps in the sigmoid and

transverse colon were also removed and found to be tubular adenomata. The patient was then referred to our institution, a safety-net hospital, where a CT scan was performed. The imaging demonstrated a 5 × 5 cm mass in the mesentery with spiculated calcifications, as well as an additional mass near the ileocecal valve that had the appearance of an intussusception (see Figure 2). Malrotation was not suspected, although later review of the imaging with a specialized CT radiologist demonstrated inversion of the normal SMA to SMV configuration (see Figure 3). Malrotation was not suspected. The liver was free of metastases. His past medical history included no prior surgery.

A laparoscopic right hemicolectomy was scheduled and commenced with introduction of a 10 mm optical trocar and two 5 mm ports. Upon entry, most of the small bowel was found plastered to the right flank, and the right colon was not visible. The left colon was visualized, but even after releasing adhesive bands holding the small bowel to the right side and mobilizing these loops to the left of midline, the ascending colon was not visible. It was decided that laparotomy was required to elucidate the findings. The abdomen was entered through a midline incision, and after mobilizing and packing off the small bowel to the left, the right paracolic gutter was found to be empty. The duodenojejunal junction, including the entirety of the duodenum, lays to the right of the vertebral

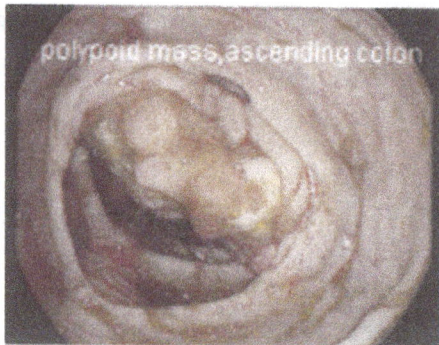

FIGURE 1: Right colon mass on colonoscopy.

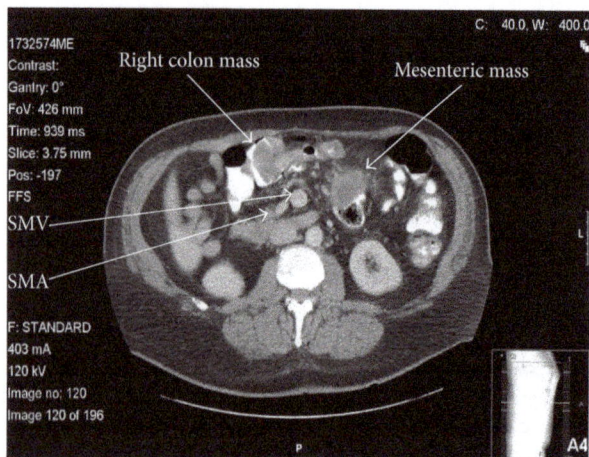

FIGURE 2: Right colon and mesenteric masses on CT.

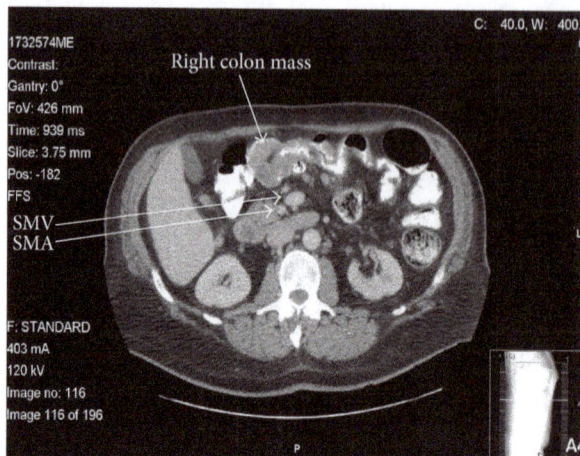

FIGURE 3: CT showing SMA dorsal to SMV.

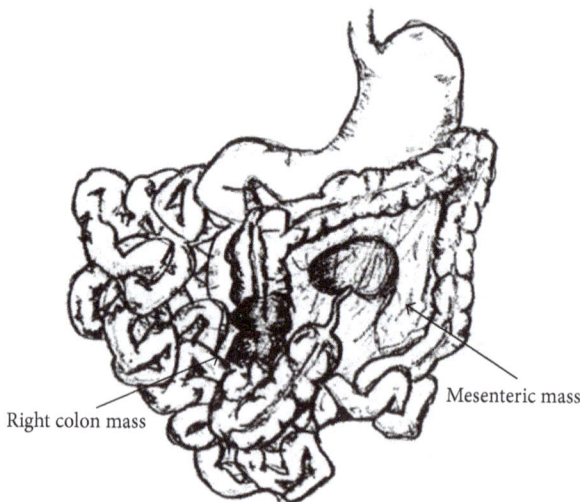

FIGURE 4: Depiction of intraoperative findings of malrotation and right colon and mesenteric masses.

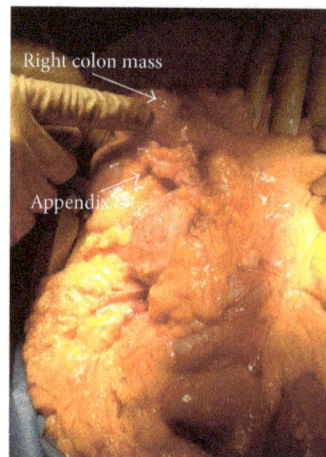

FIGURE 5: Intraoperative finding of right colon mass in setting of malrotation.

column. The right colon was tethered to the side wall of the abdomen on the right by long bands (Ladd's bands), which were eventually divided to obtain adequate mobilization. The cecum and appendix were found to occupy the left upper quadrant (see Figures 4 and 5). A tumor was palpated in the ascending colon, and a firm mass in the mesentery to its left was thought to be metastatic nodes. The superior mesenteric vessels appeared to have their usual orientation. The right colon was thereby mobilized beyond the left branch of the middle colic, and a right hemicolectomy was completed. The patient made an uneventful recovery.

Pathology revealed a 5 cm infiltrating adenocarcinoma of the ascending colon and metastatic tumor in the mesentery with no evidence of lymphatic tissue involvement. 23 lymph nodes removed were negative for metastases. The patient received chemotherapy and is doing well 12 months after surgery.

3. Discussion

Intestinal malrotation, a rare congenital disorder occurring in about 1 in 6,000 live births, results from incomplete rotation and fixation during fetal development. Rapid differential growth of the midgut, starting at gestational week five with herniation into the proximal portion of the umbilical cord, is normally followed by a 270-degree counterclockwise rotation around the superior mesenteric artery (SMA) as the intestine returns to the abdomen at week ten and fixes to the retroperitoneum [1]. Arrest of development anywhere along this process results in malrotation, which may be classified as reversed rotation, nonrotation, or varying degrees of rotation. In reversed rotation, there is an abnormal 90-degree clockwise rotation of the midgut with the cecum lying to the right of and dorsal to the SMA [2]. Nonrotation is the complete failure of midgut rotation around the SMA, whereby the duodenojejunal segment is ultimately confined to the right and the large intestine largely to the left hemi-abdomen. Our patient would seem to have had a form of nonrotation. Balthazar further classified malrotation based on involvement of duodenojejunal loops, ileocolic loops, or both [3].

Malrotation is diagnosed during the first month of life in 85–90% of cases; its presentation in adults, therefore, has traditionally been considered extremely rare. Symptomatology ranges from the asymptomatic to nebulous postprandial pain to complete obstruction, which compounds the difficulty in making the diagnosis and recognizing the true incidence of malrotation [4]. However, with increased use of advanced imaging, the diagnosis is being made more frequently in adults. A study of barium enemas on 2000 adults demonstrated a prevalence of 0.2% malrotation [5]. In a more recent report, however, 48% of 170 malrotation cases from a single institution were adults [6].

Colon cancer is statistically the third most common cancer in the U.S. It is therefore surprising that colon cancer occurring in adults with malrotation has not been reported more often. In a search of the literature, only 7 other cases of carcinoma of the colon in patients with malrotation were located [7–13]. None of the reported cases were from North America.

Even with the proliferative use of CT imaging, the diagnosis of malrotation in adults may be missed unless a high index of suspicion exists. The imaging modality of choice is the upper gastrointestinal series, which has a sensitivity of 80%. It may demonstrate an abnormal position of the duodenojejunal junction on the right side of the abdomen better than CT [14]. Ultrasonography may, furthermore, exhibit the reversal of normal superior mesenteric vessel orientation. The challenges in diagnosing appendicitis or volvulus in malrotation cases have also been well documented [7, 15]. CT scans are now the most frequently used modality for the diagnosis of malrotation. While the modality was employed in 4 of the 7 reported cases of colon carcinoma with adult malrotation, CT failed to demonstrate malrotation in 3 of 4 instances [8–11]. This mirrored our experience with the presented patient. Lymphatic mapping and angiography were used by 2 authors, which allowed for a preoperative diagnosis.

As in our patient, 5 of the 7 reported cases arose from the right colon. In this situation, right hemicolectomy obviates the need for a Ladd's procedure, but may need to be considered for left sided cancer. One case of laparoscopic right hemicolectomy for cecal carcinoma, concomitant with malrotation, was described recently [13]. When the finding is a surprise during planned laparoscopic right hemicolectomy,

failure to locate the right colon with the laparoscope may precipitate conversion to open surgery, as was our experience.

4. Conclusion

Carcinoma of the colon occurring in patients with adult malrotation is extremely rare with only a handful of cases reported. The preoperative recognition of malrotation would allow for better surgical planning and possible successful completion of a laparoscopic resection. Yet the preoperative diagnosis of malrotation has been relatively rare despite the use of CT. Greater awareness of the possibility of malrotation and use of contrast studies like upper gastrointestinal series and barium enemas may help to elucidate the diagnosis in some cases of colon cancer.

References

[1] L. Amaral, R. Quintanilha, L. Bernardo, T. Eloi, F. Bento, and V. Santos, "Intestinal malrotation in the elderly," *American Surgeon*, vol. 75, no. 7, pp. 631–633, 2009.

[2] E. T. Durkin, D. P. Lund, A. F. Shaaban, M. J. Schurr, and S. M. Weber, "Age-related differences in diagnosis and morbidity of intestinal malrotation," *Journal of the American College of Surgeons*, vol. 206, no. 4, pp. 658–663, 2008.

[3] E. J. Balthazar, "Intestinal malrotation in adults. Roentgenographic assessment with emphasis on isolated complete and partial nonrotations," *American Journal of Roentgenology*, vol. 126, no. 2, pp. 358–367, 1976.

[4] O. F. Emanuwa, A. A. Ayantunde, and T. W. Davies, "Midgut malrotation first presenting as acute bowel obstruction in adulthood: a case report and literature review," *World Journal of Emergency Surgery*, vol. 6, no. 1, article 22, 2011.

[5] J. L. Kantor, "Anomalies of the colon," *Radiology*, vol. 23, pp. 651–662, 1934.

[6] D. Nehra and A. M. Goldstein, "Intestinal malrotation: varied clinical presentation from infancy through adulthood," *Surgery*, vol. 149, no. 3, pp. 386–393, 2011.

[7] H. W. Gilbert, M. H. Thompson, and C. P. Armstrong, "The presentation of malrotation of the intestine in adults," *Annals of the Royal College of Surgeons of England*, vol. 72, no. 4, pp. 239–242, 1990.

[8] P.-T. Ren and B.-C. Lu, "Intestinal malrotation associated with colon cancer in an adult: report of a case," *Surgery Today*, vol. 39, no. 7, pp. 624–627, 2009.

[9] A. Brillantino, L. Marano, M. Schettino et al., "Report of a rare case of colon cancer complicated by anomalies of intestinal rotation and fixation: a case report," *Cases Journal*, vol. 2, no. 9, article 6555, 2009.

[10] H. Uchida, Y. J. Kawamura, K. Takegami et al., "Colon cancer complicated by vascular and intestinal anomaly," *Hepato-Gastroenterology*, vol. 51, no. 55, pp. 156–158, 2004.

[11] W. C. Torreggiani, F. Thornton, L. Lyburn, C. Brenner, and M. J. Lee, "Malrotation of the bowel resulting in a left-sided caecal carcinoma presenting as a palpable intrahernial mass," *Australasian Radiology*, vol. 45, no. 3, pp. 362–364, 2001.

[12] A. Michalopoulos, V. Papadopoulos, D. Paramythiotis et al., "Colonic cancer in a patient with intestinal malrotation: a case report," *Techniques in Coloproctology*, vol. 14, pp. S65–S66, 2010.

[13] M. Morimoto, H. Horie, H. Kumano, A. Lefor et al., "Reversed Intestinal malrotation with concurrent cecal carcinoma," *Asian Journal of Endoscopic Surgery*, vol. 5, no. 3, pp. 149–151, 2012.

[14] M. R. McVay, E. R. Kokoska, R. J. Jackson, and S. D. Smith, "The changing spectrum of intestinal malrotation: diagnosis and management," *American Journal of Surgery*, vol. 194, no. 6, pp. 712–719, 2007.

[15] T. Hanna and J. A. Akoh, "Acute presentation of intestinal malrotation in adults: a report of two cases," *Annals of the Royal College of Surgeons of England*, vol. 92, no. 7, pp. W15–W18, 2010.

28

Extragastrointestinal Stromal Tumor: A Differential Diagnosis of Compressive Upper Abdominal Tumor

Clara Kimie Miyahira [ID],[1] Miguel Bonfitto [ID],[2] Jéssyca Fernanda de Lima Farto,[1] Annelise de Figueiredo Calili,[1] Nathalia Rabello da Silva Sousa,[1] and Ana Paula de Figueiredo Calili[3]

[1]São José do Rio Preto Medical School, São José do Rio Preto, SP, Brazil
[2]Hospital de Base de São José do Rio Preto, São José do Rio Preto, SP, Brazil
[3]Marília Medical School, Marília, SP, Brazil

Correspondence should be addressed to Clara Kimie Miyahira; clara.kimie@gmail.com

Academic Editor: Christine Tunon-de-Lara

Introduction. Extragastrointestinal stromal tumors (EGIST) are rare mesenchymal tumor lesions located outside the gastrointestinal tract. A rare compressing tumor with difficult diagnosis is reported. *Presentation of the Case.* A male patient, 63 years old, was admitted in the emergency room complaining of stretching and continuous abdominal pain for one day. He took Hyoscine, with partial improvement of symptoms, but got worse due to hyporexia, and the abdominal pain persisted. The patient also reported early satiety and ten-pound weight loss over the last month. *Discussion.* EGIST could be assessed by CT-guided biopsy, leading to diagnosis and proper treatment with surgical resection or Imatinib. *Conclusion.* This case report highlights the importance of considering EGIST an important differential diagnosis of compressing upper abdominal tumors.

1. Introduction

Gastrointestinal stromal tumors (GIST) are rare lesions in the mesenchymal neoplasm, accounting for less than 1% of the primary neoplasias of the digestive tract. They may affect any segment of the gastrointestinal tract but can occur in other locations in only 10% of the cases, and, in these situations, they are called EGIST [1]. The diagnosis is hard and may be made through CT-guided puncture and immunohistochemical analysis of the biopsy.

There are three histological types: spindle (70%), epithelial (20%), and mixed-cell. In 95%, there is somatic mutation of CD117 (c-kit), and its discovery in the immunohistochemical characteristic defines the GIST [2]. Staging could be done with abdominal and pelvis tomography, MRI, or PET-CT [3].

A case of massive EGIST is reported to show a rare differential diagnosis of an upper abdominal tumor, emphasizing the proper treatment due to correct diagnosis.

2. Presentation of the Case

A male patient, 63 years old, was admitted in the emergency room complaining of stretching and continuous abdominal pain for one day. He took Hyoscine, with partial improvement of symptoms, but got worse due to hyporexia, and the abdominal pain persisted for a few hours after medication. The patient also reported early satiety and ten-pound weight loss over the last month.

He is a smoker for nearly fifty years. He has no other comorbidities, previous surgeries, nor family history. In the physical examination, the patient showed flat abdomen, pain on superficial palpation of the epigastrium, no rebound tenderness, and palpable mass approximately 12 cm wide in the left abdominal quadrant.

The laboratory assessment was normal. An acute abdominal radiography (Figure 1) was taken, showing elevated left hemidiaphragm. The abdominal tomography (Figure 2) showed a wide hypodense mass with necrosis

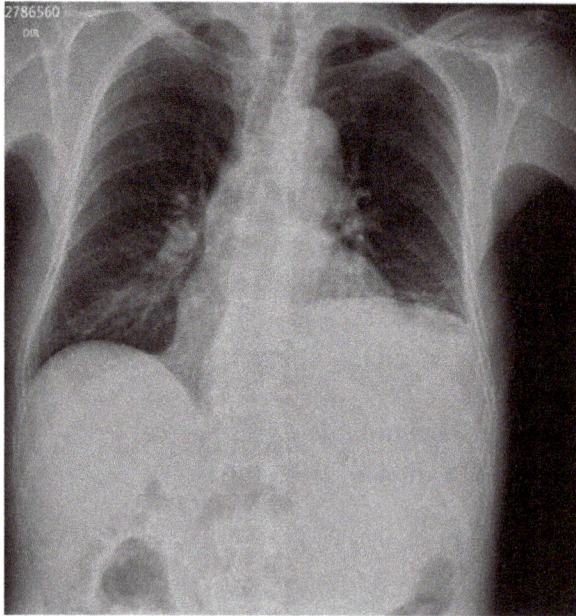

FIGURE 1: Acute abdominal X-ray showing the chest with elevated left hemidiaphragm.

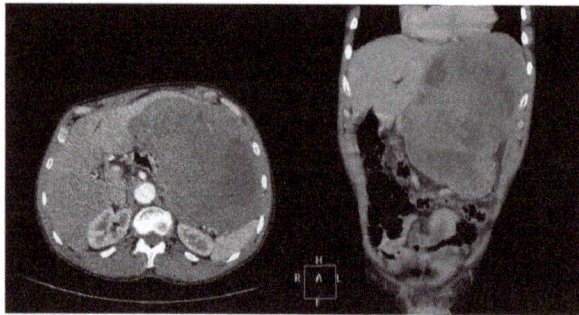

FIGURE 2: Contrast-enhanced computed tomography showing wide hypodense mass in the left hemiabdomen.

and heterogeneous absorption. The mass was posterior to the stomach and adjacent to the spleen and left kidney, without a cleavage plane between the left lobe of the liver and the pancreatic body, also compressing adjacent organs, invading the posterior wall of the stomach. The patient also underwent upper digestive endoscopy, showing bulging and gastric mucosal edema.

A CT-guided biopsy was taken, resulting in immunohistochemical analysis positive for C-Kit (Figure 3), CD34, and Ki67. These findings led to the correct diagnosis of extragastrointestinal stromal tumor (EGIST). The abdominal tomography was performed in the emergency room, also suggesting this type of tumor. The EGIST was a T4N0M0. As the tumor was greater than 2 cm and nonresectable, surgery was not suggested. The neoadjuvant therapy started with Imatinib, with weekly clinical follow-up.

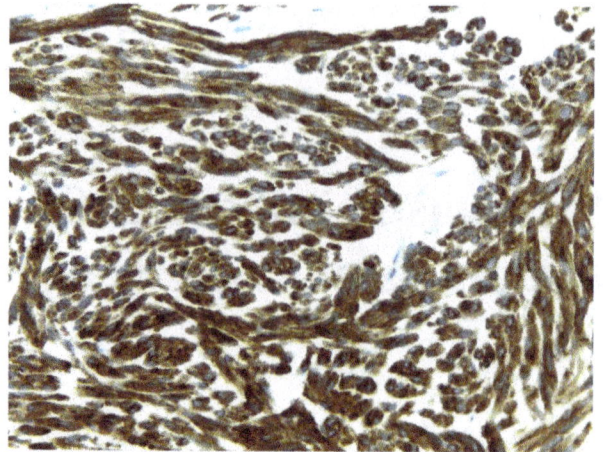

FIGURE 3: Immunohistochemical analysis positive for CD117 (C-kit) (original magnification 40x).

3. Discussion

The EGIST is a rare diagnosis regarding stromal tumors and can affect other locations in addition to the gastrointestinal tract, such as the omentum, pancreas, rectum, and small intestine. It is an important differential diagnosis of masses in the upper abdomen: leiomyoma, leiomyosarcoma, lipoma, schwannoma, carcinoids, and fibroids. CT-guided puncture or ultrasound may provide biopsy material. The immunohistochemical analysis with CD117 (C-Kit) confirms the diagnosis [4–6]. A recent study showed positive immunohistochemistry in 93.3% for CD117, 70% for CD34, and 10% for S1007. The biopsy result in this case report was positive for CD117, CD34, and Ki67.

Once the diagnosis is established, it is necessary to stage the tumor for better management [7]. The study patient was staged as T4N0M0 and nonresectable. The guidelines suggest that the first-line systemic treatment for advanced GIST cases is neoadjuvant therapy with Imatinib [3, 8, 9]. This treatment may result in 83–89% of patients responding or having the progression of the disease stabilized [8].

4. Conclusion

The EGIST should be noted as an important diagnosis of tumor masses, especially when symptomatic, such as masses in the upper abdomen. The correct diagnosis is very relevant, to the extent that it outlines the choice of clinical or surgical treatment.

Abbreviations

EGIST: Extragastrointestinal stromal tumors
GIST: Gastrointestinal stromal tumors.

Authors' Contributions

Clara Kimie Miyahira made substantial contributions to the conception and design, or data analysis and interpretation, involved in the preparation of the manuscript; Miguel Bonfitto made contributions to the data analysis and interpretation involved in the preparation of the manuscript or in the critical revision of important intellectual content; Jéssyca Fernanda de Lima Farto made substantial contributions to the design and preparation of the manuscript; Annelise de Figueiredo Calili made contributions in revising medical records and to the final revision of the case report; Nathalia Rabello da Silva Sousa was involved in the preparation of the manuscript and helped to translate the manuscript into the English language; and Ana Paula de Figueiredo Calili made contributions on data interpretation and complementary research. All authors read and approved the final manuscript.

Acknowledgments

The authors would like to thank the patient for the authorization and the employees that supported our work at the General Surgery Department.

References

[1] J. H. Yi, B.-B. Park, J. H. Kang et al., "Retrospective analysis of extra-gastrointestinal stromal tumors," *World Journal of Gastroenterology*, vol. 21, no. 6, pp. 1845–1850, 2005.

[2] D. M. Dorfman, M. M. Bui, R. R. Tubbs et al., "The CD117 immunohistochemistry tissue microarray survey for quality assurance and interlaboratory comparison - a College of American Pathologists Cell Markers Committee Study," *Archives of pathology & laboratory medicine*, vol. 130, no. 6, pp. 779–782, 2006.

[3] National Comprehensive Cancer Network, "Soft tissue sarcoma, version 2.2016, NCCN clinical practice guidelines in oncology," http://www.jnccn.org/content/14/6/758.full.

[4] M. Miettinen, W. El-Rifai, L. Sobin, and J. Lasota, "Evaluation of malignancy and prognosis of gastrointestinal stromal tumors: a review," *Human Pathology*, vol. 33, no. 5, pp. 478–483, 2002.

[5] Y. Shinomura, K. Kinoshita, S. Tsutsui, and S. Hirota, "Pathophysiology, diagnosis, and treatment of gastrointestinal stromal tumors," *Journal of Gastroenterology*, vol. 40, no. 8, pp. 775–780, 2005.

[6] P. Watal, S. G. Brahmbhatt, P. J. Thoriya, and N. U. Bahri, "Retroperitoneal extragastrointestinal stromal tumor: radiologic pathologic correlation," *Journal of Clinical Imaging Science*, vol. 4, no. 1, p. 34, 2014.

[7] N. Quezada, F. Acevedo, A. Marambio et al., "Complete pathological response to Imatinib mesylate in an extraintestinal gastrointestinal stromal tumor," *International Journal of Surgery Case Reports*, vol. 5, no. 10, pp. 681–685, 2014.

[8] H. Joensuu, P. Hohenberger, and C. L. Corless, "Gastrointestinal stromal tumour," *The Lancet*, vol. 382, no. 9896, pp. 973–983, 2013.

[9] B. P. Rubin, "Gastrointestinal stromal tumours: an update," *Histopathology*, vol. 48, no. 1, pp. 83–96, 2006.

29

Pneumatosis Intestinalis: Not Always a Surgical Indication

Haijing Zhang,[1] Stephanie L. Jun,[2] and Todd V. Brennan[1]

[1]Department of Surgery, Duke University Medical Center, Durham, NC 27710, USA
[2]Department of Radiology, University of California San Francisco, San Francisco, CA 94122, USA

Correspondence should be addressed to Todd V. Brennan, todd.brennan@duke.edu

Academic Editors: H. Kawai, G. Santori, M. Shimoda, and B. Tokar

We present a case of pneumatosis intestinalis (PI) of the colon in the setting of inflammatory bowel disease that was treated with medical management rather than emergent surgery. While the reflex response to extraluminal air in the abdomen is abdominal exploration, consideration of the clinical context in which PI is discovered and an understanding of a complete differential diagnosis of the sources of PI is critical to avoiding unnecessary surgery.

1. Introduction

Pneumatosis intestinalis (PI), also referred to as pneumatosis cystoides intestinalis, pneumatosis coli, and intestinal emphysema, is defined as the presence of extraluminal bowel gas that is confined within the bowel wall. The small intestine (42%) is most commonly involved followed by colon (36%), with involvement of both in 22% [1]. PI is an alarming radiological finding that usually prompts an emergent surgical consultation for concerns of bowel ischemia and impending bowel rupture. However, there is a wide spectrum of causes of PI ranging from the benign to the life-threatening. PI may be caused by bowel ischemia, mechanical trauma, inflammatory/autoimmune bowel disease, intestinal neoplasms, bowel infection, obstructive pulmonary disease, or drug-induced, including immunosuppression, therapy [1, 2]. Differentiating these causes is critical in directing an appropriate care plan. Complications are present in 3% of PI patients and include pneumoperitoneum, bowel obstruction, volvulus, intussusception, and hemorrhage [3]. Due to the risk of these emergent complications, suspected PI patients should be carefully evaluated for possible surgery. In a prospective review of patients with PI, bowel necrosis requiring surgery was predicted by 5 findings: an acute abdomen per history and physical, metabolic acidosis (pH < 7.3, HCO_3 < 20), elevated lactate, elevated serum amylase, and presence of portal venous gas [4]. For symptomatic PI

of mild-to-moderate severity, treatment of the underlying disease with administration of antibiotics, oxygen therapy, and elemental diet may be sufficient for PI resolution. Here we describe an elderly patient with benign PI in the setting of inflammatory bowel disease.

2. Case Presentation

A 60-year-old man was admitted for a flare of Crohn's disease, with pancolitis confirmed by colonoscopy with biopsy. He was discharged on oral prednisone, but was readmitted one week later for persistent abdominal pain, diarrhea, and a low-grade fever (38.1°C). A computed tomography (CT) scan of the abdomen on readmission showed thickening of the transverse, descending, and sigmoid colon. The right colon was normal at the time. After starting high-dose intravenous steroids (hydrocortisone 100 mg every 8 hours) and intravenous antibiotics (Cefazolin and Metronidazole), the patient defervesced and his symptoms improved. Two days later, a repeat CT performed for an elevated white blood cell count (18,000/uL) revealed extensive PI of the right colon (Figure 1(a)). Because his symptoms and physical exam findings were improving, the patient was treated with bowel rest and intravenous antibiotics while the steroids were tapered. After three days of close observation, a repeat CT scan demonstrated complete resolution of the PI

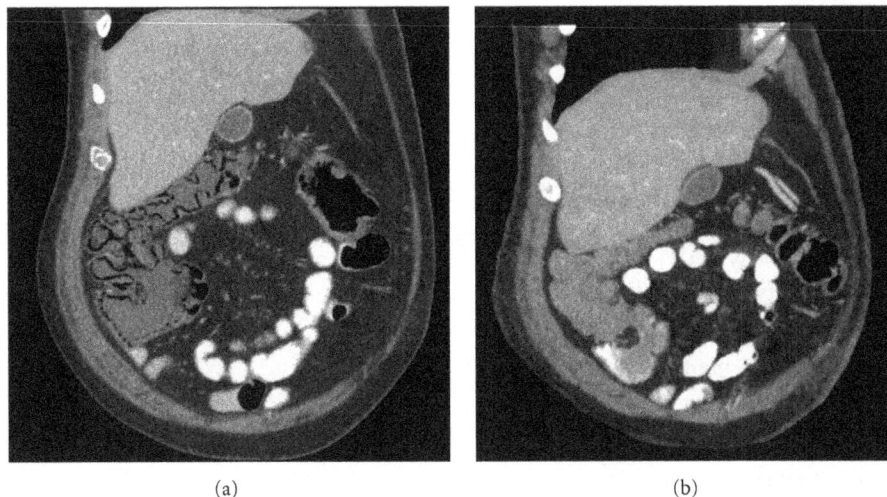

(a)

(b)

FIGURE 1: (a) CT scan of the abdomen 2 days following high-dose intravenous steroids shows extensive PI of right colon. Intramural gas tracking is visualized parallel to the bowel mucosa in the ascending and transverse colon. (b) Repeat CT scan after 3 days bowel rest and tapering of steroids and shows resolution of PI. No evidence of intramural gas along the colonic mucosa is seen.

(Figure 1(b)). The patient's symptoms resolved with medical management and he was discharged on maintenance oral prednisone.

3. Discussion

In PI, extraluminal gas predominantly localizes to the submucosal and subserosal planes of the small or large intestine, but can also localize to the muscularis propria [5]. While the pathophysiology of PI has been debated, it appears to be related to the breakdown of the mucosal and immunological barrier of the intestines, especially in the setting of increased intraluminal pressure. In our patient, the autoimmune inflammatory process of Crohn's disease and immunosuppression with high-dose steroid therapy likely contributed to PI etiology. Although the causality of high-dose corticosteroids in PI is not yet established, postulated mechanisms suggest that immunosuppression of antimicrobial defenses lead to intramural infection [6] and impairment of the intestinal wall barrier [7]. Our patient's prior colonoscopy with biopsy can be a contributing factor to developing PI as well, as recent biopsy increases risk of gas dissection into submucosa by compromising colonic mucosal integrity [8]. Based on a PubMed search, only 4 case reports [9–12] in English journals of PI associated with Crohn's disease have been presented in the past 10 years, with supportive therapy and nonsurgical resolution achieved in at least 3 of 4 cases [10–12].

Most cases of PI are asymptomatic [13] such that the diagnosis of PI may be an incidental radiographic or endoscopic finding. Patients with PI may also present only with symptoms of the underlying disease. The location of PI within the gastrointestinal tract can dictate the associated symptoms. Patients with small intestine PI most frequently present with vomiting (60%), abdominal distension (59%), weight loss (55%), and abdominal discomfort

(53%). Patients with colonic PI most commonly present with symptoms of diarrhea (56%), hematochezia (50%), abdominal discomfort (32%), and abdominal distension (28%) [14]. While multiple imaging modalities are capable of detecting PI, CT scan with or without intravenous contrast is more sensitive than plain film, MRI, or ultrasound in diagnosing and characterizing the extent of PI [15]. The radiological characteristics of PI on CT are intramural gas tracking parallel to the bowel mucosa as shown (Figure 1(a)). A review of 44 pediatric PI cases showed that additional CT features may distinguish between emergent and mild PI; these CT findings include thickening of bowel wall, free peritoneal fluid, extent of PI, and soft tissue stranding of peri-intestinal tissues [16]. Though not seen in this patient, gas in the portal and mesenteric veins is a poor prognostic factor [17], and is more frequently associated with ischemic bowel, especially in pediatric patients in the setting of acute necrotizing enterocolitis [4]. Signs of bowel ischemia, bowel necrosis, and bowel perforation resulting in intraperitoneal air indicate an emergent setting in which surgery may be appropriate. Other complications of PI such as bowel obstruction may indicate surgical intervention or endoscopic puncture and sclerotherapy of the cysts [18]. However, as in this case, PI patients with cardiovascular stability and an unimpressive abdominal exam may be closely observed and treated with bowel rest and antibiotics.

4. Conclusion

Overall, PI is a rare radiological finding and one that occurs in wide spectrum of clinical disorders. In the setting of the acute abdomen with coexisting systemic sepsis, necrotic bowel must be suspected and emergent operative management pursued. However, in the setting of a nonacute abdomen and a stable patient, benign causes of PI need to be considered in the differential diagnosis. As illustrated by the presented case, the radiological finding of PI is not always an indication for surgery and may be treated with medical therapy alone in many clinical circumstances.

References

[1] C. Braumann, C. Menenakos, and C. A. Jacobi, "Pneumatosis intestinalis—a pitfall for surgeons?" *Scandinavian Journal of Surgery*, vol. 94, no. 1, pp. 47–50, 2005.

[2] L. M. Ho, E. K. Paulson, and W. M. Thompson, "Pneumatosis intestinal is in the adult: benign to life-threatening causes," *American Journal of Roentgenology*, vol. 188, no. 6, pp. 1604–1613, 2007.

[3] S. Galandiuk and V. W. Fazio, "Pneumatosis cystoides intestinalis: a review of the literature," *Diseases of the Colon and Rectum*, vol. 29, no. 5, pp. 358–363, 1986.

[4] S. J. Knechtle, A. M. Davidoff, and R. P. Rice, "Pneumatosis intestinalis. Surgical management and clinical outcome," *Annals of Surgery*, vol. 212, no. 2, pp. 160–165, 1990.

[5] A. Koreishi, G. Y. Lauwers, and J. Misdraji, "Pneumatosis intestinalis: a challenging biopsy diagnosis," *American Journal of Surgical Pathology*, vol. 31, no. 10, pp. 1469–1475, 2007.

[6] A. John, K. Dickey, J. Fenwick, B. Sussman, and W. Beeken, "Pneumatosis intestinalis in patients with Crohn's disease," *Digestive Diseases and Sciences*, vol. 37, no. 6, pp. 813–817, 1992.

[7] Y. Shimojima, W. Ishii, M. Matsuda, K. Tojo, R. Watanabe, and S. I. Ikeda, "Pneumatosis cystoides intestinalis in neuropsychiatric systemic lupus erythematosus with diabetes mellitus: case report and literature review," *Modern Rheumatology*, vol. 21, no. 4, pp. 415–419, 2011.

[8] M. A. Meyers, G. G. Ghahremani, J. L. Clements Jr., and K. Goodman, "Pneumatosis intestinalis," *Gastrointestinal Radiology*, vol. 2, no. 2, pp. 91–105, 1977.

[9] V. Arena, I. Pennaccia, L. Abenavoli et al., "... And suddenly a tree!," *International Journal of Surgical Pathology*, vol. 19, no. 6, p. 776, 2011.

[10] A. Breitinger, R. Kozarek, and E. Hauptman, "Pneumatosis cystoides intestinalis in Crohn's disease," *Gastrointestinal Endoscopy*, vol. 57, no. 2, p. 241, 2003.

[11] J. Hwang, V. S. Reddy, and K. W. Sharp, "Pneumatosis cystoides intestinalis with free intraperitoneal air: a case report," *American Surgeon*, vol. 69, no. 4, pp. 346–349, 2003.

[12] D. Gelfond, S. S. Blanchard, and A. Malkani, "Pneumatosis intestinalis: a rare presentation of Crohn disease exacerbation," *Journal of Pediatric Gastroenterology and Nutrition*, vol. 52, no. 2, pp. 225–226, 2011.

[13] Y. Heng, M. D. Schuffler, R. C. Haggitt, and C. A. Rohrmann, "Pneumatosis intestinalis: a review," *American Journal of Gastroenterology*, vol. 90, no. 10, pp. 1747–1758, 1995.

[14] J. Jamart, "Pneumatosis cystoides intestinalis. A statistical study of 919 cases," *Acta Hepato-Gastroenterologica*, vol. 26, no. 5, pp. 419–422, 1979.

[15] B. L. Pear, "Pneumatosis intestinalis: a review," *Radiology*, vol. 207, no. 1, pp. 13–20, 1998.

[16] D. E. Olson, Y. W. Kim, J. Ying, and L. F. Donnelly, "CT predictors for differentiating benign and clinically worrisome pneumatosis intestinalis in children beyond the neonatal period," *Radiology*, vol. 253, no. 2, pp. 513–519, 2009.

[17] S. W. Nelson, "Extraluminal gas collections due to diseases of the gastrointestinal tract," *The American Journal of Roentgenology*, vol. 115, no. 2, pp. 225–248, 1972.

[18] K. Johansson and E. Lindstrom, "Treatment of obstructive pneumatosis coli with endoscopic sclerotherapy: report of a case," *Diseases of the Colon and Rectum*, vol. 34, no. 1, pp. 94–96, 1991.

30

Sentinel Bleeding as a Sign of Gastroaortic Fistula Formation after Oesophageal Surgery

M. Uittenbogaart, M. N. Sosef, and J. van Bastelaar

Department of Surgery, Atrium Medical Centre, Henri Dunantstraat 5, 6419 PC Heerlen, The Netherlands

Correspondence should be addressed to J. van Bastelaar; j.v.bastelaar@atriummc.nl

Academic Editor: Oded Olsha

Gastroaortic fistula formation is a very rare complication following oesophageal resection and, in most cases, leads to sudden death. We report the case of a 65-year-old male with an adenocarcinoma of the oesophagus who underwent neoadjuvant chemoradiation followed by a minimally invasive transthoracic oesophagectomy with gastric tube reconstruction and intrathoracic anastomosis. After an uneventful postoperative course and hospital discharge, the patient reported blood regurgitation on postoperative day 23. Endoscopy revealed an adherent blood clot on the oesophageal wall, which after dislocation caused exsanguination. Autopsy determined the cause of death being massive haemorrhage due to a gastroaortic fistula. The sudden onset of haemorrhage makes this condition particularly difficult to treat. Recognition of warning signs such as thoracic or epigastric pain, regurgitation of blood, or the passing of bloody stools or melena is crucial in the early detection of fistula and may improve patient outcome.

1. Introduction

The development of an aortic fistula after oesophagectomy is a life threatening condition mostly due to its lethal nature even when diagnosed at an early stage. This rare complication generally occurs 2-3 weeks after oesophagectomy [1] and often forces surgeons to perform emergency salvage surgery in order to prevent exsanguination. However, in most cases, this diagnosis only becomes apparent at postmortem examination of patients after sudden, unexplained death has occurred [2].

We report a case in which there was in fact a small sentinel or herald bleed, as a prelude to massive exsanguination. Early recognition of a sentinel bleed may be essential to improve patient outcome.

2. Case Presentation

A 65-year-old male presented to our outpatient clinic with a three-week history of dysphagia and weight loss. Workup revealed an eT3N3M0 adenocarcinoma of the lower third of the oesophagus. The patient was treated with neoadjuvant chemoradiation, consisting of a five-week course of carbo-platin/paclitaxel combined with radiotherapy consisting of

23 fractions of 1.8 Gy, 41.4 Gy in total. Following neoadjuvant therapy a minimally invasive transthoracic oesophagectomy was performed with gastric tube reconstruction with an intrathoracic end-to-side circular stapled anastomosis according to the Ivor-Lewis technique. The postoperative course was uneventful and a postoperative contrast swallow on postoperative day 7 showed no sign of anastomotic leak. The patient was discharged in good condition on the 13th postoperative day.

Histological examination of the resection specimen showed a significant response to the neoadjuvant chemoradiation (tumor regression grade 2 according to Mandard) with a small residual adenocarcinoma invading the submucosa and 11 negative lymph nodes (ypT1N0).

Ten days after hospital discharge, the patient reported regurgitation of small amounts of blood and mild dysphagia. Dietary intake was reduced to fluids only and the patient was scheduled for endoscopy the following day.

Endoscopy of the upper oesophagus and gastric tube showed an intact anastomosis with an adherent blood clot. Dislocation of the clot revealed an uncontrollable massive arterial bleeding and caused severe haemorrhagic shock. Despite endoscopic attempts to control the bleeding and administered advanced life support, the patient succumbed due to exsanguination in the endoscopy suite.

Postmortem examination revealed a 1.5 centimetre diameter dehiscence at the level of the intrathoracic anastomosis with a closely adherent aortic wall, revealing a gastroaortic fistula at the level of the intrathoracic anastomosis without signs of aneurysmal widening of the aortic diameter. The gastrointestinal tract was full of blood, supporting the cause of death being exsanguination due to the gastroaortic fistula. No signs of residual malignancy were found during examination.

3. Discussion

Formation of fistulae between the aorta and the gastric tube after oesophagectomy is a very rare phenomenon. The first report of the occurrence of an aortoesophageal fistula was by Dubrueil [3] in 1818, reporting a case of a perforation of the aorta due to ingestion of an avian bone. Ingestion of foreign bodies, most commonly animal bones or dentures, is thought to cause mediastinitis due to pressure necrosis and perforation of the oesophagus, eventually leading to aortitis and fistula formation [4].

3.1. Possible Causes of Gastroaortic Fistula. Our case describes a fistula secondary to oesophageal surgery, but in general, aetiology of secondary fistula is diverse, including foreign body perforation, peptic ulceration of the gastric tube, and anastomotic leakage [5]. Most commonly, fistulae are caused by aneurysms of the descending aorta, rupturing into the adjacent oesophagus and thereby causing a fistula between the aorta and the oesophagus [6]. Expansion of the aneurysm increases wall tension, damaging the vasa vasorum of the aorta and thereby gradually weakening the aortic wall. This is thought to cause necrosis of the oesophagus due to the pressure applied on the oesophageal wall. Perforation of the oesophageal wall subsequently causes adherence and inflammation of the aortic wall, resulting in fistula formation [2].

3.1.1. Surgery: Oesophageal Resection and Intrathoracic Stapled Anastomosis. Previous reports have suggested that the degree and method of dissection might predispose for aortic erosion [1]. However, if the cause of massive exsanguination was iatrogenic injury to the vascular wall, one would expect symptoms of blood loss to occur within hours after surgery. In this case, the patient developed symptoms after discharge from the hospital, thus making iatrogenic injury to the vascular wall unlikely the underlying cause of bleeding.

Another possibility is the presence of continuous contact pressure between the linear staples at the level of the anastomosis and the aortic wall causing an erosion of the aorta and eventually resulting in gastroaortic fistula. This mechanism has been previously described as being responsible for formation of tracheogastric fistulae [7]. Thus far there are 23 reports of aortoesophageal fistulae as a complication of oesophagectomy [1]. Up to 60% of patients with a postsurgical gastroaortic fistula develop bleeding between the 9th and 21th days after surgery; 82% occurs between the 2nd and 6th weeks [1].

3.1.2. Neoadjuvant Radiotherapy. The contribution of neoadjuvant therapy to the formation of fistula is to be considered. Our patient was treated with a five-week course of carboplatin/paclitaxel combined with radiation therapy consisting of 23 fractions of 1.8 Gy (total 41.4 Gy). As shown in Figure 1, along with the oesophagus, the anterior wall of the descending aorta is embedded in the radiation field. It is possible that radiation caused relative ischemia of the oesophagus causing partial destruction of the mucosal barrier. Histological studies have shown that mainly the submucosal layer is affected by the radiation, resulting in teleangiectasia, fibrosis, and neovascularization [8]. Besides causing damage to the epithelium of the intestinal tract, damage to the arterial wall could be expected following radiotherapy. Previous reports have shown the possibility of aortic rupture due to subclinical perivascular infection following radiation therapy [9].

Although this phenomenon is mostly observed six months to five years after radiation therapy [10], it is possible that radiation might contribute to formation of fistulae. Retrospective studies in patients who developed aortaduodenal fistulae and who underwent radiation therapy prior due to malignancy showed that radiation dosis starting at 50 to 60 Gy was associated with chronic intestinal radiation damage and formation of fistula [11].

3.2. Diagnosis. The sudden onset of haemorrhage makes this condition particularly difficult to treat. Recognition of warning signs such as thoracic or epigastric pain, regurgitation of blood, or passing of bloody stools or melena is crucial in the early detection of fistula and may improve patient outcome.

Our patient reported dysphagia and regurgitation of blood, in retrospect being the first sign of the underlying pathology. This type of sentinel bleeding has been reported in other types of gastrointestinal surgery, such as pylorus preserving pancreaticoduodenectomy and classic Whipple surgery [12]. Sentinel bleeding as a prelude of an aortoesophageal fistula was first described in the nineteenth century by Chiari-Strassburgh [13], wherein he reported a triad of midthoracic pain or dysphagia, followed by a herald bleed and finally massive hematemesis after a lucid interval. The herald bleed presents mostly 2 to 6 weeks after surgery and the subsequent asymptomatic interval may vary from 30 minutes to 3 days [1]. This symptom-free window of opportunity might be explained by activation of the coagulation cascade due to erosion of the aortic wall, resulting in clot formation, which functions as a plug in the defect. Corrosion by the gastrointestinal contents or even bacterial activity might weaken the clot, as such causing the catastrophic bleed [1].

Although early recognition of this sequence of events seems essential in order to maximize the survival, there is no apparent consensus on the optimal diagnostic strategy. Endoscopy of the upper gastrointestinal tract might aid in the detection of fistula. Endoscopic findings may be directly due to visualization of pulsatile blood into the oesophagus or a pulsatile adherent blood clot. More subtle findings during endoscopy might point in direction of a fistula, such as submucosal hematoma shown as a blue-gray discoloration of the oesophageal wall [5]. However, the sensitivity of detection of fistulae via endoscopy is a mere 38% [14]; therefore

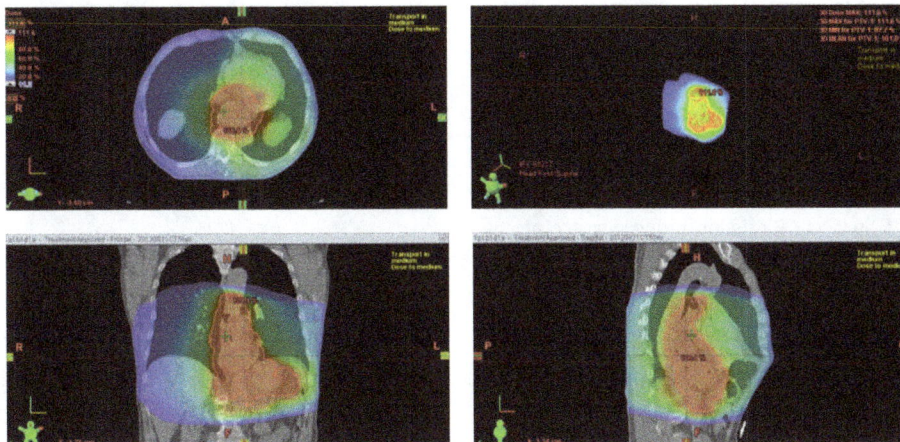

FIGURE 1: Images of radiation field showing embedding of the anterior wall of the descending aorta and of the oesophagus.

endoscopy might be of more use to exclude other common causes of upper gastrointestinal bleeding, such as Mallory-Weiss lesions and peptic ulcers [1]. Arterial contrast studies, such as aortography or even computed tomography scans with arterial contrast, are potentially useful in the detection of fistula, but during the symptom-free interval radiological evidence of the fistula may be absent due to the transient clot formation [15].

3.3. Treatment. The literature reports twenty-three cases of gastroaortic fistula following oesophageal surgery, all but three reporting a fatal outcome despite surgical efforts [1]. The main problem is the delay in diagnosis resulting in a limited time frame in which salvage surgery can be performed; the majority of patients will perish before reaching the operating theatre. Therefore the solution has to be sought in temporary measures to prolong the interval between diagnosis and exsanguination. Use of the Sengstaken-Blakemore tube was first described in 1966 as being a successful as a bridge to definite surgical repair [16], but the much disputed pressure necrosis of the oesophageal wall [17] has caused this device to become obsolete. With the ongoing advancements in endovascular as well as endoscopic techniques, stenting the aorta or even oesophagus might be helpful in case of haemorrhagic shock, functioning as a bridge to definitive and major surgical repair [18].

4. Conclusion

Patients reporting regurgitation of blood or hematemesis following an oesophagectomy should raise suspicion of a gastroaortic fistula. This sentinel or herald bleed should prompt us to actively "seek the leak." It is essential to recognise the lucid interval between the sentinel bleed and the massive hematemesis and utilize it to rapidly confirm diagnosis and create a treatment plan. Depending on the extent of the bleeding, we would advise to start with a computed tomography scan with arterial contrast to visualise the origin of the bleeding and determine the best surgical approach, either endovascular, endoscopic, or invasive salvage surgery. In case of an inconclusive scan, a subsequent endoscopy of

the upper gastrointestinal tract might confirm the suspicion. However, despite early diagnosis and extensive surgical effort, reported patient outcome is poor.

Learning Points

(i) Regurgitation of blood or hematemesis should be recognised as a possible sentinel bleed due to a gastroaortic fistula. (ii) Sentinel or herald bleed after oesophagectomy should prompt us to actively "seek the leak" and treat it. (iii) Computed tomography scanning with arterial contrast or endoscopy of the upper gastrointestinal tract should be used to confirm diagnosis. (iv) Despite early diagnosis and surgical effort, patient outcome is poor.

References

[1] C. Molina-Navarro, S. W. Hosking, S. J. Hayward, and A. D. S. Flowerdew, "Gastroaortic fistula as an early complication of esophagectomy," *The Annals of Thoracic Surgery*, vol. 72, no. 5, pp. 1783–1788, 2001.

[2] R. W. Byard, "Lethal aorto-oesophageal fistula—characteristic features and aetiology," *Journal of Forensic and Legal Medicine*, vol. 20, no. 3, pp. 164–168, 2013.

[3] Dubrueil, "Observations sur la perforation de l'oesophage et de l'aortethoracique par une potion d'os avale: avec des reflexions," *J Univ Sci Med*, vol. 9, pp. 357–365, 1818.

[4] S. Amin, J. Luketich, and A. Wald, "Aortoesophageal fistula: case report and review of the literature," *Digestive Diseases and Sciences*, vol. 43, no. 8, pp. 1665–1671, 1998.

[5] R. L. Heckstall and J. E. Hollander, "Aortoesophageal fistula: recognition and diagnosis in the emergency department," *Annals of Emergency Medicine*, vol. 32, no. 4, pp. 502–505, 1998.

[6] J. E. Hollander and G. Quick, "Aortoesophageal fistula: a comprehensive review of the literature," *The American Journal of Medicine*, vol. 91, no. 3, pp. 279–287, 1991.

[7] Y. Y. Chen, J. M. Chang, and W. W. Lai, "Tracheo-neo-esophageal fistula caused by exposed metallic staples erosion," *Annals of Thoracic Surgery*, vol. 94, no. 4, pp. 1375–1376, 2012.

[8] O. Drognitz, J. Pfeiffenberger, and W. Schareck, "Primäre aorto-duodenale Fistel als Spätkomplikation nach paraaortaler Radiatio Ein Fallbericht," *Der Chirurg*, vol. 73, no. 6, pp. 633–637, 2002.

[9] R. A. McCready, G. L. Hyde, B. A. Bivins, S. S. Mattingly, and W. O. Griffen Jr., "Radiation-induced arterial injuries," *Surgery*, vol. 93, no. 2, pp. 306–312, 1983.

[10] R. B. Galland and J. Spencer, "Radiation-induced gastrointestinal fistulae," *Annals of the Royal College of Surgeons of England*, vol. 68, no. 1, pp. 5–7, 1986.

[11] M. Berthrong and L. F. Fajardo, "Radiation injury in surgical pathology. Part II. Alimentary tract," *The American Journal of Surgical Pathology*, vol. 5, no. 2, pp. 153–178, 1981.

[12] E. F. Yekebas, L. Wolfram, G. Cataldegirmen et al., "Postpancreatectomy hemorrhage: diagnosis and treatment—an analysis in 1669 consecutive pancreatic resections," *Annals of Surgery*, vol. 246, no. 2, pp. 269–280, 2007.

[13] H. Chiari-Strassburgh, "Injury of the esophagus with perforation of the aorta produced by a foreign body (Ueber Fremdkorperverletzung des Oesophagus mit Aortenperforation)," *Berliner klinische Wochenschrift*, vol. 51, pp. 7–9, 1914.

[14] G. D. Perdue, R. B. Smith, J. D. Ansley, and M. J. Costantino, "Impending aortoenteric hemorrhage: the effect of early recognition on improved outcome," *Annals of Surgery*, vol. 192, no. 3, pp. 237–243, 1980.

[15] F. I. Khawaja and M. K. Varindani, "Aortoesophageal fistula: review of clinical, radiographic, and endoscopic features," *Journal of Clinical Gastroenterology*, vol. 9, no. 3, pp. 342–344, 1987.

[16] E. J. Valtonen and A. Koivuniemi, "Aortoesophageal fistula complicating carcinoma of the esophagus. Report of observations in two cases," *Journal of Thoracic and Cardiovascular Surgery*, vol. 53, no. 3, pp. 448–452, 1967.

[17] P. Vlavianos, A. E. S. Gimson, D. Westaby, and R. Williams, "Balloon tamponade in variceal bleeding: use and misuse," *British Medical Journal*, vol. 298, no. 6681, article 1158, 1989.

[18] Y. Okita, K. Yamanaka, K. Okada et al., "Strategies for the treatment of aorto-esophageal fistula," *European Journal Cardio-Thoracic Surgery*, vol. 46, no. 5, pp. 894–900, 2014.

31

Removal of Eroded Gastric Bands using a Transgastric SILS Device

C. Spitali, K. De Vogelaere, and G. Delvaux

UZ Brussel, Brussels 1090, Belgium

Correspondence should be addressed to C. Spitali; carmelaspitali@hotmail.com

Academic Editors: A. Cho, B. Kirshtein, and G. Rallis

Background. Laparoscopic adjustable gastric banding (LAGB) is a popular method for the treatment of morbid obesity. One of the most feared complications is gastric band erosion which occurs with a reported incidence of 0.3 to 14%. Intragastric migrated bands are best managed by endoscopic removal. Recent case studies reported successful endoscopic removal of intragastric migrated bands, but it is not always possible. We report our first experience with a transgastric removal of eroded bands using a Single Incision Laparoscopic Surgery (SILS) device. *Methods*. A patient who underwent gastric banding in the past (2007) presented with symptoms of epigastric pain and weight gain. Preoperative gastroscopy revealed stomach wall erosion with the gastric band partially (2/3) migrated into the gastric lumen. Attempts to remove the band by endoscopy were not successful. A laparoscopy was performed and multiple adhesions with evidence of inflammation was seen in the upper abdomen around the band. A SILS port was inserted through a 2 cm incision in the left hypochondrium with the internal ring of the port placed into the stomach through a small anterior gastrotomy. The band was cut in the stomach and removed. The anterior gastrotomy was closed. We had a perfect intragastric view of the gastric banding. *Results*. There were no intra- or postoperative complications. The patient was discharged on the fifth postoperative day on a gastric adapted diet. *Conclusion*. Removal of a gastric band after gastric erosion by SILS is feasible, safe, and effective. This is the first reported case of transgastric removal of eroded bands using an SILS device.

1. Introduction

Laparoscopic adjustable gastric banding (LAGB) is an effective treatment for morbid obesity.

One of the most serious complications associated with LAGB is intragastric band migration or band erosion through the stomach wall.

The best management of band erosion is unclear in the current published literature.

We present a case of gastric band erosion 4 years after placement.

We removed the band using an SILS device placed transgastrically.

2. Case Report

A 31-year-old female underwent laparoscopic gastric banding for morbid obesity 4 years ago.

A Lap band (Bio Entererics) was placed laparoscopically utilizing the pars flacida technique. Preoperatively there were no problems. The patient recovered well and was discharged one day after the intervention.

One year following the procedure, the patient presented to the emergency room with abdominal pain.

A abdominal CT scan was negative for leak or free air, but showed an inflammation around the port.

The band was deflated and the patient was admitted for observation. The patient recovered well and was discharged after 4 days.

The band was adjusted with saline several times, without any problem.

Four years following the procedure, the patient presented to our consultation with symptoms of epigastric pain and weight gain.

A UGI contrast study showed a slippage of the band.

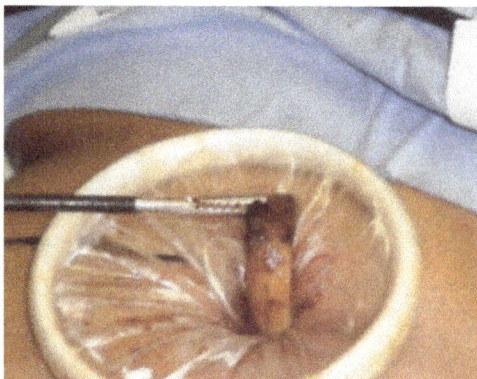

FIGURE 1: Endoscopy revealed stomach wall erosion with the gastric band partially (2/3) migrated into the gastric lumen.

Endoscopy revealed stomach wall erosion with the gastric band partially (2/3) migrated into the gastric lumen (Figure 1).

We decided to remove the eroded band.

The procedure was performed in the operating room with the patient under general anesthesia with endotracheal intubation.

Peroperative a gastroscopy was performed. Removal of the band by endoscopy was impossible because the band could not be cut with the material available for endoscopy.

A laparoscopy was performed and multiple adhesions with evidence of inflammation were seen in the upper abdomen around the band. There was no visualisation of the band.

A 2 cm skin incision was made at the left hypochondrium. The stomach was grasped at the anterior site with straight forward instruments and brought outside the abdomen (Figure 2). The stomach was opened at the anterior site and the edge of the stomach was sutured at the edge of the skin with interrupted stiches. The internal ring of the SILS port (Allergan) was placed into the stomach, while the external ring was outside. Insufflation was started at 15 mmHg. We had a perfect view of the internal site of the stomach.

A standard 10 mm laparoscope was used for visualization and two 5 mm straight forward working instruments were inserted through the SILS port.

The band was cut in the stomach with scissors and removed (Figure 3).

The SILS port was removed and the supporting stiches of the stomach were removed. The anterior gastrotomy was closed outside with a running suture of PDS 3.0 (Ehicon). The stomach was pulled back into the abdomen.

Methylene blue and air tests were performed during the operation to rule out leaks, and they were negative.

A Blake drain 19Fr (Ethicon) was placed near the gastrotomy.

A nasogastric tube was also left in place postoperatively.

The operation time was 60 minutes. There was no blood loss.

There were no intra- or postoperative complications.

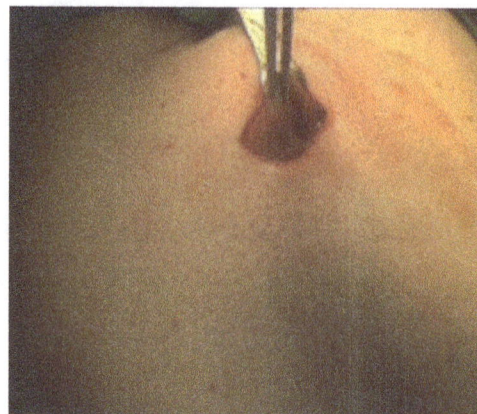

FIGURE 2: Stomach was grasped at the anterior site and brought outside the abdomen.

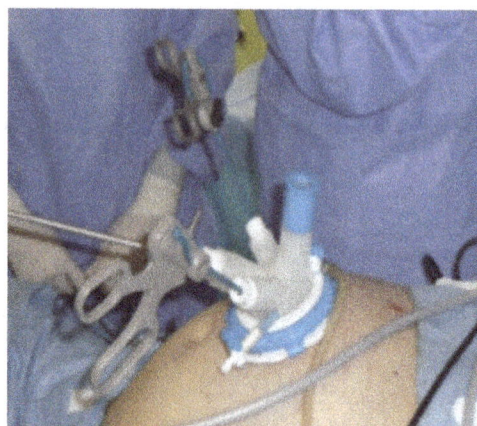

FIGURE 3: The band was cut in the stomach with scissors and removed.

The nasogastric tube and drain were removed on postoperative day 2 and the patient resumed oral dieting beginning by liquids.

The patient was discharged from the hospital on postoperative day 5.

At the postoperative control no complications were seen after 1 month.

3. Discussion

Laparoscopic adjustable gastric banding (LAGB) is an effective treatment for morbid obesity.

The complications reported for LAGB are infections of the port site, band slippage, pouch dilatation, and intragastric band migration or band erosion.

Gastric band erosion has a highly reported incidence of 0.3 to 14% [1].

Erosion usually presents as a late complication (1–3 years after intervention) but some series report erosion within the first weeks.

Early erosion is generally a technical problem due to unrecognized gastric perforation during surgery or an early infection.

Other theories for erosion as a late complication are gastric wall ischemia secondary to a tight band, peptic ulcer perforation, implantation of a contaminated device, binge eating, and purging [2].

A large spectrum of clinical presentations is possible. From loss of restrictive effect, unexplained weight gain to life threatening sepsis and multiorgan failure.

Diagnosis can be confirmed by upper gastrointestinal endoscopy. CT findings can be suggestive, if there is extraluminal air or periprosthetic infection [1].

Intragastric migrated bands are best managed by endoscopic removal. Recent case studies reported successful endoscopic removal of intragastric migrated bands, but it is not always possible [3]. The timing of removal is still unclear.

It is also recommended to wait at least 3 months before reinsertion of another band [1, 3].

Removal of a gastric band after erosion by an SILS port introduced in the stomach has never been reported before.

We report the first case of the use of transgastric SILS port to remove eroded gastric bands.

Removal of a gastric band after gastric erosion is feasible, safe, and effective.

References

[1] P. T. Cherian, G. Goussous, F. Ashori, and A. Sigurdsson, "Band erosion after laparoscopic gastric banding: a retrospective analysis of 865 patients over 5 years," *Surgical Endoscopy and Other Interventional Techniques*, vol. 24, no. 8, pp. 2031–2038, 2010.

[2] E. Chousleb, S. Szomstein, E. Lomenzo et al., "Laparoscopic removal of gastric band after early gastric erosion: case report and review of the literature," *Surgical Laparoscopy, Endoscopy and Percutaneous Techniques*, vol. 15, no. 1, pp. 24–27, 2005.

[3] E. Mozzi, "Treatment of band erosion: feasibility and safety of endoscopic band removal," *Surgical Endoscopy*, vol. 25, no. 12, pp. 3918–01122, 1820.

32

Multivisceral Resection with Performing a Double Roux-en-Y Reconstruction for Advanced Gastric Cancer

Zijah Rifatbegovic,[1] **Zlatan Mehmedovic,**[1] **Majda Mehmedovic,**[2]
Jasmin Hasanovic,[1] **and Amra Mestric**[1]

[1]*Department of General Abdominal Surgery, Clinic for Surgery, University Clinical Center Tuzla,*
Tuzla, Bosnia and Herzegovina
[2]*Department of Gastroenterology and Hepatology, Clinic for Internal Diseases, University Clinical Center Tuzla,*
Tuzla, Bosnia and Herzegovina

Correspondence should be addressed to Zijah Rifatbegovic; drzooro@gmail.com

Academic Editor: Dimitrios Mantas

Background. The role of multivisceral resection, in the setting of locally advanced gastric cancer, is still debated. Previous studies have reported a higher risk for perioperative morbidity and mortality, with limited objective benefit in terms of survival. *Patient.* A male patient, 55 years old, was admitted to the clinic of surgery for surgical treatment of bleeding gastric ulceration. Preoperative diagnostic evaluation was performed, and patient had undergone a surgical treatment which revealed a large mass in head of the pancreas, infiltrating the hepatoduodenal ligament and transverse mesocolon. Total gastrectomy, duodenopancreatectomy, and right hemicolectomy were performed. The digestive tube continuity was reestablished by deriving the double Roux limbs. *Conclusion.* The aim of this case presentation is to demonstrate a method of digestive tube reconstruction by performing the double Roux-en-Y reconstruction in advanced gastric cancer when the multivisceral resection is performed.

1. Introduction

Although the incidence of gastric carcinoma is declining, it is still one of the leading causes of death from malignant tumors worldwide. Despite improved diagnostic techniques, most patients present with an advanced stage tumor [1].

The role of multivisceral resection, in the setting of locally advanced gastric cancer, is still debated. Previous studies have reported a higher risk for perioperative morbidity and mortality, with limited objective benefit in terms of survival. Conversely, recent studies have shown the feasibility of enlarged resection for clinical stage T4b gastric adenocarcinoma with good long-term results [2].

For patients undergoing curative surgery for gastric cancer R0 resection (negative microscopic and macroscopic margins) is the most powerful predictor of outcome. Unfortunately, gastric cancer typically presents at an advanced stage,

and tumor invasion into adjacent structures is present in many of these patients [3].

After the multivisceral resection is performed the digestive tube continuity can be made by the Roux-en-Y reconstruction, or the double Roux-en-Y, as an alternative reconstruction after the pancreaticoduodenectomy. When the pancreaticojejunostomy and hepaticojejunostomy due to pancreaticoduodenectomy are performed, the double Roux-en-Y digestive tract reconstruction can be addressed to decrease the liquid flow and pressure in the duodenal lumen and reduce not only the distance between the pancreaticojejunostomy and choledochojejunostomy but also the risks of traction, twisting, and angularity of the jejunal loop associated with common reconstruction methods [4].

We aim to present a case of 56-year-old male who underwent surgery for an advanced gastric cancer, as well as the optimal method of digestive tube reconstruction following a multivisceral resection.

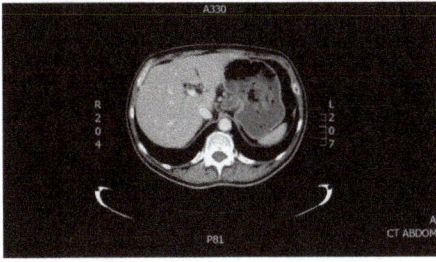

FIGURE 1: Computed tomography scan (CT) showed a structure of 2.0 × 3.5 cm in diameter on a lesser gastric curvature that could stand for large penetrating ulcer.

2. Case Presentation

A male patient, 55 years of age, was admitted to surgery clinic for surgical treatment of bleeding gastric ulcer. His major complaints were fatigue, abdominal pain, and tarry stool. Physical examination revealed painful abdomen in the region of epigastrium. During esophagogastroduodenoscopy gastric lumen was filled with multiple coagulum and revealed an elongated deep ulcer that stretched out from lesser gastric curvature to middle and lower third of gastric body. Its borders reddened and its bottom was filled with fibrin and coagula. Computed tomography scan (CT) showed a structure of 2.0 × 3.5 cm in diameter on a lesser gastric curvature that could stand for large penetrating ulcer (Figure 1).

After preoperative diagnostics was performed, patient underwent a surgical treatment and a large tumour that infiltrates head of pancreas, hepatoduodenal ligament, and transverse mesocolon was found. Total gastrectomy, duodenopancreatectomy, and right hemicolectomy were performed. The procedure took five hours and thirty minutes.

The pathohistological analysis showed margins which are tumor-free and confirmed that the R0 resection was performed. Due to pathological T4 (TNM stage) of the tumor omentectomy and D1 lymphadenectomy were also performed.

The continuity of digestive tube was reestablished by deriving double Roux limbs. Jejunal limb was isolated by Roux method and end-to-side esophagojejunal anastomosis by circular stapler was made. The limb was then resected on 60 cm from esophagojejunal anastomosis. Digestive tube continuity was reestablished by creating hepaticojejunal, pancreaticojejunal, and jejunojejunal anastomoses. Ileum-transversum anastomosis was created as well (Figures 2(a) and 2(b)).

Complications such as bile leakage, pancreatic leakage, and digestive tract obstruction were not observed during the follow-up period.

3. Discussion

The overall 5-year survival rate for all patients with gastric carcinoma who underwent surgery is only 20–30%. Even after a curative resection, only 30–50% of the patients are still alive after 5 years, with local recurrence being the main

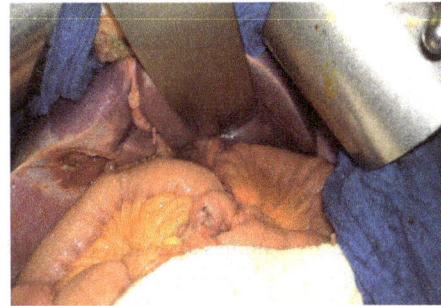

(a)

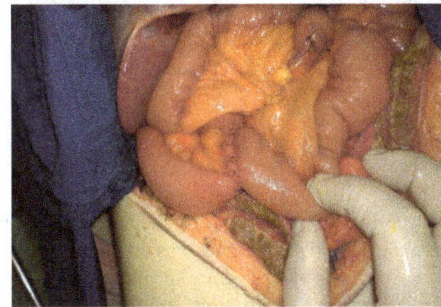

(b)

FIGURE 2: (a) and (b) show esophagojejunal anastomosis, hepaticojejunal, pancreaticojejunal, and jejunojejunal anastomoses.

cause of treatment failure. The surgical management of T4 gastric carcinoma remains controversial and the benefits of an extended resection are still doubtful [5].

The prognosis of patients with gastric cancer with invasion to adjacent organs (T4) was reported to be poor. However, some patients treated by radical surgery can survive for a long time after surgery [6].

For gastric carcinoma, standard therapy included subtotal/total gastrectomy, D2 lymphadenectomy, and omentectomy. The extent of the resection performed depended on tumor site and histological type. If safe resection margins could be achieved, subtotal gastrectomy was performed. If pancreatic infiltration was suspected intraoperatively, en bloc gastrectomy with pancreatic resection was performed. Splenectomy was done in patients with proximal carcinoma invading the spleen, in cases of enlarged lymph nodes in the splenic hilum, or in cases with invasion of the pancreas tail or body (in combination with pancreatic resection) [1].

Method for digestive tube reconstruction after multivisceral resection remains an open question. There are different ways to create reconstruction. In our case, we decided for a double Roux limb to avoid performing all the necessary anastomoses on a single loop.

When compared to single Roux limb, double Roux-en-Y reconstruction of the digestive tube is not beneficial in terms of surgical outcome and postoperative morbidity and mortality and should be avoided due to unnecessarily prolonged surgery [7].

We believe that in certain cases performing the double Roux-en-Y reconstruction can be a successful way to address the digestive tube continuity.

4. Conclusion

Even though the previous studies about the double Roux-en-Y showed no beneficial surgical outcome, in our case report it was a successful way for digestive tube reconstruction. We believe that the double Roux-en-Y should be considered as a way for reconstruction in certain cases with a multivisceral resection.

References

[1] P. Piso, T. Bellin, H. Aselmann, H. Bektas, H. J. Schlitt, and J. Klempnauer, "Results of combined gastrectomy and pancreatic resection in patients with advanced primary gastric carcinoma," *Digestive Surgery*, vol. 19, no. 4, pp. 281–285, 2002.

[2] F. Pacelli, G. Cusumano, F. Rosa et al., "Multivisceral resection for locally advanced gastric cancer: an italian multicenter observational study," *JAMA Surgery*, vol. 148, no. 4, pp. 353–360, 2013.

[3] S. S. Brar, R. Seevaratnam, R. Cardoso et al., "Multivisceral resection for gastric cancer: a systematic review," *Gastric Cancer*, vol. 15, no. 1, pp. S100–S107, 2012.

[4] C.-K. Jia, X.-F. Lu, Q.-Z. Yang, J. Weng, Y.-K. Chen, and Y. Fu, "Pancreaticojejunostomy, hepaticojejunostomy and double Roux-en-Y digestive tract reconstruction for benign pancreatic disease," *World Journal of Gastroenterology*, vol. 20, no. 36, pp. 13200–13204, 2014.

[5] D. Y. Kim, J. K. Joo, K. W. Seo et al., "T4 gastric carcinoma: the benefit of non-curative resection," *ANZ Journal of Surgery*, vol. 76, no. 6, pp. 453–457, 2006.

[6] H. Isozaki, N. Tanaka, N. Tanigawa, and K. Okajima, "Prognostic factors in patients with advanced gastric cancer with macroscopic invasion to adjacent organs treated with radical surgery," *Gastric Cancer*, vol. 3, no. 4, pp. 202–210, 2000.

[7] F. G. Uzunoglu, M. Reeh, and R. Wollstein, "Single versus double Roux-en-Y reconstruction techiques in pancreaticoduodenectomy: a comparative single-center study," *World Journal of Surgery*, vol. 38, no. 12, pp. 3228–3234, 2014.

33

Large Enterolith Complicating a Meckel Diverticulum Causing Obstructive Ileus in an Adolescent Male Patient

Constantinos Nastos,[1] **Dimitrios Giannoulopoulos,**[1] **Ioannis Georgopoulos,**[2] **Christos Salakos,**[3] **Dionysios Dellaportas,**[1] **Ioannis Papaconstantinou,**[1] **Theodosios Theodosopoulos,**[1] **and Georgios Polymeneas**[1]

[1]*Second Department of Surgery, National and Kapodistrian University of Athens, School of Medicine, Aretaieion University Hospital, Athens, Greece*
[2]*First Department of Pediatric Surgery, National and Kapodistrian University of Athens, School of Medicine, Agia Sofia University Hospital, Athens, Greece*
[3]*Department of Pediatric Surgery, National and Kapodistrian University of Athens, School of Medicine, Attikon University Hospital, Athens, Greece*

Correspondence should be addressed to Dimitrios Giannoulopoulos; dimitris.giannoulopoulos@hotmail.com

Academic Editor: Tahsin Colak

We present a unique case of a 16-year-old male patient who was eventually diagnosed with a large enterolith arising from a Meckel's diverticulum. The enterolith had caused intermittent intestinal symptoms for three years before resulting in small bowel obstruction requiring surgical intervention. Meckel's enterolith ileus is very rare with only few cases described in the literature. To our knowledge, this is only the second case of Meckel's enterolith which had caused intermittent symptoms over a period of time, before resulting in ileus, and the first case where the intermittent symptoms lasted several years before bowel obstruction. The patient had been evaluated with colonoscopy, computerized tomography (CT), and magnetic resonance imaging enterography (MRIE); a calcified pelvic mass had been found, but no further diagnosis other than calcification was established. The patient presented at our emergency department, with symptoms of obstructive ileus and underwent exploratory laparotomy, where a large enterolith arising from a Meckel's diverticulum (MD) was identified, causing the obstruction. A successful partial enterectomy, enterolith removal, and primary end-to-end anastomosis took place; the patient was permanently relieved from his long-standing symptoms. Consequently, complications of Meckel's diverticulum and enterolithiasis have to be included in the differential diagnosis of abdominal complaints.

1. Introduction

Meckel's diverticulum is a common embryological remnant that can be found incidentally during surgery for other pathology, or may manifest as acute abdomen, most commonly due to diverticular inflammation. More rare complications of Meckel's diverticulum, including bleeding, herniation, intussusception, and enterolithiasis, have also been reported [1, 2]. We present a rare case of a large enterolith formed inside a Meckel's diverticulum that was diagnosed in adolescence after having caused intermittent abdominal symptoms and finally small bowel obstruction.

2. Case Presentation

A 16-year-old patient presented to our outpatient clinic for evaluation of a pelvic calcified mass, initially found three years earlier in an abdominal X-ray, during investigation of an episode of lower right quadrant pain (Figure 1).

At that time, the patient did not require any surgical intervention and was managed conservatively. He was

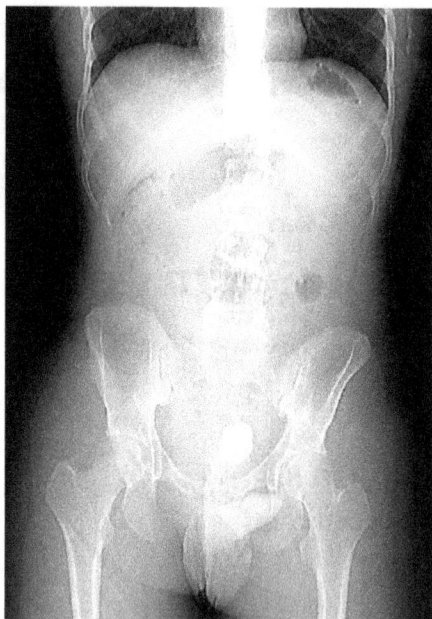

FIGURE 1

advised to have an outpatient workup of this mass. He was evaluated by a gastroenterologist and underwent an MRI enterography and colonoscopy. The MRI enterography revealed a calcified lesion in the distal ileum, located inside the pelvis, while the colonoscopy failed to recognize any lesion or inflammation in the terminal ileum. Meanwhile, the patient occasionally complained of nonspecific abdominal symptoms, which did not prompt him to seek further medical attention and resolved automatically.

Two years later, we scheduled an abdomen computerized tomography (CT), as a follow up. Contrast-enhanced abdominal CT revealed the same calcified lesion, 5 cm in diameter, that was in contact with the small bowel in the pelvis. The lesion had not grown in size during the last years.

Three years after the first onset of symptoms, the patient presented in our emergency department with symptoms of small bowel obstruction, namely, vomiting, intense colicky abdominal pain, and gas/flatus retention for 48 hours. Clinical examination revealed abdominal tenderness, distension, and hyperactive bowel sounds upon auscultation. Lab studies revealed mild leukocytosis. Plain X-ray showed multiple air-fluid levels. A new CT scan of the abdomen revealed obstruction of the small intestine, by the aforementioned mass (Figure 2).

The patient underwent an emergency laparotomy, where a loop of small bowel was found to be adherent to the pelvic wall. Upon dissection and mobilization of this loop from the pelvic wall, an enlarged and inflamed Meckel's diverticulum was identified. The diverticulum contained an enterolith, which was obstructing the bowel lumen. A partial enterectomy and an end-to-end anastomosis of the small bowel were performed.

The operation led to resolution of the obstruction, and the postoperative course was uneventful.

The pathology report confirmed the presence of a large enterolith, 5 cm in diameter, and ulcerative transmural inflammation of the resected part of the small intestine.

Six months following the operation, the patient was completely relieved from his occasional abdominal complaints and remained totally asymptomatic.

Informed consent was obtained from the patient for publication of this case report.

3. Discussion

Meckel's diverticulum is usually asymptomatic (85–95%), but clinical presentations associated with Meckel's diverticulum are diverticulitis, rectal bleeding, and small intestinal obstruction [3]. Small bowel obstruction can be the result of intussusception, volvulus around a fibrous band between Meckel's diverticulum and umbilicus, internal hernia through a fibrous band or an aberrant vitelline artery, prolapse of Meckel's diverticulum through a persistent omphalomesenteric effect, Littre's hernia, and rarely, enterolithiasis [1, 2, 4].

Meckel's diverticulum is complicated with enterolithiasis in 3–10% of cases [1]. In a large study by Park et al. involving 1476 patients with Meckel's diverticulum, it was found that 0.7% of asymptomatic patients and 6% of symptomatic patients had enterolithiasis at laparotomy [5]. The differential diagnosis of enterolithiasis includes calcified abscess, possibly due to Crohn's disease, possibly ingested foreign body, phytobezoar, trichobezoar, lactobezoar or pharmacobezoar, calcified neoplasm, undescendant testicle, teratoma, and abscess due to Crohn's disease [1].

Enteroliths can cause obstruction [1], diverticulitis [6], injury to the bowel mucosa [1], perforation [1], afferent loop syndrome [7], intussusception [8], gangrene [1], hemorrhage [1], and iron deficiency anemia. Meckel's diverticulum-related enterolith intestinal obstruction has rarely been reported [4].

To our knowledge, our case is only the second to describe a Meckel associated large enterolith that had been causing intermittent-type bowel symptoms for a certain period of time, before resulting in acute abdomen, due to obstructive ileus, thus requiring immediate surgical intervention [9]. Interestingly, this is the first case that the intermittent symptoms had lasted for several years, without a definite diagnosis regarding the cause of the symptoms being made in the meanwhile, before eventually producing small bowel obstruction.

In conclusion, enterolithiasis is an entity that can be a diagnostic challenge for the clinician. Meckel diverticulum-associated enterolithiasis can produce bowel obstruction. The clinician should include Meckel's diverticulum complications and enterolithiasis in the differential diagnosis of abdominal symptoms, either acute or chronic.

4. Conclusions

Meckel diverticulum-associated enterolithiasis is a rare condition that can be either asymptomatic or produce nonspecific symptoms but can also manifest itself as acute

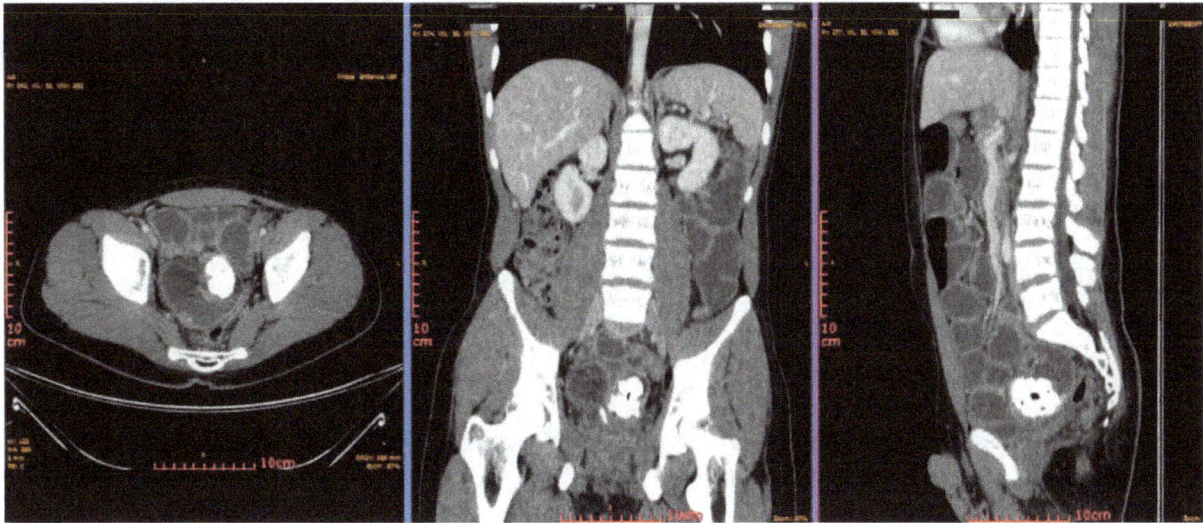

FIGURE 2

abdomen. Intestinal obstruction due to Meckel's enterolithiasis is very rare, with only few cases described in the literature. Our patient experienced intermittent symptoms for a course of several years before developing intestinal obstruction. Our case underlines that complications of Meckel's diverticulum and Meckel diverticulum-associated enterolithiasis need to be included in the differential diagnosis of abdominal complaints, as this diagnosis can be particularly challenging.

References

[1] G. E. Gurvits and G. Lan, "Enterolithiasis," *World Journal of Gastroenterology*, vol. 20, no. 47, pp. 17819–17829, 2014.

[2] G. Morris, A. Kennedy Jr., and W. Cochran, "Small bowel congenital anomalies: a review and update," *Current Gastroenterology Reports*, vol. 18, no. 4, p. 16, 2016.

[3] K. M. Elsayes, C. O. Menias, H. J. Harvin, and I. R. Francis, "Imaging manifestations of Meckel's diverticulum," *American Journal of Roentgenology*, vol. 189, no. 1, pp. 81–88, 2007.

[4] V. Demetriou, D. McKean, J. Briggs, and N. Moore, "Small bowel obstruction due to a liberated Meckel's enterolith," *BMJ Case Reports*, vol. 2013, no. 31, p. bcr2013008868, 2013.

[5] J. J. Park, B. G. Wolff, M. K. Tollefson, E. E. Walsh, and D. R. Larson, "Meckel diverticulum: the Mayo Clinic experience with 1476 patients (1950-2002)," *Annals of Surgery*, vol. 241, no. 3, pp. 529–533, 2005.

[6] N. Agaoglu, "Meckel's diverticulum enterolith: a rare cause of acute abdomen," *Acta Chirurgica Belgica*, vol. 109, no. 4, pp. 513–515, 2009.

[7] C. Cartanese, G. Campanella, E. Milano, and M. Sacco, "Enterolith causing acute afferent loop syndrome after Billroth II gastrectomy: a case report," *Il Giornale Di Chirurgia*, vol. 34, no. 5-6, p. 1646, 2013.

[8] H. J. Kim, J. H. Moon, H. J. Choi et al., "Endoscopic removal of an enterolith causing afferent loop syndrome using electrohydraulic lithotripsy," *Digestive endoscopy*, vol. 22, no. 3, pp. 220–222, 2010.

[9] R. P. Jones and D. McWhirter, "Intermittent small bowel obstruction caused by Meckel's enterolith," *Annals of the Royal College of Surgeons of England*, vol. 92, no. 5, pp. e16–e17, 2010.

34

Gigantic GIST: A Case of the Largest Gastrointestinal Stromal Tumor Found to Date

Abdalla Mohamed ⓘ,[1] **Youssef Botros,**[2] **Paul Hanna ⓘ,**[3] **Sang Lee,**[3] **Walid Baddoura,**[2] **Jamshed Zuberi,**[3] **and Tanuja Damani**[3]

[1]*Department of Medicine, St. Joseph's University Medical Center, Paterson, NJ, USA*
[2]*Division of Gastroenterology and Hepatology, St. Joseph's University Medical Center, Paterson, NJ, USA*
[3]*Department of Surgery, St. Joseph's University Medical Center, Paterson, NJ, USA*

Correspondence should be addressed to Abdalla Mohamed; r_mohamedab@sjhmc.org

Academic Editor: Dimitrios Mantas

Gastrointestinal stromal tumors are uncommon when compared to all gastrointestinal neoplasms but are the most common mesenchymal tumors of the gastrointestinal tract. The largest gastrointestinal stromal tumor ever recorded in literature weighed approximately 6.1 kg and measured 39 cm × 27 cm × 14 cm. About two-thirds of GISTs are malignant. The tumor size, mitotic rate, cellularity, and nuclear pleomorphism are the most important parameters when considering prognosis and recurrence. The definitive treatment for these tumors is resection. In the year 2000, the first patient was treated with the tyrosine kinase inhibitor imatinib and since then, gastrointestinal stromal tumors with high-risk features have been treated successfully with tyrosine kinase inhibitors. We present the largest gastrointestinal stromal tumor recorded in medical literature measuring 42.0 cm × 31.0 cm × 23.0 cm in maximum dimensions and weighing in at approximately 18.5 kg in a 65-year-old African-American male who presented with increased abdominal distention. The mass was successfully excised, and the patient was treated with imatinib without local or distant recurrence 1.5 years postoperatively.

1. Introduction

Although GISTs are relatively uncommon (<1% of all gastrointestinal neoplasms) compared with adenocarcinoma, they are the most common mesenchymal tumors of the gastrointestinal tract [1, 2]. According to SEER (Surveillance, Epidemiology, and End Results) data from 1992 to 2000, the estimated incidence in the USA is 6.8 per million. The incidence of occult micro-GISTs smaller than 1 cm is actually much higher [3].

The majority of cases present as symptomatic disease. Small GISTs are usually asymptomatic and are incidentally found during radiologic evaluation, endoscopy, or at the time of surgery for another cause. Although a GIST is not a mucosa-based tumor, like adenocarcinoma, but instead grows from the muscle layer of the bowel wall, it still may

be accompanied by bleeding in up to 25% of patients due to erosion of the mucosa resulting in melena, hematemesis, or symptomatic anemia. Other signs and symptoms include abdominal fullness, early satiety, a palpable mass, or abdominal pain [4]. To our knowledge, the largest reported GIST in the literature measured 39 cm × 27 cm × 14 cm and weighed 6.1 kg [5].

Tumor size and the mitotic count are the most commonly used prognostic factors to estimate the outcome and risk of recurrence of the tumor. Tumors arising from the stomach have a more favorable prognosis compared to other sites [6]. Treatment strategy for GIST will depend on the tumor site, size, and presence or absence of metastasis. Small GIST (less than 2 cm) can be conservatively observed [7]. Surgical resection is the mainstay for nonmetastatic tumors, most commonly in the form of a wedge

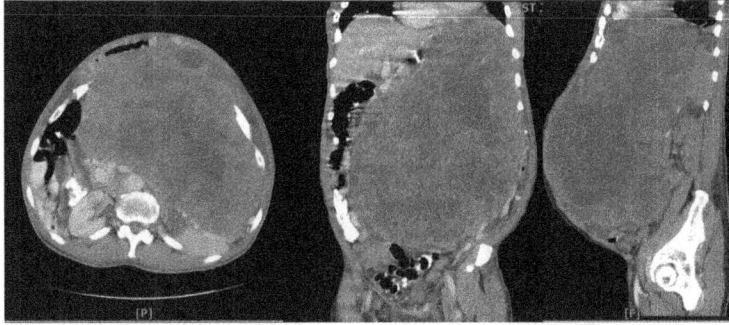

FIGURE 1: Coronal, transverse, and sagittal views of CT of the abdomen and pelvis showing heterogeneous, partially necrotic mass.

resection. Another modality for treating small tumors is endoscopic resection [8].

We present a rare case of a gastric GIST larger in size than any previously documented, rapidly growing and invading into the surrounding structures that was successfully treated with surgical resection with total gastrectomy as well as en bloc resection of the pancreas, spleen, and colon with ostomy creation.

GISTs are encountered frequently in the surgical clinical setting with varying sizes, invasion, and treatment modalities. We present this case for a review of GISTs and review of the surgical decision-making and to highlight the patient's success despite massive resection of major abdominal organs.

2. Case Presentation

A 65-year-old African-American male with no significant past medical history presented to facility with complaints of worsening abdominal distention for approximately one year, associated with dyspnea, early satiety, and weight loss of about 23 pounds. He denied chest pain, melena, or hematochezia. He had never had an endoscopy or colonoscopy performed. The patient did have a remote history of smoking of about a half pack of cigarettes per day for 10 years; however, he had quit 15 years prior. Family history was significant for a brother with lung cancer, otherwise noncontributory.

On physical examination, he was noted to have bitemporal wasting and marked abdominal distension secondary to a large firm mass with ill-defined margins.

A contrast-enhanced CT scan of the abdomen and pelvis showed a large, heterogeneous, partially necrotic mass measuring 38 cm × 25 cm, arising from the left upper quadrant with no evidence of metastases seen. There was displacement of the stomach and duodenum to the right and the left kidney was displaced inferiorly. The mass was suggestive of a sarcoma or possibly a GIST tumor with malignant degeneration (Figure 1). Chest radiograph was done which confirmed no pulmonary pathology or metastatic disease.

Preoperative laboratory analysis showed a white blood cell count of 5.9 K/mm^3 with 80% neutrophils. Hemoglobin of 10 G/dl and hematocrit 31.2% with a platelet count of 328 K/mm^3. Basic metabolic panel and liver function tests and PT/INR were unremarkable.

The patient was taken for an exploratory laparotomy, which revealed a large mass arising from the posterior gastric wall with a giant omental vessel as well as dilated gastroepiploic vessels. The mass was invading the spleen, distal pancreas, and the mesentery of the transverse colon. Over the next 7 hours, the mass was completely resected with a total gastrectomy, esophagojejunostomy and feeding jejunostomy, distal pancreatectomy, and splenectomy. Resection required division of the mesentery of the transverse colon, which resulted in ischemia of the transverse colon warranting resection with end colostomy creation. The tumor, spleen, distal pancreas, and transverse colon were all sent for frozen section. As expected of GISTs, pathology reports showed that the 6 harvested lymph nodes as well as the surgical margins were all negative for malignancy. During the 7-hour procedure, the patient lost nearly 3 l of blood and received 6 l of IV fluids, 12 units of packed red blood cells, 4 units of fresh-frozen plasma, 1 unit of single donor platelets, and 4 units of albumin with intermittent pushes of vasopressive medications. The patient was taken to the surgical intensive care unit postoperatively, was weaned off vasopressive medications, extubated, and started on tube feeds, and eventually fed orally. The remainder of his hospital course was uneventful, and the patient was discharged to home on postoperative day 14. The patient was started on imatinib at this time and has been maintained on that with no recurrence approximately 1.5 years postoperatively. The patient returned 8 months later for a planned colostomy take-down, which was successful and uneventful.

Macroscopically, the mass was irregularly shaped, attached to the posterior-inferior aspect of the stomach, weighed 18,500 grams, and measured 42.0 × 31.0 × 23.0 cm in maximum dimensions (Figure 2).

Histopathology showed gastric stromal tumor cells staged as high grade with >5 mitoses per high power field (hpf).

Immunohistochemistry confirmed GIST with strong positive staining for CD117, DOG1, and CD34 (Figure 3). Postoperative recovery was uneventful.

3. Discussion

Our patient presented with progressively worsening abdominal distension for 9 months, weight loss, and was found to have a giant GIST causing early satiety, anemia, and locally invading into adjacent organs such as the spleen, distal pancreas, and the mesentery of the transverse colon. Despite the enormous size and weight of the tumor, our patient denied

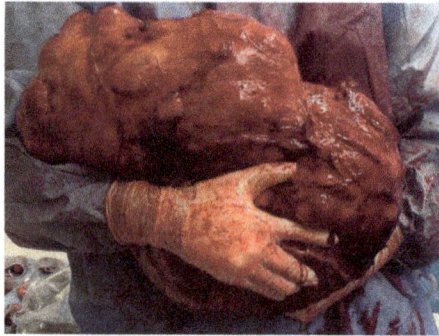

FIGURE 2: Gross image of the resected mass measuring $42 \times 31 \times 23$ cm and weighing 18.5 kg.

any severe abdominal pain or other associated symptoms other than abdominal distention with decreased diet tolerance.

We report the largest GIST tumor reported to date. The size of our tumor measured 42.0 cm $\times 31.0$ cm $\times 23.0$ cm in dimensions. The largest tumor reported prior to our tumor measured 39 cm $\times 27$ cm $\times 14$ cm. The weight of our tumor was 18.5 kg, which is about 3 times heavier than the heaviest tumor previously reported, 6.1 kg.

The treatment strategy for GIST depends on the tumor site, size, and presence or absence of metastasis. In this case, surgery was unavoidable due to the complex nature and size of the tumor as well as the associated early gastrointestinal obstruction identified by patient's decreased diet tolerance and findings on the imaging. For this reason, the decision was made to proceed with surgical intervention as opposed to neoadjuvant therapy with imatinib. Achieving an adequate en bloc resection was difficult due to the multivisceral involvement. The patient underwent a total gastrectomy, esophagojejunostomy and feeding jejunostomy, distal pancreatectomy, and splenectomy. The added difficulty during the case was after resection of the transverse mesocolon, finding evidence of a nonviable segment of bowel from the transverse colon to mid descending colon which was resected and a temporary ostomy was created. It was not advisable to create a primary anastomosis at this time given the patient's hypotension, significant blood loss, and transfusion requirement. There is no consensus on the use of neoadjuvant therapy for the treatment of GISTs. There have been approximately seven trials in which neoadjuvant chemotherapy was studied and utilized [9]. RTOG (Radiation Therapy Oncology Group) 0132 was the first trial of preoperative imatinib in GIST [9, 10]. Thirty-one primary GIST patients were analyzed as the neoadjuvant group. The median tumor size was 8.7 cm. Imatinib was administered at 600 mg/day for 8 to 12 weeks before surgery, and imatinib administration also continued for 2 years after surgery. In the primary GIST group, the progression-free survival, which was the primary end point of this trial, was calculated as 83.9% for 2 years and 56.7% for 5 years [9, 10]. This was the first trial to show some use of neoadjuvant imatinib, but unfortunately, the same trial failed to show any superiority of adding neoadjuvant chemotherapy compared to adjuvant alone [9, 10]. Kurokawa et al. had similar results in a recent study published in 2017 that showed that neoadjuvant therapy

along with surgery may be beneficial long term [10, 11]. As mentioned previously, the decision was made to forego neoadjuvant imatinib therapy due to the development of gastrointestinal obstruction.

As investigated preoperatively, there was also no evidence of hematogenous spread to distal organs on the imaging. As evidenced in previous studies, markers of hepatic invasion by GIST are tumor size of >5 cm and the presence of nodal metastasis or mitotic count greater than 5/hpf [12]. The tumor was confirmed to be a GIST, and approximately 0.5 cm from the closest margin and less than one hpf from the serosa.

Because GISTs often demonstrate an exophytic pattern of growth toward the peritoneal cavity [13], the patient probably remained asymptomatic until the tumor reached a quite large size. Exophytic GISTs can invade structures such as the pancreas or colon and may result in bowel obstruction or adjacent organ dysfunction [13]. Imatinib, a tyrosine kinase inhibitor, could have been used as a neoadjuvant therapy if the tumor pathology was known earlier [10]. Although neoadjuvant therapy may have decreased the magnitude of the surgery, the biopsy would also increase the risk of tumor rupture which is associated with inevitable peritoneal recurrence [14].

Postoperatively, the patient has been monitored for recurrence and basic hematologic parameters because the massive size of the tumor is known to be associated with a higher recurrence rate [13]. Nearly half of patients with GISTs present with metastatic disease, most commonly to the liver and peritoneum [15]. Fortunately, however, our patient's histopathology showed T4N0M0 and pathology from colostomy take-down remained to be negative.

The most important immunohistological features of GIST are as follows: (i) the tumor cells are whorls of spindle-shaped cells with eosinophilic cytoplasm and elongated nuclei; (ii) mitotic figures indicate high risk of progression; and (iii) immunoreactivity to c-KIT, CD117, or DOG1 confirms the diagnosis [16]. Heinrich et al. reported that five percent of GISTs do not demonstrate c-KIT immunoreactivity, and these tumors usually harbor mutations in platelet-derived growth factor receptor [17]. Our immunohistochemistry included DOG1, CD34, CD117, actin, and S100, and the tumor was strongly positive for DOG-1, CD34, and CD117.

In 1998, Hirota et al. described the underlying gain function mutation leading to the development of GIST tumors, the c-kit proto-oncogene (CD117) coding the KIT receptor—a tyrosine kinase transmembrane receptor that controls crucial cell functions in tumor genesis, including proliferation, adhesion, apoptosis, and differentiation. The KIT gene mutation leads to uncontrolled cell proliferation due to stimulation of downstream signaling pathways [18].

Different markers are used to identify KIT-negative GISTs including: calcium-dependent and receptor-activated chloride channel protein, known as DOG1 and protein kinase C theta [19, 20]. Carbonic anhydrase II is another sensitive biomarker for GIST [21]. The importance of distinguishing GIST from other mesenchymal tumors arises from their notorious resistance to conventional chemotherapy

(a)

(b)

(c)

(d)

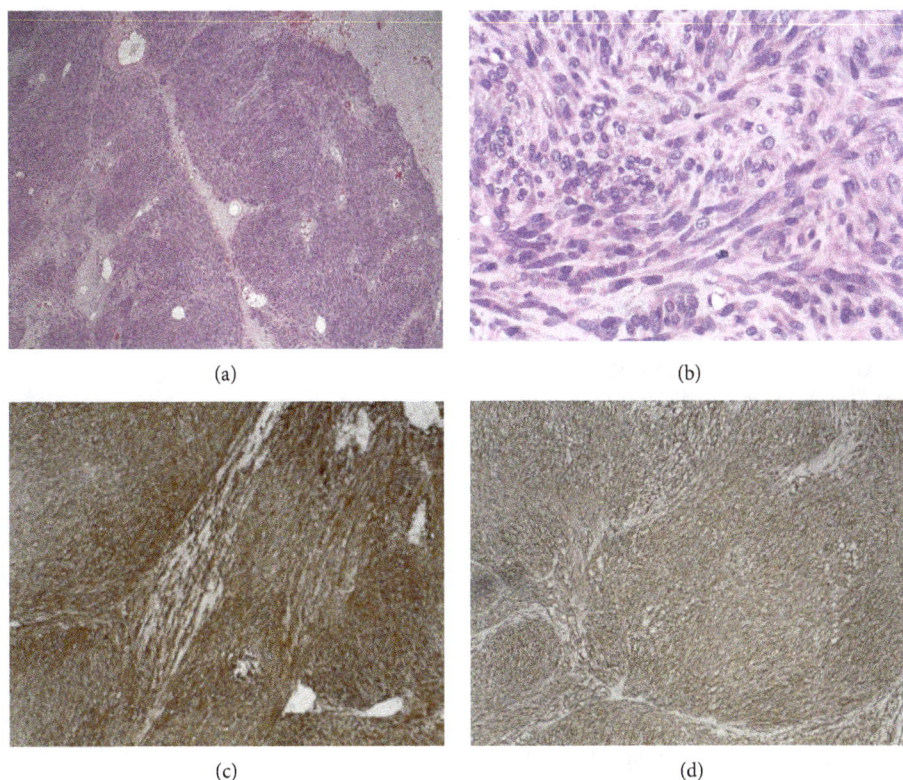

FIGURE 3: (a) Low-power H&E stain. (b) High-power H&E stain showing gastric stromal tumor cells with mitosis. (c) DOG-1 stain: strongly positive. (d) CD117 stain: strongly positive.

and radiation and their good response to the targeted treatment, e.g., imatinib [22].

Adjuvant therapy along with surgery is the preferred method of treatment when it comes to GIST. Imatinib for adjuvant treatment was approved based on the ACOSOG Z9001 study in 2008 in the USA and in 2009 in Europe. In this study, eligible patients had complete resection of a primary GIST of at least 3 cm in size. The median follow-up was 19.7 months. Adjuvant treatment for one year led to a RFS of 98% [23, 24].

Most GIST patients will achieve the clinical benefits with imatinib, but an estimated 10% will progress within 3 to 6 months of initiating therapy. Such cases are described as showing primary resistance to treatment. Another 40% to 50% of patients will go on to develop resistance within the first two years [25]. Primary resistance is observed in approximately 10% of patients. Tumors that are most likely to show primary resistance are those that are KIT and PDGFRA wild-type, those that have a KIT exon 9 mutation, and those that have a PDGFRA D842V substitution [25]. Delayed imatinib resistance most often is associated with the expansion of tumor clones with secondary KIT or PDGFRA mutations [25]. Our patient was started on imatinib shortly after the postoperative period and has not shown any recurrence or resistance to date, approximately 1.5 years postoperatively.

We present this case to demonstrate a successful management of the largest GIST recorded in literature with invasion into the surrounding structures requiring en bloc resection and a multidisciplinary-staged approach to treatment.

References

[1] B. P. Rubin, M. C. Heinrich, and C. L. Corless, "Gastrointestinal stromal tumour," *The Lancet*, vol. 369, no. 9574, pp. 1731–1741, 2007.

[2] T. Nishida and S. Hirota, "Biological and clinical review of stromal tumours in the gastrointestinal tract," *Histology and Histopathology*, vol. 15, no. 4, pp. 1293–1301, 2000.

[3] T. Tran, J. A. Davila, and H. B. El-Serag, "The epidemiology of malignant gastrointestinal stromal tumors: an analysis of 1,458 cases from 1992 to 2000," *The American Journal of Gastroenterology*, vol. 100, no. 1, pp. 162–168, 2005.

[4] A. D. Levy, H. E. Remotti, W. M. Thompson, L. H. Sobin, and M. Miettinen, "Gastrointestinal stromal tumors: radiologic features with pathologic correlation," *Radiographics*, vol. 23, no. 2, pp. 283–304, 2003, 456.

[5] A. Koyuncuer, L. Gönlüşen, and A. V. Kutsal, "A rare case of giant gastrointestinal stromal tumor of the stomach involving the serosal surface," *International Journal of Surgery Case Reports*, vol. 12, pp. 90–94, 2015.

[6] C. D. Fletcher, J. J. Berman, C. Corless et al., "Diagnosis of gastrointestinal stromal tumors: a consensus approach," *Human Pathology*, vol. 33, no. 5, pp. 459–465, 2002.

[7] G. D. Demetri, M. von Mehren, C. R. Antonescu et al., "NCCN task force report: update on the management of patients with gastrointestinal stromal tumors," *Journal of the National Comprehensive Cancer Network*, vol. 8, Supplement 2, pp. S-1–S-41, 2010.

[8] F. Feng, Z. Liu, X. Zhang et al., "Comparison of endoscopic and open resection for small gastric gastrointestinal stromal tumor," *Translational Oncology*, vol. 8, no. 6, pp. 504–508, 2015.

[9] T. Ishikawa, T. Kanda, H. Kameyama, and T. Wakai, "Neoadjuvant therapy for gastrointestinal stromal tumor," *Translational Gastroenterology and Hepatology*, vol. 3, p. 3, 2018.

[10] B. L. Eisenberg, J. Harris, C. D. Blanke et al., "Phase II trial of neoadjuvant/adjuvant imatinib mesylate (IM) for advanced primary and metastatic/recurrent operable gastrointestinal stromal tumor (GIST): early results of RTOG 0132/ACRIN 6665," *Journal of Surgical Oncology*, vol. 99, pp. 42–47, 2009.

[11] Y. Kurokawa, H. K. Yang, H. Cho et al., "Phase II study of neoadjuvant imatinib in large gastrointestinal stromal tumours of the stomach," *British Journal of Cancer*, vol. 117, no. 1, pp. 25–32, 2017.

[12] A. Gaitanidis, M. Alevizakos, A. Tsaroucha, C. Simopoulos, and M. Pitiakoudis, "Incidence and predictors of synchronous liver metastases in patients with gastrointestinal stromal tumors (GISTs)," *The American Journal of Surgery*, vol. 216, no. 3, pp. 492–497, 2018.

[13] H. C. Kang, C. O. Menias, A. H. Gaballah et al., "Beyond the GIST: mesenchymal tumors of the stomach," *Radiographics*, vol. 33, no. 6, pp. 1673–1690, 2013.

[14] J. Cameron and A. M. Cameron, *Cameron's Surgical Therapy*, Elsevier, Philadelphia, PA, USA, 12th edition, 2017.

[15] R. P. DeMatteo, J. J. Lewis, D. Leung, S. S. Mudan, J. M. Woodruff, and M. F. Brennan, "Two hundred gastrointestinal stromal tumors: recurrence patterns and prognostic factors for survival," *Annals of Surgery*, vol. 231, no. 1, pp. 51–58, 2000.

[16] I. Espinosa, C. H. Lee, M. K. Kim et al., "A novel monoclonal antibody against DOG1 is a sensitive and specific marker for gastrointestinal stromal tumors," *The American Journal of Surgical Pathology*, vol. 32, no. 2, pp. 210–218, 2008.

[17] M. C. Heinrich, C. L. Corless, A. Duensing et al., "PDGFRA activating mutations in gastrointestinal stromal tumors," *Science*, vol. 299, no. 5607, pp. 708–710, 2003.

[18] S. Hirota, K. Isozaki, Y. Moriyama et al., "Gain-of-function mutations of c-kit in human gastrointestinal stromal tumors," *Science*, vol. 279, no. 5350, pp. 577–580, 1998.

[19] H. Joensuu, P. Hohenberger, and C. L. Corless, "Gastrointestinal stromal tumour," *The Lancet*, vol. 382, no. 9896, pp. 973–983, 2013.

[20] P. Blay, A. Astudillo, J. M. Buesa et al., "Protein kinase C θ is highly expressed in gastrointestinal stromal tumors but not in other mesenchymal neoplasias," *Clinical Cancer Research*, vol. 10, no. 12, pp. 4089–4095, 2004.

[21] S. Parkkila, J. Lasota, J. A. Fletcher et al., "Carbonic anhydrase II. A novel biomarker for gastrointestinal stromal tumors," *Modern Pathology*, vol. 23, no. 5, pp. 743–750, 2010.

[22] H. Joensuu, P. Roberts, M. Sarlomo-Rikala et al., "Effect of the tyrosine kinase inhibitor STI571 in a patient with a metastatic gastrointestinal stromal tumor," *The New England Journal of Medicine*, vol. 344, no. 14, pp. 1052–1056, 2001.

[23] R. P. de Matteo, K. V. Ballman, C. R. Antonescu et al., "Adjuvant imatinib mesylate after resection of localised, primary gastrointestinal stromal tumour: a randomised, double-blind, placebo-controlled trial," *The Lancet*, vol. 373, no. 9669, pp. 1097–1104, 2009.

[24] S. Cameron, "Long-term adjuvant treatment of gastrointestinal stromal tumors (GIST) with imatinib—a comment and reflection on the PERSIST-5 study," *Translational Gastroenterology and Hepatology*, vol. 3, p. 16, 2018.

[25] A. W. Gramza, C. L. Corless, and M. C. Heinrich, "Resistance to tyrosine kinase inhibitors in gastrointestinal stromal tumors," *Clinical Cancer Research*, vol. 15, no. 24, pp. 7510–7518, 2009.

35

A Case of Midgut Volvulus Associated with a Jejunal Diverticulum

Joseph Gutowski,[1] **Rachel NeMoyer,**[2] **and Glenn S. Parker**[3]

[1]*Rutgers Robert Wood Johnson Medical School, Piscataway Township, NJ 08854, USA*
[2]*Rutgers Robert Wood Johnson Medical School, New Brunswick, NJ 08901, USA*
[3]*Jersey Shore University Medical Center, Neptune City, NJ 07753, USA*

Correspondence should be addressed to Rachel NeMoyer; rachel.nemoyer@gmail.com

Academic Editor: Cheng-Yu Long

Midgut volvulus in adults is a rare entity that may present with intermittent colicky abdominal pain mixed with completely asymptomatic episodes. This small bowel twist may result in complications of obstruction, ischemia, hemorrhage, or perforation. With a midgut volvulus, complications may be life-threatening, and emergent surgical intervention is the mainstay of treatment. This current case involves an 80-year-old woman with intermittent abdominal pain with increasing severity and decreasing interval of time to presentation. A CAT scan revealed mesenteric swirling with possible internal hernia. A diagnostic laparoscopy followed by laparotomy revealed a midgut volvulus, extensive adhesions involving the root of the mesentery, and a large jejunal diverticulum. The adhesions were lysed enabling untwisting of the bowel, allowing placement of the small bowel in the correct anatomic position and resection of the jejunal diverticulum. This is a rare case of midgut volvulus with intermittent abdominal pain, associated with jejunal diverticulum managed successfully. A midgut volvulus should be considered in the differential diagnosis of a patient who present with a small bowel obstruction secondary to an internal hernia, especially when a swirl sign is present on the CAT scan.

1. Introduction

In the adult patient population, small bowel obstruction is a relatively common diagnosis. However, obstruction due to small bowel volvulus is quite rare, and most cases have been documented in newborns. Current literature suggests the annual incidence of small bowel volvulus to be 1.7–5.7 per 100,000 adults in Western countries [1]. Most commonly, it is attributed to congenital abnormalities or prior abdominal surgeries [1]. If left untreated, ischemia and subsequent infarction may ensue [2]. Here, we present a case of a patient undergoing an exploratory laparotomy for recurrent abdominal pain and imaging suggestive of an obstructive pathology who was found to have small bowel volvulus with a diverticulum.

2. Case Report

The patient is an 80-year-old female with a history of recurrent abdominal pain. Permission was obtained from the patient to allow discussion and publication of his case. The patient had a history of coronary artery disease, atrial fibrillation (on anticoagulation), multiple cerebral vascular accidents, chronic obstructive pulmonary disease, an aortic and mitral valve replacement, and a prior hysterectomy. The patient was noted to have presented to the hospital three times in the prior month with similar complaints of vague, diffuse abdominal pain that would last a few hours and resolve. The patient did note nausea and vomiting with these episodes. The patient re-presented to the emergency room, where a CAT scan was performed (Figure 1) which showed mesenteric swirling secondary to possible internal hernia. The patient underwent a small bowel follow through with gastrografin, which demonstrated no abnormalities. The patient then underwent an obstructive series that was also noted to be normal. The patient's symptoms, however, did not subside. Due to the chronicity and the unresolving symptoms, the patient was brought to the operating room after a long discussion of possible outcomes with the patient.

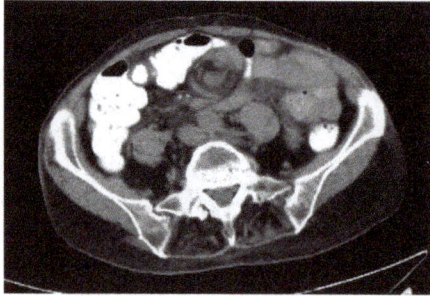

FIGURE 1: Axial view of CAT scan. Mesenteric swirl sign.

The operation was started laparoscopically but was soon converted to an open laparotomy due to a large mass of small bowel swirled onto itself that was adhered together (Figure 2). In mobilizing the small bowel, blunt dissection was used to lyse adhesions and untwist the mesentery. The small bowel mesentery was observed, and no mesenteric defects were noted. It was seen that the mesentery had swirled and twisted upon itself (Figure 3). While running the bowel, a large, proximal jejunal diverticulum was present. The diverticulum was excised using a 60 mm stapler. The bowel was run from the ligament of Treitz down to the ileocecal valve with no mesenteric defects noted, and all bowel was viable. The small bowel was returned to the abdomen. The patient did well postoperatively and was seen in follow-up without complication.

3. Discussion

Small bowel obstruction is a fairly common diagnosis in the adult population of the United States, with the most common causes being postoperative adhesions, masses, and hernias. Patients typically experience severe and intermittent abdominal pain, nausea, vomiting, and the inability to pass stool or flatus. A small bowel volvulus can occur if a portion of the bowel twists on itself and its mesentery, effectively causing an obstruction. If the obstruction is a closed-loop obstruction, which includes small bowel volvulus, the CAT scan can demonstrate a swirl sign. This finding represents mesenteric soft-tissue and fat attenuation with adjacent loops of bowel surrounding the rotated intestinal vessels [3]. A relatively recent study suggested that the swirl sign has a sensitivity of 64% and a PPV of 21% in diagnosing a small bowel volvulus [3].

The differential diagnosis for a patient presenting with symptoms of a small bowel obstruction may include adhesions, hernia, neoplasm, intussusception, small bowel hematoma, or pathology relating to the patency of the lumen such as a bezoar or a gallstone [4]. Volvulus accounts for only 4 to 15% of mechanical small bowel obstructions in the United States and Western Europe [5]. More common is volvulus of the large intestine, specifically at the sigmoid, which makes up 70 to 80% of large intestine cases, followed by the cecum, which makes up 10 to 20% of large intestine cases [2].

Small bowel volvulus may be classified as primary or secondary. Primary volvulus occurs in patients with a virgin

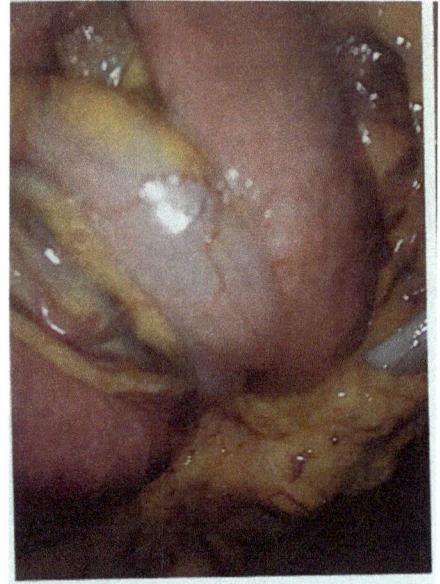

FIGURE 2: Laparoscopic view of adherent small bowel.

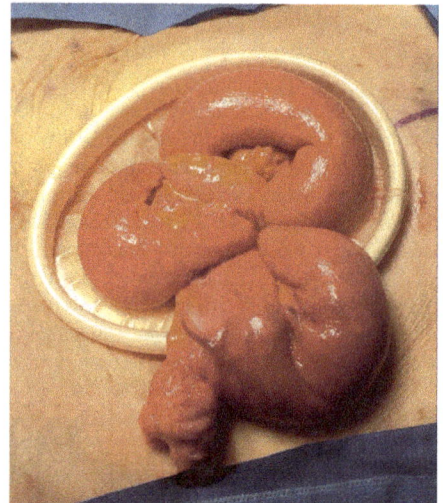

FIGURE 3: Open view of volvulized small bowel.

abdomen who possess no anatomic abnormalities that would predispose them to develop a volvulus [2]. These represent 10 to 22% of all volvulus cases in the Western world [2]. Secondary volvulus is much more common in the United States. It occurs in patients who have congenital or acquired pathology of the abdomen such as adhesions, tension bands, or anatomic malformations [2]. Diverticulum of the small bowel, such as the one seen in our patient, has also been associated with the development of volvulus, as one study found the incidence of small bowel diverticulum in patients with small bowel volvulus to be as high as 35% [6].

The primary determinant in reducing the morbidity and mortality of small bowel volvulus is early diagnosis and treatment [2]. If the obstruction becomes advanced, vascular compromise can occur thus increasing the risk of intestinal necrosis and subsequent intestinal perforation. Unfortunately, it is difficult to accurately diagnose ischemic bowel on CAT scan [4]. The best indicators of gangrenous bowel are peritoneal signs, a palpable mass, fever, and leukocytosis [7]. In addition to the metabolic alkalosis that can result from excessive vomiting, a metabolic acidosis can occur if the bowel is ischemic due to the accumulation of lactic acid [8]. Early surgical intervention remains the best form of treatment for small bowel volvulus. Manually untwisting the volvulus may be sufficient if the bowel appears healthy and viable after the maneuver. However, gangrenous bowel must be resected to minimize the risk of infection and perforation [2].

This is a rare case of midgut volvulus with intermittent abdominal pain, associated with jejunal diverticulum managed successfully. A midgut volvulus should be considered in the differential diagnosis of a patient who presents with a small bowel obstruction secondary to an internal hernia, especially when a swirl sign is present on the CAT scan to minimize morbidity and possible mortality of the patient.

Disclosure

This paper was presented as a poster at the American Society of Colon and Rectal Surgeons at the annual meeting in Seattle, WA, June 2017.

References

[1] T. M. Coe, D. C. Chang, and J. K. Sicklick, "Small bowel volvulus in the adult populace of the United States: results from a population-based study," *The American Journal of Surgery*, vol. 210, no. 2, pp. 201–210.e2, 2015.

[2] A. Roggo and L. W. Ottinger, "Acute small bowel volvulus in adults. A sporadic form of strangulating intestinal obstruction," *Annals of Surgery*, vol. 216, no. 2, pp. 135–141, 1992.

[3] J. B. Duda, S. Bhatt, and V. S. Dogra, "Utility of CT whirl sign in guiding management of small-bowel obstruction," *American Journal of Roentgenology*, vol. 191, no. 3, pp. 743–747, 2008.

[4] C. P. Mullan, B. Siewert, and R. L. Eisenberg, "Small bowel obstruction," *American Journal of Roentgenology*, vol. 198, no. 2, pp. W105–W117, 2012.

[5] G. McEntee, D. Pender, D. Mulvin et al., "Current spectrum of intestinal obstruction," *British Journal of Surgery*, vol. 74, no. 11, pp. 976–980, 1987.

[6] C. K. Chou, C. W. Mark, R. H. Wu, and J. M. Chang, "Large diverticulum and volvulus of the small bowel in adults," *World Journal of Surgery*, vol. 29, no. 1, pp. 80–82, 2005.

[7] E. Valsdottir and J. H. Marks, "Volvulus: small bowel and colon," *Clinics in Colon and Rectal Surgery*, vol. 21, no. 2, pp. 91–93, 2008.

[8] K. Takeuchi, Y. Tsuzuki, T. Ando et al., "Clinical studies of strangulating small bowel obstruction," *The American Surgeon*, vol. 70, no. 1, pp. 40–44, 2004.

36

Perforated Duodenal Diverticulum Treated Conservatively: Another Two Successful Cases

Jad A. Degheili,[1] **Mohammed H. Abdallah,**[1] **Ali A. Haydar,**[2]
Ahmad Moukalled,[1] **and Ali H. Hallal**[1]

[1]*Division of General Surgery, Department of Surgery, American University of Beirut Medical Center, Riad El-Solh,
Beirut 1107 2020, Lebanon*
[2]*Division of Interventional Radiology, Department of Diagnostic Radiology, American University of Beirut Medical Center,
Riad El-Solh, Beirut 1107 2020, Lebanon*

Correspondence should be addressed to Ali H. Hallal; ah05@aub.edu.lb

Academic Editor: Dimitrios Mantas

Diverticula of the duodenum proceed those of the colon in respect to frequency of location. Incidence at times of autopsy ranges from 15 to 23%. Despite the fact that more than 90% of duodenal diverticulum cases are asymptomatic, complications if they do occur can be calamitous. Perforation is one of these rare complications. Surgical intervention has always been the mainstay for symptomatic/complicated duodenal diverticula, but with the advancement of imaging, medical treatment, and proper intensive observation, conservative treatment came forth. We hereby present two cases of duodenal diverticula, complicated by perforation and fistulization into the retroperitoneal cavity, both treated conservatively by Taylor's approach of upper gastrointestinal tract perforation. Review of other cases of duodenal diverticulum perforation has also been presented.

1. Introduction

Diverticulum of the duodenum is the second most common location after that of the large bowel. It has been on the bottom differential for chronic epigastric pain, abdominal bloating, nausea, and hyporexia, yet, almost 90% are asymptomatic. Complications if they do occur can lead to pancreatitis, hemorrhage, diverticulitis with or without perforation, and other biliopancreatic manifestations including cholidocholithiasis and cholangitis. Surgery has always been the mainstay approach for symptomatic diverticula. With the advent of new medical treatments and the high rate of morbidity postop, physicians are now trending more toward more conservative approach. What follows are another two successful cases of perforated duodenal diverticula treated conservatively.

2. Case One

An 81-year-old male was admitted to the Emergency Department with a sudden onset complaint of severe epigastric pain for the past four hours, high grade fever of 39,3°C, nausea, and vomiting. Albeit hemodynamically stable, he was tachycardic with a 105 bpm heart rate. Isolated epigastric tenderness without any signs of peritoneal irritation was elicited upon palpation. Laboratory workup revealed leucocytosis of 28,100 white blood cells with 95% left shift and lactic acid of 3.80 mmol/L. Remaining blood studies were normal, including liver function tests and amylase.

A Computed Tomography (CT) scan of the abdomen/pelvis with intravenous and oral contrast showed the presence of a duodenal diverticulum measuring 4.5×3.0 cm, surrounded by fat streaking and multiple pockets of free air (Figures 1(a) and 1(b)), a constellation of findings consistent with a perforated duodenal diverticulum.

Patient was started on total parenteral nutrition (TPN) and broad-spectrum antibiotics. His clinical status improved gradually. Gastrografin swallow imaging followed by a CT scan, one week later, revealed contrast accumulation within a duodenal pouch, corresponding to the previously described diverticulum, with absence of contrast extravasation (Figures

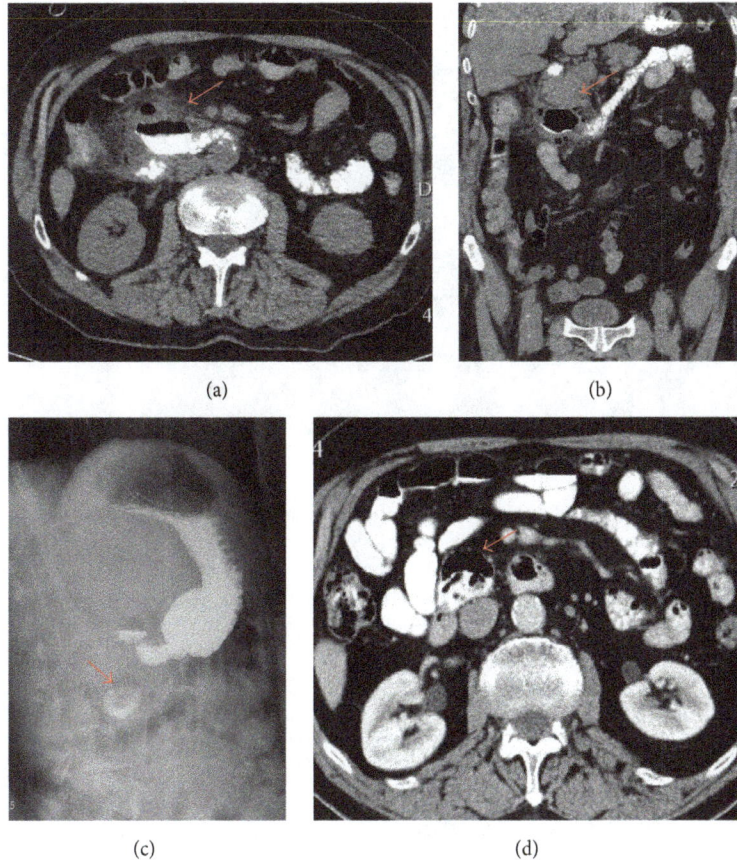

(a)

(b)

(c)

(d)

FIGURE 1: (a & b) Computed Tomography of the abdomen, with PO contrast, showing the evidence of a duodenal diverticulum with contrast extravasation, surrounded by fat stranding and air pockets (arrow), suggestive of perforation ((a) axial; (b) coronal). (c) Gastrografin swallow fluoroscopy, upon follow-up, showing the presence of contrast within the diverticulum (arrow) and absence of any extravasation. (d) Enhanced CT scan with IV and PO contrast showing the diverticulum with absence of extravasation and minimal air pocket with fat stranding (arrow).

1(c) and 1(d)). Clear fluid diet was started and advanced gradually as tolerated. He was discharged two weeks later with stable conditions.

3. Case Two

53-year-old female, with no antecedent medical or surgical history, recalled chronic episodes of epigastric pain, for which an esophagogastroduodenoscopy (EGD) and colonoscopy were done, 10 days prior to presentation, revealing a large duodenal diverticulum and multiple sigmoid diverticula. Two days after endoscopy, she underwent urgent surgical drainage of a large retroperitoneal collection with insertion of a Penrose drain within the right lower quadrant (RLQ). Upon transfer to our medical center, she was clinically stable, yet reporting occasional low-grade fever and alteration in consistency of the RLQ discharge to bilious in nature, over the past few days, with significant increase in its amount to around 1200 mL per 24 hrs. Physical examination was insignificant for any signs of peritonitis, but rather significant for biliary discharge from the RLQ drain.

Laboratory workup showed leukocytosis of 17,200 with 86% left shift; serum liver and pancreatic function tests were normal. Amylase and lipase level, from the draining fluid, were significantly elevated, measuring 482 IU/Lit and 11243 U/Lit, respectively.

Fluoroscopic guided drainogram showed delineation of a retroperitoneal collection in the RLQ, with a fistulous tract in junction with a duodenal segment (Figure 2(a)), suggestive of a high output duodenal-retroperitoneal fistula. The fistula is likely secondary to diverticular perforation, after endoscopy. Patient was started on broad-spectrum antibiotics and TPN.

Gradually, her clinical status improved, and the output drainage started to decrease to around 350 mL/day. A feeding jejunostomy tube was then inserted and enteral feeding initiated (Figure 2(b)). Follow-up CT and gastrografin swallow imaging showed the evidence of two outpouching structures within the D2 and D3 segments of the duodenum with layering of contrast (Figure 2(c)), representing two wide-neck duodenal diverticula. Neither contrast collection within the peritoneal cavity nor any persistent fistulous tract was noted. She was then started on PO diet, which was advanced as tolerated. Forty days later, she was discharged home, off any drains.

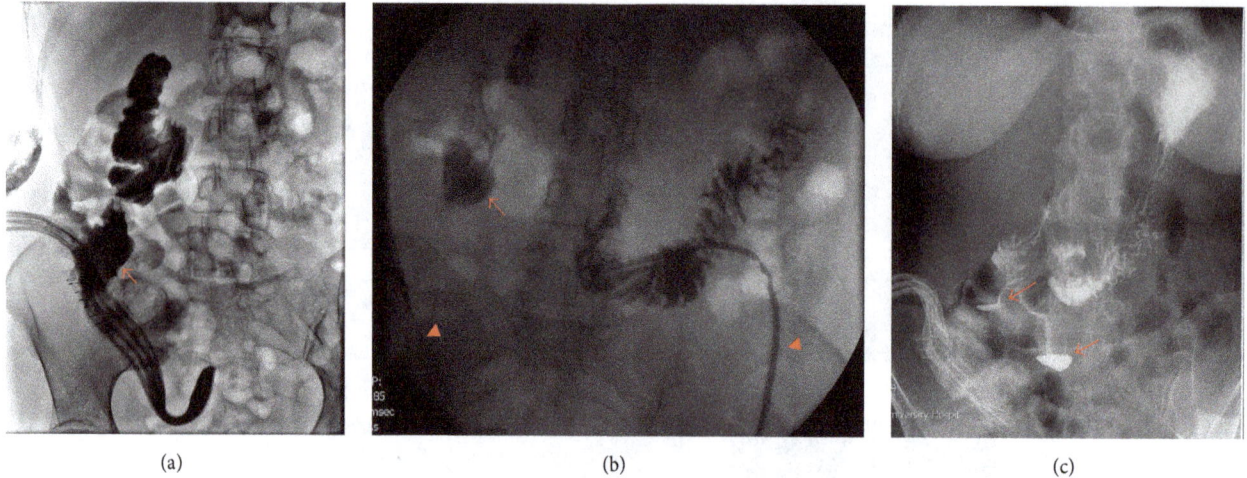

(a)   (b)   (c)

FIGURE 2: (a) Drainogram showing a fistulous tract (arrow) between the retroperitoneal cavity and the duodenum, secondary to a perforated duodenal diverticulum. (b) Gastrografin swallow fluoroscopy, upon follow-up, with absence of any contrast extravasation from within the duodenal diverticulum (arrow). Note the jejunostomy feeding tube and the retroperitoneal drain in place (arrow heads). (c) Layering of contrast, during a gastrografin swallow, into two duodenal diverticula (arrows), without any contrast extravasation, seen upon follow-up.

4. Discussion

Duodenal diverticulum (DD) has first been described by the French pathologist Pierre Chomel in 1710, containing 22 gallstones [1]. Because of its rarity and because most are asymptomatic, it has been identified in only 5–10% of patients undergoing radiological or endoscopic procedures for other etiologies and in 15–23% at times of autopsy [2]. Around 60% of these diverticula are located in the second portion of the duodenum, within 2 to 3 cm from ampulla of Vater, referred to as perivaterian or periampullary diverticula. This is followed by 30% of diverticula located in the D3 portion, and around 8% present in the D4 segment [3]. Nearly 90% of diverticula are present on the medial surface (along the pancreatic or mesenteric border) of the duodenum, with multiple diverticula present in 10–15% of patients with this entity [4].

Two types of duodenal diverticula have been identified: the most common include the acquired extraluminal pseudo-diverticulum, consisting of around 90% of duodenal diverticula, and the congenital intraluminal type which is rarer than the former type and occurs during early development [5]. 40% of cases having intraluminal diverticula are associated with other congenital malformations [6].

A surgical consensus states that intervention is only required for symptomatic duodenal diverticula, constituting only 1–5% of total cases [7]. This is attributed to the high complication rate that might occur after excision of the diverticulum [8]. For history, the first who performed diverticulectomy were Forssell and Key in 1915 [9].

Complications necessitating intervention for such diverticula can be categorized as follows: the most common are those related to biliopancreatic manifestations mainly cholidocholithiasis mostly pigmented stones [10], which may result in obstructing jaundice and cholangitis; mechanical

obstruction of the common bile duct (CBD) by the diverticulum itself (Lemmel's syndrome) [8], or even acute pancreatitis if the pancreatic duct has been obstructed. Stasis of the bile within the CBD can thus result in malabsorption of vitamin B12 and steatorrhea. A second important complication includes inflammation or diverticulitis that may or may not end up with perforation: a fearful complication. Hemorrhage is also a serious complication of DD, especially if erosion occurs at the site of the pancreaticoduodenal arcade [11].

Searching the world English literature will reveal a near 171 cases [12–15] of perforated duodenal diverticula, since the first case described by Bassett in 1907. Most of these perforations (78%) are seen within the second portion of the duodenum, mainly along the medial wall, within 2 cm from the ampulla of Vater. Diverticulitis is the most common cause of perforation representing 62%, followed by enterolithiasis (~10%) [12]. Ulceration, iatrogenic causes [16], trauma [17], or even foreign bodies [14] are all rarer causes of perforation.

It is with great difficulty to differentiate between a perforated duodenal diverticulum and perforated duodenal ulcer; the former mostly involves distal portion of duodenum, whereas the later mostly involves the duodenal bulb [18]. Other differentials include peptic ulcer disease, colitis, retrocecal appendicitis, pancreatitis, or even cholecystitis [19].

In regard to treatment of duodenal diverticula, we should note that the clinical condition and hemodynamic stability of the patient guide the treatment: whether conservative versus surgical, and with surgical, this includes several options. A great importance and attention in case one decided for a surgical option is the location of the diverticulum in relation to the biliary system especially the ampulla of Vater. This can be aided by inserting a catheter through the ampulla by doing either a cholecystostomy or cholidostomy, intraoperatively [20, 21].

Given the high morbidity and mortality for the surgical options reaching as high as 30% [8], including duodenal leak and fistulization, the option of conservative treatment has become more and more implicated. The first nonoperative management of perforated DD had been reported by Shackleton in 1963 [22]. From 1963 to 1989, five new cases have been treated conservatively, two of which had duodenocolic fistulas. From 1989 to 2011, 14 (23%) out of 61 patients with perforated DD were successfully treated without operative interventions [12], the so-called "Taylor's approach for upper GI perforation," mainly applied for duodenal ulcer perforation, which includes bowel rest with or without nasogastric tube suction, intravenous hydration and antibiotics, total parenteral nutrition, and, when needed, percutaneous catheter drainage of retroperitoneal collections [23].

In the Thorson et al. series [12] of 61 patients presenting with perforated DD, 47 (77%) underwent operative treatment versus 14 (23%) who underwent successful nonoperative management. The complication in the surgical group was reported in 17 (36%) out of 47 patients, versus only 1 (7%) complication seen in patients undergoing nonoperative management. Mortality in surgical group was 3 (6%) out of 47 versus null in the conservative group.

5. Conclusion

We hereby reported another two successful cases of conservative management of a perforated duodenal diverticulum. Surgical approach has long been the preferred option for most surgeons, yet with advancements in all medical specialties, physicians are leaning more toward less invasive approaches, given the more info we had from previous case series, aiming for avoiding any drastic postop complications.

Abbreviations

DD: Duodenal diverticulum(a)
CT: Computed Tomography
TPN: Total parenteral nutrition
EGD: Esophagogastroduodenoscopy
CBD: Common bile duct.

Authors' Contributions

Jad A. Degheili and Mohammed H. Abdallah have contributed equally to this manuscript. Both were involved in the literature review and writing of the initial draft. Ali A. Haydar is the senior radiologist, who performed the radiological procedures, and provided the images and legends, accordingly. Ahmad Moukalled assisted in literature review. Ali H. Hallal is the senior surgeon and author of the manuscript and has been involved in the revision of the different manuscript's versions.

References

[1] J. Chomel, "Report of a case of duodenal diverticulum containing gallstones," *Histoire de l'Académie Royale des Sciences (Paris)*, vol. 1710, pp. 48–50.

[2] B. M. Evers, "Small intestine," in *Sabiston Textbook of Surgery: the Biological Basis of Modern Surgical Practice*, C. M. TownSend, R. D. Beauchamp, B. M. Evers, and K. L. Mattox, Eds., pp. 1318–1319, WB Saunders Company, Philadelphia, Pa, USA, 18th edition, 2008.

[3] M. P. Vullierme, V. Vilgrain, and Y. Menu, "Imagerie des syndromes tumoraux du duodénum chez l'adulte," *Encyclopédie médico-chirurgicale*, vol. 33-155, no. A-10, article 15, 1999.

[4] T. W. Jones and K. A. Merendino, "The perplexing duodenal diverticulum," *Surgery*, vol. 48, no. 6, pp. 1068–1084, 1960.

[5] N. Oukachbi and S. Brouzes, "Management of complicated duodenal diverticula," *Journal of Visceral Surgery*, vol. 150, no. 3, pp. 173–179, 2013.

[6] M. J. D'Alessio, A. Rana, J. A. Martin, and J. Moser, "Surgical management of intraluminal duodenal diverticulum and coexisting anomalies," *Journal of the American College of Surgeons*, vol. 201, no. 1, pp. 143–148, 2005.

[7] I. A. Chitambar and C. Springs, "Duodenal diverticula," *Surgery*, vol. 33, no. 5, pp. 768–791, 1953.

[8] C. M. Teven, E. Grossman, K. K. Roggin, and J. B. Matthews, "Surgical management of pancreaticobiliary disease associated with juxtapapillary duodenal diverticula: case series and review of the literature," *Journal of Gastrointestinal Surgery*, vol. 16, no. 7, pp. 1436–1441, 2012.

[9] G. Forssell and E. Key, "Ein divertikel an der pars descendens duodeni mittels Röntgenuntersuchung diagnostiziert und operativ entfernt," *Fortschr. A. d. Geb. der Röntgenstrahlen*, vol. 24, pp. 48–57, 1916.

[10] J. Fritsch, F. Prat, G. Pelletier, and C. Buffet, "Anomalies anatomiques de la région papillaire et pathologie biliopancréatique," *Gastroentérologie Clinique et Biologique*, vol. 23, pp. 717–729, 1999.

[11] H. T. Debas and S. H. Carvajal, "Surgical management of duodenal diverticula," in *Surgery of the Upper Gastrointestinal Tract*, pp. 537–547, Springer Science, 1994.

[12] C. M. Thorson, P. S. Paz Ruiz, R. A. Roeder, D. Sleeman, and V. J. Casillas, "The perforated duodenal diverticulum," *Archives of Surgery*, vol. 147, no. 1, pp. 81–88, 2012.

[13] I. Barillaro, V. Grassi, A. De Sol et al., "Endoscopic rendez-vous after damage control surgery in treatment of retroperitoneal abscess from perforated duodenal diverticulum: a techinal note and literature review," *World Journal of Emergency Surgery*, vol. 8, no. 1, article 26, 2013.

[14] J. Favre Rizzo, E. López-Tomassetti Fernández, J. Ceballos Esparragón, L. Santana Cabrera, and J. R. Hernández Hernández, "Duodenal diverticulum perforated by foreign body," *Revista Española de Enfermedades Digestivas*, vol. 105, no. 6, pp. 368–369, 2013.

[15] A. Rossetti, B. N. Christian, B. Pascal, D. Stephane, and M. Philippe, "Perforated duodenal diverticulum, a rare complication of a common pathology: a seven-patient case series," *World Journal of Gastrointestinal Surgery*, vol. 5, no. 3, pp. 47–50, 2013.

[16] A. Fichera and F. Michelassi, "Diverticular disease of the small bowel," in *Current Surgical Therapy*, J. L. Cameron, Ed., pp. 124–126, Mosby, St. Louis, MO, SA, 8th edition, 2004.

[17] M. J. Metcalfe, T. G. Rashid, and R. L. R. Bird, "Isolated perforation of a duodenal diverticulum following blunt abdominal

trauma," *Journal of Emergencies, Trauma and Shock*, vol. 3, no. 1, pp. 79–81, 2010.

[18] J. T. Ames, M. P. Federle, and K. M. Pealer, "Perforated duodenal diverticulum: clinical and imaging findings in eight patients," *Abdominal Imaging*, vol. 34, no. 2, pp. 135–139, 2009.

[19] B. Coulier, P. Maldague, A. Bourgeois, and B. Broze, "Diverticulitis of the small bowel: CT diagnosis," *Abdominal Imaging*, vol. 32, no. 2, pp. 228–233, 2007.

[20] D. O. J. Volchok, T. Massimi, S. Wilkins, and E. Curletti, "Duodenal Diverticulum: case report of a perforated extraluminal diverticulum containing ectopic pancreatic tissue," *Archives of Surgery*, vol. 144, no. 2, pp. 188–190, 2009.

[21] G. Miller, C. Mueller, D. Yim et al., "Perforated duodenal diverticulitis: a report of three cases," *Digestive Surgery*, vol. 22, no. 3, pp. 198–202, 2005.

[22] M. E. Shackleton, "Perforation of a duodenal diverticulum with massive retroperitoneal emphysema," *The New Zealand Medical Journal*, vol. 62, pp. 93–94, 1963.

[23] R. M. Gore, G. G. Ghahremani, M. D. Kirsch, A. A. Nemcek, and M. P. Karoll, "Diverticulitis of the duodenum: clinical and radiological manifestations of seven cases," *The American Journal of Gastroenterology*, vol. 86, no. 8, pp. 981–985, 1991.

37

Spontaneous Intramural Duodenal Hematoma: Pancreatitis, Obstructive Jaundice, and Upper Intestinal Obstruction

Chalerm Eurboonyanun,[1] **Kulyada Somsap,**[2] **Somchai Ruangwannasak,**[1] **and Anan Sripanaskul**[1]

[1]*Department of Surgery, Faculty of Medicine, Khon Kaen University, Khon Kaen 40002, Thailand*
[2]*Department of Radiology, Faculty of Medicine, Khon Kaen University, Khon Kaen 40002, Thailand*

Correspondence should be addressed to Chalerm Eurboonyanun; chaleu@kku.ac.th

Academic Editor: Reza Mofidi

Nontraumatic intramural duodenal hematoma can cause upper gastrointestinal tract obstruction, upper gastrointestinal hemorrhage, jaundice, and pancreatitis and may be present in patients with normal coagulation. However the pathogenesis of the condition and its relationship with acute pancreatitis remain unknown. We present a case of spontaneous intramural duodenal hematoma and a case of successful nonoperative treatments.

1. Introduction

Intramural duodenal hematoma was first described by McLauchlan in 1838 [1]. Intramural duodenal hematoma usually occurs secondary to blunt abdominal injury [2, 3]. Spontaneous intramural duodenal hematoma has been associated with coagulopathy, coagulating drugs, and endoscopic procedures [4–8]. However, there are many reports regarding intramural duodenal hematoma's association, with acute pancreatitis and pancreatic malignancy [9–13]. However, the association between intramural duodenal hematoma and acute pancreatitis is still unclear. In this paper, we discuss a case in which a patient presented with obstructive jaundice, upper gastrointestinal obstruction, and upper gastrointestinal hemorrhage complicated by acute pancreatitis.

2. Ethical Consideration

This retrospective case report was approved by the Ethics Committee for Human Research based on the declaration of Helsinki and the ICH good clinical practice guidelines. Clinical data were obtained by reviewing medical records.

3. Case Report

A 27-year-old Thai male was admitted to the hospital after experiencing one day of epigastric pain, hematemesis, and jaundice without evidence of previous trauma. His symptoms also resulted in upper gastrointestinal obstruction, which caused 2 kilograms of weight loss (70 to 68 kilograms) in one week. He had no history of warfarin or aspirin therapy. However, he was a heavy drinker consuming 500 mL of liquor per day.

A physical examination revealed jaundice and mild tenderness over the epigastric region. Blood tests showed a hemoglobin level of 12.3 g/dL, white blood cell count of 13,960/μL, platelet count of 669,000/μL, prothrombin time of 12.10 sec, INR of 1.14, activated partial thromboplastin time of 31.40 sec, lipase level of 477 U/L, and total bilirubin level of 12.1 mg/d.

Contrast-enhanced abdominal computed tomography revealed hematoma in the whole duodenum with duodenitis. Localized acute pancreatitis was found in the uncinate process and head of the pancreas with a small pancreatic pseudocyst causing distal common bile duct obstruction with biliary dilatation (Figures 1(a)-1(b)).

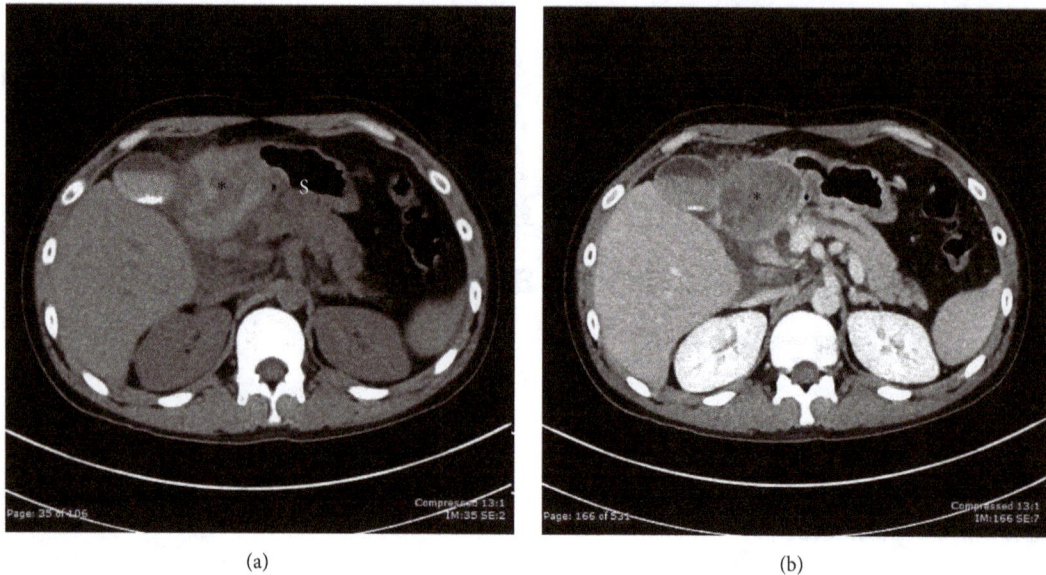

(a)   (b)

FIGURE 1: (a) Noncontrast CT scan shows a heterogeneously high-attenuation mass (∗) along the course of 1st, 2nd, and 3rd part of duodenum, which is compatible with duodenal hematoma. Note the surrounding fat stranding. S = stomach. (b) Contrast-enhanced CT shows the lack of enhancement within the mass (asterisk). Note the displacement of gas in gastric lumen secondary to mass.

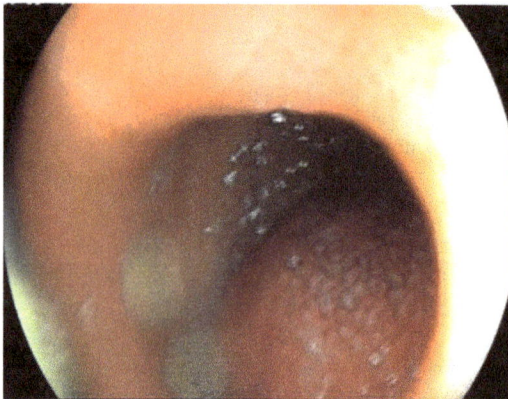

FIGURE 2: Submucosal swelling with erythematous surface extending from the duodenal bulb to the 3rd part of the duodenum causing partial duodenal obstruction: suspected intramural duodenal hematoma.

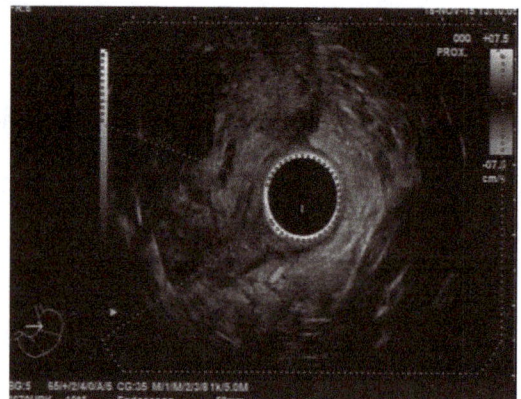

FIGURE 3: Endoscopic ultrasonography revealed avascular a heteroechoic submucosal mass at the posterolateral wall of the duodenum.

Esophagogastroduodenoscopy showed bulging, inflammation, and swelling of mucosa at the posterolateral wall of second to third part of the duodenum with partial obstruction of the duodenal lumen (Figure 2). Endoscopic ultrasonography showed a heteroechoic mass at the posterolateral wall of the duodenum (Figure 3).

The patient was diagnosed with acute pancreatitis, intramural duodenal hematoma, acute cholangitis, and upper gastrointestinal obstruction. He was conservatively treated with intravenous antibiotics and fluid replacement therapy, restricting the oral intake of food/liquids.

17 days after admission the patient was able to consume a low residual diet orally without abdominal discomfort. His jaundice had also improved. He discontinued intravenous antibiotics after 10 days of therapy. He was discharged on the 21st day after admission.

Three months after admission follow-up esophagogastroduodenoscopy showed normal duodenal mucosa with a mild narrowing of the lumen at the second part of the duodenum. Magnetic resonance cholangiopancreatography revealed a distal common bile duct obstruction and revealed that the intramural duodenal hematoma, pancreatitis of head, and uncinate process had resolved (Figures 4(a)-4(b)).

4. Discussion

Spontaneous intramural duodenal hematoma is usually associated with coagulation abnormalities resulting from anticoagulating drugs [4–7]. If spontaneous intramural duodenal hematoma occurs in patients with normal coagulation, pancreatic diseases should be investigated [9–14].

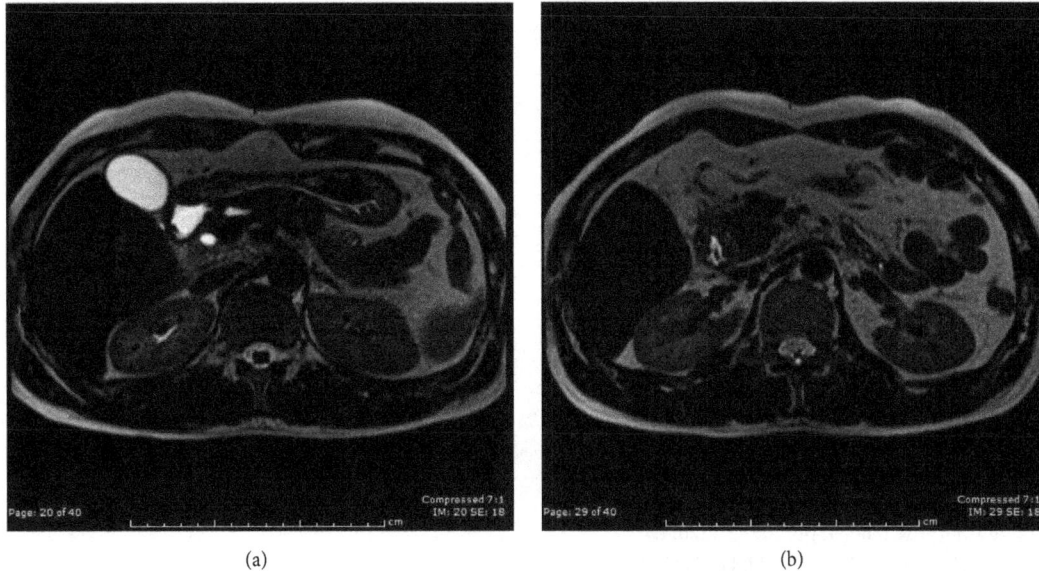

(a)   (b)

FIGURE 4: A follow-up MRI after 3 months of conservative treatment shows a nearly complete resolution of the duodenal hematoma.

In cases of spontaneous intramural small bowel hematoma, the rates of abdominal pain and emesis are high (84.6–100%). However, hematemesis and fever are only occasionally present (15.3–23.1%) [6]. In this case, the patient presented with abdominal pain, hematemesis, and jaundice. The only positive findings upon physical examination were jaundice and mild tenderness over the epigastric region.

CT scans, gastroduodenoscopy, and endoscopic ultrasonography revealed evidence of duodenal hematoma, pancreatitis, biliary obstruction, and a gallstone.

He was successfully treated using conservative methods. Although there has been a case report of endoscopic decompression for intramural duodenal hematoma with gastric outlet obstruction to relieve the symptoms of the obstruction [15], this procedure requires further investigation.

In this case, the disease may have developed from either alcoholic pancreatitis due to patient's history of heavy drinking or biliary pancreatitis, as there was evidence of a gallstone. It is also possible that spontaneous intramural duodenal hematoma of unknown origin caused the acute pancreatitis. But pancreatitis is likely to be the leading cause in this case, based on the patient's history of alcohol consumption and evidence of a gallstone without any coagulation abnormalities. However, it is difficult to explain the true pathophysiology.

In conclusion, the patient who presented with spontaneous intramural duodenal hematoma with acute pancreatitis with clinical jaundice, upper gastrointestinal obstruction, and upper gastrointestinal hemorrhage was able to be treated conservatively. However, the relationship between the disease and pathophysiology remains unclear.

Competing Interests

The authors declare that there is no conflict of interests regarding the publication of this paper.

Acknowledgments

The authors would like to thank Mr. Dylan Southard and the Research Affairs for helping with the English in this manuscript.

References

[1] J. McLauchlan, "False aneurysmal tumour occupying nearly the whole of the duodenum," *The Lancet*, pp. 2203–2205, 1838.

[2] K. Hayashi, S. Futagawa, S. Kozaki, K. Hirao, and Z. Hombo, "Ultrasound and CT diagnosis of intramural duodenal hematoma," *Pediatric Radiology*, vol. 18, no. 2, pp. 167–168, 1988.

[3] T. C. Jewett Jr., V. Caldarola, M. P. Karp, J. E. Allen, and D. R. Cooney, "Intramural hematoma of the duodenum," *Archives of Surgery*, vol. 123, no. 1, pp. 54–58, 1988.

[4] C. Polat, A. Dervisoglu, H. Guven et al., "Anticoagulant-induced intramural intestinal hematoma," *American Journal of Emergency Medicine*, vol. 21, no. 3, pp. 208–211, 2003.

[5] C.-Y. Tseng, J.-S. Fan, S.-C. Yang et al., "Anticoagulant-induced intramural intestinal hemorrhage," *The American Journal of Emergency Medicine*, vol. 28, no. 8, pp. 937–940, 2010.

[6] M. A. Abbas, J. M. Collins, K. W. Olden, and K. A. Kelly, "Spontaneous intramural small-bowel hematoma: clinical presentation and long-term outcome," *Archives of Surgery*, vol. 137, no. 3, pp. 306–310, 2002.

[7] M. A. Abbas, J. M. Collins, and K. W. Olden, "Spontaneous intramural small-bowel hematoma: imaging findings and outcome," *American Journal of Roentgenology*, vol. 179, no. 6, pp. 1389–1394, 2002.

[8] C. Grasshof, A. Wolf, F. Neuwirth, and C. Posovszky, "Intramural duodenal haematoma after endoscopic biopsy: case report and review of the literature," *Case Reports in Gastroenterology*, vol. 6, no. 1, pp. 5–14, 2012.

[9] N. Veloso, P. Amaro, M. Ferreira, J. M. Romãozinho, and C. Sofia, "Acute pancreatitis associated with a nontraumatic, intramural duodenal hematoma," *Endoscopy*, vol. 45, supplement 2, pp. E51–E52, 2013.

[10] K. Shiozawa, M. Watanabe, Y. Igarashi, Y. Matsukiyo, T. Matsui, and Y. Sumino, "Acute pancreatitis secondary to intramural duodenal hematoma: case report and literature review," *World Journal of Radiology*, vol. 2, no. 7, pp. 283–288, 2010.

[11] J. D. Silva, N. Veloso, R. Godinho, L. Gonçalves, I. Medeiros, and C. Viveiros, "Fatal acute pancreatitis following sclerosis of a bleeding duodenal ulcer complicated by an intramural duodenal hematoma," *Revista Espanola de Enfermedades Digestivas*, vol. 104, no. 11, pp. 603–604, 2012.

[12] C.-M. Chang, H.-H. Huang, and C.-K. How, "Acute pancreatitis with an intramural duodenal hematoma," *Internal Medicine*, vol. 54, no. 7, pp. 755–757, 2015.

[13] T. Khurana, "Intramural duodenal hematoma with acute pancreatitis in a patient with an overt pancreatic malignancy," *ACG Case Reports Journal*, vol. 1, no. 4, pp. 209–211, 2014.

[14] W. R. Jones, W. J. Hardin, J. T. Davis, and J. D. Hardy, "Intramural hematoma of the duodenum: a review of the literature and case report," *Annals of Surgery*, vol. 173, no. 4, pp. 534–544, 1971.

[15] J. Y. Lee, J. S. Chung, and T. H. Kim, "Successful endoscopic decompression for intramural duodenal hematoma with gastric outlet obstruction complicating acute pancreatitis," *Clinical Endoscopy*, vol. 45, no. 3, pp. 202–204, 2012.

38

Syncope with Surprise: An Unexpected Finding of Huge Gastric Diverticulum

Mauro Podda, Jenny Atzeni, Antonio Messina Campanella, Alessandra Saba, and Adolfo Pisanu

Department of Surgical Science, General, Emergency and Laparoscopic Surgery, University of Cagliari, Blocco G, 09042 Monserrato, Italy

Correspondence should be addressed to Mauro Podda; mauropodda@ymail.com

Academic Editor: Shin-ichi Kosugi

A gastric diverticulum is a pouch protruding from the gastric wall. The vague long clinical history ranging between dyspepsia, postprandial fullness, and upper gastrointestinal bleeding makes this condition a diagnostic challenge. We present a case of large gastric diverticulum that has been diagnosed during clinical investigations for suspected cardiovascular issues in a patient admitted at the medical ward for syncope. A 51-year-old man presented to the medical department due to a syncopal episode occurring while he was resting on the beach after having his lunch, with concomitant vague epimesogastric gravative pain without any other symptom. A diagnosis of neuromediated syncopal episode was made by the cardiologist. Due to the referred epimesogastric pain, an abdominal ultrasound scan was carried out, showing perisplenic fluid. A CT scan of the abdomen was performed to exclude splenic lesions. The CT scan revealed a large diverticulum protruding from the gastric fundus. The upper gastrointestinal endoscopy visualized a large diverticular neck situated in the posterior wall of the gastric fundus, partially filled by undigested food. The patient underwent surgery, with an uneventful postoperative course. Histologic examination showed a full-thickness stomach specimen, indicative of a congenital diverticulum. At the 2nd month of follow-up, the patient was asymptomatic.

1. Introduction

A gastric diverticulum (GD) is a pouch protruding from the gastric wall, first described by Moebius in 1661 and later by Roax in 1774 [1]. Although it is the least common diverticulum of the gastrointestinal tract, GD has similar characteristics to duodenal, jejunal, and colonic diverticula [2]. It is a rare and uncommon clinical condition, with a prevalence of 0.03–0.1% in contrast upper gastrointestinal radiographs, 0.01–0.1% in upper gastrointestinal endoscopy, and 0.03–0.3% in autoptical reports [3]. Incidence is equally distributed between males and females. Most symptomatic diverticula are found in patients between 20 and 60 years of age [4]. Typical diverticula are 1–3 cm in diameter, but larger types can occur [5]. The lack of pathognomonic symptoms and the vague long clinical history ranging between dyspepsia, postprandial fullness, and upper gastrointestinal bleeding make this condition a diagnostic challenge for physicians and surgeons [6]. We present the case of a large GD that has

been diagnosed during clinical investigations for suspected cardiovascular issues in a patient admitted at the medical ward for syncope.

2. Case Report

A 51-year-old Caucasian policeman was admitted at the medical department of the University of Cagliari Hospital (Italy) due to a syncopal episode occurring while he was resting on the beach after eating his lunch, with concomitant vague epimesogastric gravative pain without any other symptoms. In the anamnesis he reported a previous similar episode, occurring 10 years earlier, during a walk in a shopping center after having a carbonated beverage (cola). For this reason, he underwent cardiovascular and neurological investigations. The electrocardiogram, echocardiogram, and stress test on the treadmill were unremarkable. The head-up tilt-table test reproduced the original symptoms, with objective evidence of a sudden drop in blood pressure without a decrease in heart

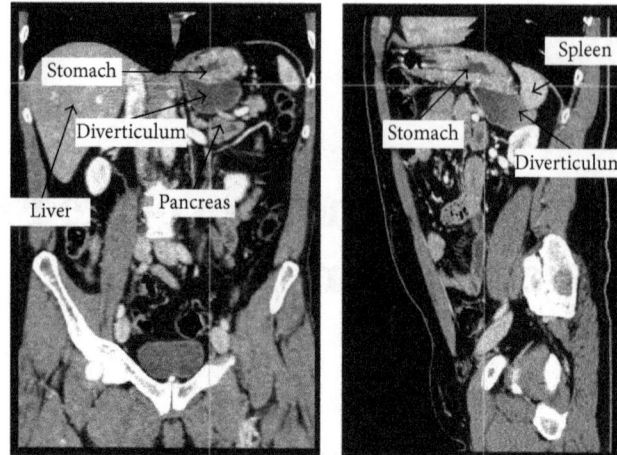

FIGURE 1: Arterial phase CT scan (frontal and sagittal planes) showing a large diverticulum of the size of 52 × 68 × 72 millimeters protruding from the gastric fundus, with fluid content. The retroperitoneal location of the pouch is well visible in the sagittal scan, as well as its tight adhesions with the inferomedial surface of the spleen, the ipsilateral adrenal gland, and the upper posterior surface of the body and tail of the pancreas.

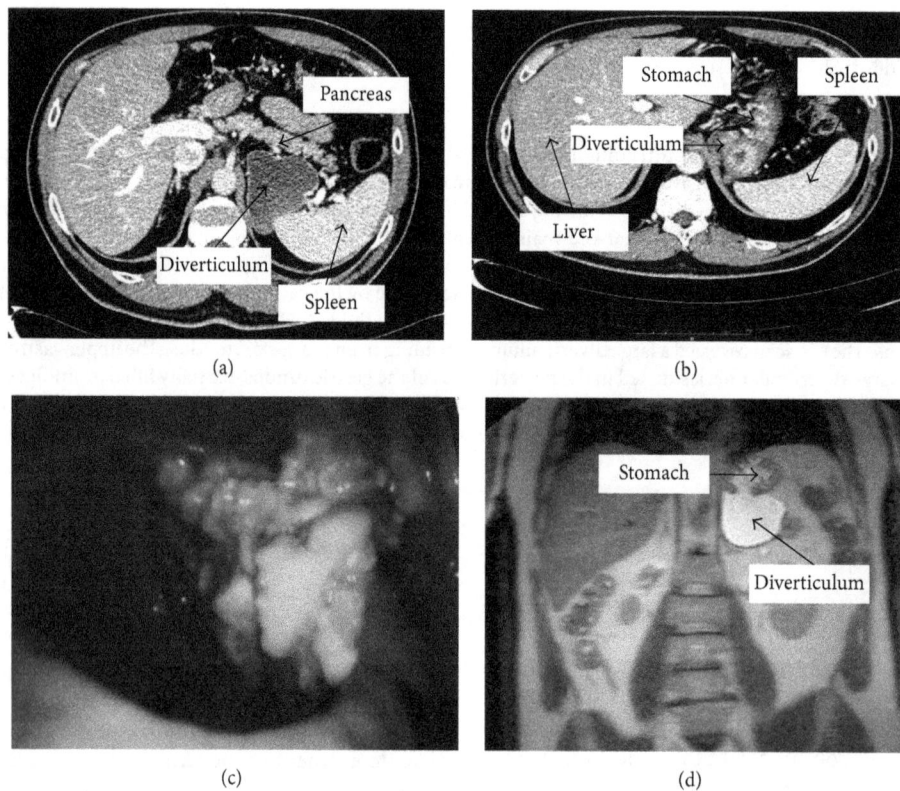

(a)

(b)

(c)

(d)

FIGURE 2: Arterial phase CT scan, transverse planes (a-b). Endoscopic image of a large diverticular neck (30 × 20 millimeters) situated in the posterior wall of the gastric fundus, with the pouch partially filled by undigested food (c). T2-weighted MRI image (d).

rate. Therefore, a final diagnosis of neuromediated syncopal episode was carried out. Due to the referred epimesogastric pain, an abdominal US scan was carried out, showing a small amount of perisplenic fluid. A CT scan and an MRI scan of the abdomen were performed in order to exclude splenic lesions. The CT scan revealed a large diverticulum of the size of 52 × 68 × 72 millimeters protruding from the gastric fundus showing tight adhesions with the inferomedial surface of the spleen, the ipsilateral adrenal gland, and the upper posterior surface of the body and tail of the pancreas (Figures 1 and 2). The patient was therefore referred to our surgical team. When a deeper anamnesis was carried out, the

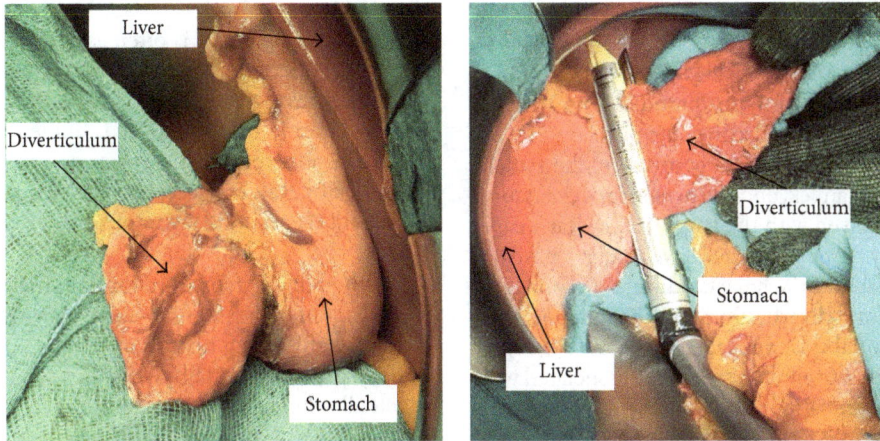

FIGURE 3: Intraoperative view. The gastrocolic ligament and the short gastric vessels have been released and the stomach is rotated to expose the superior-posterior wall. The adhesions between the diverticulum and the posterior surface of the pancreatic body have been dissected. Exposure of the neck of the diverticulum for preparation of diverticulectomy and resection of the neck with the linear stapler.

patient reported a two-year symptomatology characterized by recurrent dyspepsia, postprandial fullness, and frequent burping with fetor ex ore.

On physical examination the hemodynamics were stable, and the patient had a mild epigastric tenderness. Abdominal and thoracic examination was otherwise unremarkable. Blood tests and chest and abdominal X-rays were normal. The upper gastrointestinal endoscopy visualized a large diverticular neck (30 × 20 millimeters) situated in the posterior wall of the gastric fundus. After further exploration, a pouch partially filled by undigested food was discovered (Figure 2). Due to the large volume of the diverticulum and its retroperitoneal location patient underwent open surgery. The resection of the gastric diverticulum was performed using an Echelon Flex Powered Endopath 60 mm gold reload (Ethicon Endo-Surgery, Cincinnati, Ohio, USA). The stapler line was oversewn by a running suture with resorbable coated polyclacin 2-0 suture (Vicryl™, Ethicon) (Figure 3). The patient had an uneventful postoperative course. On postoperative day one, a barium study showed normal anatomy and no leaks. He was placed on a fluid diet on postoperative day one and regular diet on postoperative day three. The patient was discharged on postoperative day five. Histologic examination showed a full-thickness stomach specimen, indicative of a congenital diverticulum, with slight chronic inflammation and diffuse hyperplasia and hypertrophy of the oxyntic cells. At the 2nd month of follow-up appointment, both epigastric pain and halitosis had disappeared.

3. Discussion

According to the hypothesis suggested by Schmidt and Walters, GD can by classified into congenital and acquired types, with congenital types being more common [5, 7, 8]. As reported in the literature, congenital gastric diverticula are true diverticula, mostly located in the posterior wall of the fundus, 2 cm below the oesophagogastric junction and 3 cm from the lesser curve (70%). They contain all layers of the gastric wall, and it is believed that they occur as a result of splitting of the longitudinal muscular fibers at the cardia level, leaving only circular muscle fibers in the gastric wall through which a diverticulum can develop during the fetal period [9, 10]. Conversely, false diverticula are acquired, less common and typically located in the antrum. Acquired diverticula can develop either with a traction or pulsion mechanism and usually present with a background history of chronic gastrointestinal inflammatory disease, such as peptic ulcer, pancreatitis, malignancy, or gastric outlet obstruction [5, 8, 11, 12]. The development of congenital GD within the retroperitoneal space can be explained by the analysis of the embryogenesis of the stomach in the period between the 20th and the 50th day of gestation. At this time, a 90° rotation of the stomach, together with the duodenum, the pancreas, and the dorsal mesentery, occurs and a diverticulum of the posterior wall of the gastric fundus could hypothetically herniate through an area of dorsal mesentery before its fusion with the left posterior body wall. Therefore, with further extension, the diverticulum could project posterior to the pancreas [6, 13].

Being a rare and mostly asymptomatic condition, a high clinical index of suspicion is needed to diagnose and effectively manage patients with GD [6]. When symptoms occur, they can vary and imitate those of other common upper gastrointestinal disorders. Indeed, the most common complaint reported by symptomatic patients is a vague upper abdominal pain (18–30%), possibly due to food retention inside the diverticulum and subsequent distension of the pouch [14]. Other complaints include vomiting, vague sensation of fullness or discomfort in the upper abdomen, dysphagia, eructation, and halitosis, which could be explained by the bacterial overgrowth on the food retained inside the GD [15, 16]. Moreover, this condition can evolve to dramatic scenarios, such as massive bleeding or perforation following the digestive process of the retained food by gastric juices. This causes possible ulceration of the mucosa or complicated diverticulitis [17]. Two cases of invasion with adenocarcinoma in gastric diverticulum were also reported in the literature [18, 19].

GD is considered as a great mime: Palmer found that in 30 of 49 symptomatic patients with GD the symptomatology was ascribable to other gastrointestinal diseases [20].

Our patient presented with postprandial loss of consciousness, with no remarkable cardiogenic problem proved. Carbonated beverages ingestion, as reported by the patient before his first syncopal attack, and the presence of eructation have already been involved with the triggering in some cases of neuromediated syncope [21]. Moreover, many gastroesophageal diseases such as achalasia, diffuse oesophageal spasm, hiatal hernia, and diverticulum have been reported to be the trigger of syncopal episodes called "Swallow Syncope," which is defined as a dysautonomic syndrome associated with intense vagal afferent activation [21–25].

In the majority of cases GD are incidental findings during the investigation of their common symptoms. The condition can be diagnosed by endoscopic or radiological examinations. Upper gastrointestinal contrast radiographic studies, as well as oesophagogastroduodenoscopy, are the most performed diagnostic investigations. However, it is worth emphasizing that, especially in case of diverticulum with a narrow neck, they can give false negative results. Indeed, as reported by Palmer in his review, 5% of GD are missed during contrast radiographic study [20].

Upper gastrointestinal endoscopy is the gold standard investigation to achieve a precise diagnosis. It useful not only to confirm the location and the size of the pouch, but also to perform a biopsy if a concurrent pathology is found. This diagnostic tool may be able to reproduce symptoms with distension of the diverticulum, indicating which patients would benefit from a resection [5, 12].

More authors have reported their experience on the use of CT scan as part of the diagnostic work-up for patients with gastric diverticulum. However, CT and/or MRI findings in GD have been published only as case reports in the literature [3, 26–28]. CT and MRI scans can provide a complete overview on the relationships between the diverticulum and the pancreatic gland, the spleen, and the left adrenal gland. These diagnostic tools are necessary during the planning of the surgical strategy, as proven by our case report.

The appropriate treatment for both symptomatic and asymptomatic GD is still a matter of debate. It is well documented that there is no specific therapeutic strategy for asymptomatic diverticula [10, 20].

Although Proton Pump Inhibitors (PPIs) have been suggested to alleviate the vague symptoms of gastric diverticulum, this treatment is not able to resolve the underlying pathology. Endoscopy can play an important role in the management of active upper gastrointestinal bleeding due to GD, as reported by Chen et al. [2]. Surgical resection is the recommended approach when the diverticulum is large (>4 cm in diameter), patients are still symptomatic after PPIs administration, and complications such as bleeding, perforation, or suspicion of malignancy occur [6]. Both open and laparoscopic resections achieve good results. Since Fine in 1998 described the first successful laparoscopic resection of a large proximal gastric diverticulum, this approach is now considered safe and feasible, with excellent outcomes [29].

Access to the retrogastric space by dividing the gastrocolic/gastrosplenic ligament is often easier to achieve laparoscopically in experienced hands, although in other cases the minimally invasive approach can be challenging because the diverticulum is often collapsed, hidden in the splenic bed, or deeply adherent to the posterior surface of the pancreas [6, 9, 20, 30]. Rate of success is very high, with over two-thirds of patients remaining symptom-free after surgical resection [20].

Although GD remains a rarity in the etiology of abdominal pain, a high index of suspicion should be kept in mind for patients with a long history of vague upper abdominal pain and dyspepsia, especially when not subsided with PPIs and when all other more common diseases, such as gastritis and gastric cancer, have been ruled out.

Abbreviations

GD: Gastric diverticulum
CT: Computed tomography
MRI: Magnetic resonance imaging
US: Ultrasound
PPI: Proton Pump Inhibitors.

Competing Interests

The authors declare that there are no competing interests regarding the publication of this paper.

Authors' Contributions

Mauro Podda, M.D., contributed to conception, design, and draft of the paper. Jenny Atzeni, M.D., contributed to conception, draft, and revision of the paper. Antonio Messina Campanella, M.D., contributed to writing the paper and doing literature review. Alessandra Saba, M.D., contributed to writing the paper and doing literature review. Adolfo Pisanu, M.D. and Ph.D., contributed to revision of the paper critically for important intellectual content. All authors read and approved the final paper.

Acknowledgments

The authors thank Dr. Giorgio Carta, Ph.D. (Trinity College, Dublin, Ireland), and Ms. Tanya Marie Castagna (University of Maryland, USA), for revising the English. This study was supported by a grant from the University of Cagliari, Italy (CAR 2015).

References

[1] W. R. Moses, "Diverticula of the stomach," *Archives of Surgery*, vol. 52, pp. 59–65, 1946.

[2] J.-H. Chen, W.-C. Su, C.-Y. Chang, and H. Lin, "Education and imaging. Gastrointestinal: bleeding gastric diverticulum," *Journal of Gastroenterology and Hepatology*, vol. 23, no. 2, article 336, 2008.

[3] N. L. Simstein, "Congenital gastric anomalies," *The American Surgeon*, vol. 52, no. 5, pp. 264–268, 1986.

[4] I. Gockel, D. Thomschke, and D. Lorenz, "Gastrointestinal: gastric diverticula," *Journal of Gastroenterology and Hepatology*, vol. 19, no. 2, p. 227, 2004.

[5] V. M. Wolters, P. G. J. Nikkels, D. C. Van Der Zee et al., "A gastric diverticulum containing pancreatic tissue and presenting as congenital double pylorus: case report and review of the literature," *Journal of Pediatric Gastroenterology and Nutrition*, vol. 33, no. 1, pp. 89–91, 2001.

[6] F. Rashid, A. Aber, and S. Y. Iftikhar, "A review on gastric diverticulum," *World Journal of Emergency Surgery*, vol. 7, article 1, 2012.

[7] H. W. Schmidt and W. Walters, "Diverticula of stomach," *Surgery, Gynecology & Obstetrics*, vol. 60, p. 106, 1935.

[8] D. A. Rodeberg, S. Zaheer, C. R. Moir, and M. B. Ishitani, "Gastric diverticulum: a series of four pediatric patients," *Journal of Pediatric Gastroenterology and Nutrition*, vol. 34, no. 5, pp. 564–567, 2002.

[9] L. Marano, G. Reda, R. Porfidia et al., "Large symptomatic gastric diverticula: two case reports and a brief review of literature," *World Journal of Gastroenterology*, vol. 19, no. 36, pp. 6114–6117, 2013.

[10] N. E. Reich, "Gastric diverticula," *The American Journal of Digestive Diseases*, vol. 8, no. 3, pp. 70–76, 1941.

[11] M. Meeroff, J. R. Gollán, and J. C. Meeroff, "Gastric diverticulum," *The American Journal of Gastroenterology*, vol. 47, no. 3, pp. 189–203, 1967.

[12] D. Anaise, D. L. Brand, N. L. Smith, and H. S. Soroff, "Pitfalls in the diagnosis and treatment of a symptomatic gastric diverticulum," *Gastrointestinal Endoscopy*, vol. 30, no. 1, pp. 28–30, 1984.

[13] P. Mohan, M. Ananthavadivelu, and J. Venkataraman, "Gastric diverticulum," *Canadian Medical Association Journal*, vol. 182, no. 5, article E226, 2010.

[14] J. W. Kilkenny, "Gastric diverticula: it's time for an updated review," *Gastroenterology*, vol. 108, no. 4, Article ID A1226, 1995.

[15] F. Rashid, R. Singh, A. Cole, and S. Y. Iftikhar, "Troublesome belching with fetor odour," *Gut*, vol. 59, no. 3, pp. 310–324, 2010.

[16] S. C. Donkervoort, L. C. Baak, J. L. Blaauwgeers, and M. F. Gerhards, "Laparoscopic resection of a symptomatic gastric diverticulum: a minimally invasive solution," *Journal of the Society of Laparoendoscopic Surgeons*, vol. 10, no. 4, pp. 525–527, 2006.

[17] S. Elliott, A. D. Sandler, J. J. Meehan, and J. P. Lawrence, "Surgical treatment of a gastric diverticulum in an adolescent," *Journal of Pediatric Surgery*, vol. 41, no. 8, pp. 1467–1469, 2006.

[18] F.-T. Fork, E. Toth, and C. Lindström, "Early gastric cancer in a fundic diverticulum," *Endoscopy*, vol. 30, no. 1, article S2, 1998.

[19] Y. Adachi, M. Mori, Y. Haraguchi, and K. Sugimachi, "Gastric diverticulum invaded by gastric adenocarcinoma," *The American Journal of Gastroenterology*, vol. 82, no. 8, p. 807, 1987.

[20] E. D. Palmer, "Gatric diverticula," *International Abstracts of Surgery*, vol. 92, pp. 417–428, 1951.

[21] B. Olshansky, "A pepsi challenge," *The New England Journal of Medicine*, vol. 340, no. 25, article 2006, 1999.

[22] T. Maekawa, M. Suematsu, T. Shimada, G. O. Masayoshi, and T. Shimada, "Unusual swallow syncope caused by huge hiatal hernia," *Internal Medicine*, vol. 41, no. 3, pp. 199–201, 2002.

[23] A. N. Kalloo, J. H. Lewis, K. Maher, and S. B. Benjamin, "Swallowing. An unusual cause of syncope," *Digestive Diseases and Sciences*, vol. 34, no. 7, pp. 1117–1120, 1989.

[24] B. J. Carey, J. de Caestecker, and R. B. Panerai, "More on deglutition syncope," *The New England Journal of Medicine*, vol. 341, no. 17, pp. 1316–1317, 1999.

[25] A. Farb and S. A. Valenti, "Swallow syncope," *Maryland Medical Journal*, vol. 48, no. 4, pp. 151–154, 1999.

[26] A. N. Schwartz, R. C. Goiney, and D. O. Graney, "Gastric diverticulum simulating an adrenal mass: CT appearance and embryogenesis," *American Journal of Roentgenology*, vol. 146, no. 3, pp. 553–554, 1986.

[27] T. Tsitsias and J. G. Finch, "Gastric diverticulum of the prepyloric region: a rare presentation of gastric diverticulum," *Case Reports in Gastroenterology*, vol. 6, no. 1, pp. 150–154, 2012.

[28] M. O. Muis, K. Leitao, J. Havnen, T. B. Glomsaker, and J. A. Søreide, "Gastric diverticulum and halitosis—a case for surgery?" *International Journal of Surgery Case Reports*, vol. 5, no. 7, pp. 431–433, 2014.

[29] A. Fine, "Laparoscopic resection of a large proximal gastric diverticulum," *Gastrointestinal Endoscopy*, vol. 48, no. 1, pp. 93–95, 1998.

[30] M. MacCauley and E. Bollard, "Gastric diverticulum: a rare cause of refractory epigastric pain," *American Journal of Medicine*, vol. 123, no. 5, pp. e5–e6, 2010.

39

Duodenal Diverticular Perforation after Small Bowel Obstruction

Khuram Khan ⓘ,[1] **Saqib Saeed,**[1] **Haytham Maria,**[1] **Mohammed Sbeih,**[1] **Farhana Iqbal,**[2] **Alexius Ramcharan,**[1] **and Brian Donaldson**[1]

[1]*Department of Surgery, Harlem Hospital Center, Columbia University, New York, NY, USA*
[2]*Department of Medicine, Richmond University Medical Center, Staten Island, New York, NY, USA*

Correspondence should be addressed to Khuram Khan; khurram112@gmail.com

Academic Editor: Dimitrios Mantas

Introduction. Duodenal diverticulum is a rare disease that can be easily missed. The incidence of duodenal diverticulum diagnosed by upper GI study is approximately 5%. Autopsy results show that 22% of the population have duodenum diverticulum. Most patients with duodenal diverticulum are asymptomatic. However, complications like inflammation, perforation with retroperitoneal abscess, sepsis, pancreatitis, bile duct obstruction, and bleeding can occur. Approximately 162 cases of perforated duodenal diverticulum have been reported in the literature. *Case Presentation.* We present a rare case of an 82-year-old female with perforation of a duodenal diverticulum caused by small bowel obstruction; in addition to this, there was a synchronous colonic tumor. *Conclusion.* Diagnosis and management of this rare disorder are controversial. Nonoperative management is advocated in some cases. Some of the cases require early aggressive surgical intervention. The mortality rate remains approximately 45% in all these patients.

1. Introduction

Perforation of the duodenum diverticulum (DD) is a rare disease that can be easily missed as it can be a clinical diagnosis. Management of the perforation requires urgent surgical intervention for favorable outcomes. Perforation can be caused by infections such as diverticulitis, ulceration, foreign body, trauma, and iatrogenic perforation after ERCP and would require CT scan of the abdomen for diagnosis and treatment in some cases, while diagnosis of duodenal diverticulum can be made with upper gastrointestinal series.

2. Case Presentation

An 82-year-old African American female with history of hypertension, chronic active smoker for 60 years along with prior surgical history significant for a laparotomy more than 20 years previously for unknown reason who was initially admitted to the medical service after a fall. She had a long history of nonspecific lower abdominal pain. As per her family,

she had not seen a doctor for 10 years and never had a colonoscopy. She reported unintentional weight loss. Vital signs at the time of presentation were stable. On physical examination, she appeared cachectic and dehydrated. Her abdomen was soft, non-tender with audible bowel sounds. Mild right lower quadrant tenderness was noted. Labs were significant for microcytic hypochromic anemia and urine analysis positive for leukocyte esterase. Liver function test was normal. Chest X-ray showed cardiomegaly. Abdominal US revealed mild ascites and dilated common bile duct to 1 cm. The patient was admitted to medical service with a diagnosis of dehydration, failure to thrive, and for work-up of an occult gastrointestinal malignancy. She was scheduled for EGD and colonoscopy by gastroenterology team. In addition to all of this, her CEA was 12.2 ng/ml (normal less than 3 ng/ml). While the patient was on the medical service, her hemoglobin dropped to 6.2 gm/dL requiring blood transfusions. During the second unit of blood transfusion, the patient became hypoxemic and tachypneic. She was transferred to Medical Intensive Care Unit (MICU) and subsequently intubated for acute respiratory failure. Chest X-ray at this point showed bilateral infiltrates, and the patient was started on IV antibiotics for possible pneumonia. The scheduled GI procedures were cancelled due to critical health status. She had echocardiography in MICU which revealed mitral stenosis and severe pulmonary hypertension, with normal ejection fraction. Her respiratory status improved, and she was transferred back to medical floor after staying four days in MICU. She also had urine culture which grew klebsiella. Three days later after being transferred from MICU, she developed abdominal distension. A CT scan of the abdomen without contrast was obtained which revealed gastric, small bowel, and colonic distension. There was copious amount of stool in the colon. She was transferred to the surgical service for management of possible ileus/stool impaction pending colonoscopy to rule out colonic lesion. She was managed with nil per os, nasogastric tube suction, intravenous fluid hydration, and enemas. Nasogastric tube output was minimal but the patient's abdomen remained distended while on surgical service. The patient became hypotensive and tachycardic and less responsive. After fluid resuscitation, another CT of the chest and abdomen with oral and intravenous contrast was performed one week from prior CT, which revealed persistent dilation of the stomach, small bowel, and large bowel, a left colonic mass, and large amount of retroperitoneal free fluid in the region of the duodenum and pancreas (Figures 1 and 2). She was taken to the operating room for exploratory laparotomy. A midline laparotomy was performed, and numerous adhesions from the previous laparotomy were seen. The patient had a high-grade small bowel obstruction with a transition point in the mid ileum caused by adhesions. Lysis of adhesions was performed. There was a large left descending colonic mass invading the lateral abdominal wall causing partial large bowel obstruction. The transverse colon was attached to the left colon mass with adhesions, creating a space through which there was herniation of dilated small bowel. However, this did not cause an obstruction. These dilated bowel loops were reduced. Because of the finding of free air in the retroperitoneum of the upper abdomen, we decided to explore that area. Generous kocherization of the duodenum was performed. The head of the pancreas and hepatic flexure were mobilized and found to be normal. With further mobilization of the duodenum, a perforated duodenal diverticulum was noticed in the third part of the duodenum. There was a leak of bile in the area. There was extensive retroperitoneal necrosis extending across the upper abdomen to the tail of the pancreas. The duodenal diverticulum was broad based, inflamed, and closely attached to the superior mesenteric artery. The diverticulum was dissected off, stapled, and sent for pathology (Figure 3). The third part of the duodenum became dusky, and we decided to resect it with a GIA. At this point, the patient was hypotensive and acidotic. A decision was made to perform damage control and a temporary abdominal closure and to transfer the patient to ICU for resuscitation. In the ICU, she was aggressively resuscitated with correction of her acidosis, coagulopathy, and hypothermia. She was brought back to the OR the following day. There

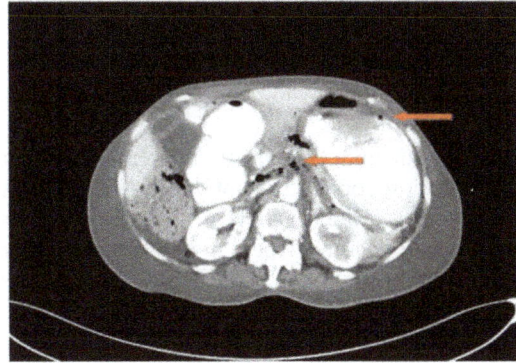

FIGURE 1: CT scan of the abdomen. Retroperitoneal free air.

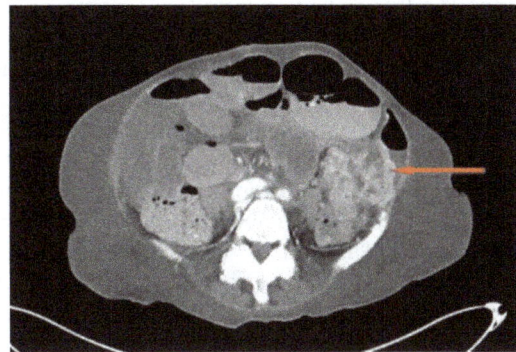

FIGURE 2: CT scan of the abdomen. Image shows dilated small bowel loops with air fluid level and small bowel obstruction.

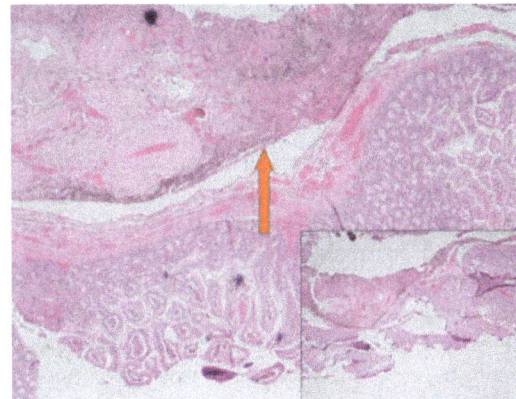

FIGURE 3: Histology slide. Small intestinal tissue with acute serositis (red arrow) consistent with perforated viscus.

were no signs of bowel ischemia, and the small bowel obstruction had resolved. An end to side duodenojejunostomy was performed using an EEA. The anastomosis was protected with a Stamm's gastrostomy through which a feeding jejunostomy was passed distal to the anastomosis. A drain was left in the right upper quadrant. We then performed a transverse colon loop colostomy to divert the colonic tumor. Blood cultures later grew pseudomonas and yeast. The patient subsequently developed multiorgan failure, and the family requested DNI/DNR. Their after family requested terminal extubation 12 days after the last operation.

3. Discussion

Duodenal diverticulum complications are rarely seen, and it is the second most common site of diverticula of the gastrointestinal tract after the colon [1]. DD can be congenital or acquired [2]. The acquired type is usually a pseudodiverticulum where there is herniation of the mucosa through the wall of the duodenum. Most of these occur along the mesenteric border of the duodenum [3]. Duodenal diverticulum is not rare, but complications like perforation, bleeding, pancreatitis, and bile duct obstruction are very rare. Less than 200 cases of perforated duodenal diverticulitis have been reported in the literature [2]. Causes of perforation include diverticulitis, ulceration, foreign body, trauma, and iatrogenic perforation after ERCP. In our case, we believe that the perforation occurred secondary to duodenal distension as a result of back pressure from associated bowel obstruction. The diagnosis is difficult as patients present with nonspecific signs and symptoms. Usually, there is no tenderness on abdominal exam because of retroperitoneal perforation. Computerized tomography plays an important role in diagnosis by showing free retroperitoneal air and phlegmon. Upper GI studies and endoscopy can be used in stable patients. The diagnosis is usually made with intraoperative exploration, as in our case. Because of rarity of the disease, there are no clear guidelines regarding conservative versus surgical management. Some cases of known perforated duodenal diverticulum in stable patients were managed conservatively by nil per os, intravenous fluid hydration, intravenous antibiotics, parenteral nutrition, and percutaneous drains for the localized collections.

Many operative techniques have been described. After adequate mobilization of the duodenum, the diverticulum should be dissected completely down to the base and either handsewn or stapled diverticulectomy can be performed. The defect can be closed in layers [3]. The relation of the neck of the diverticulum to the common bile duct must be ascertained to avoid bile duct injury. The bile duct should be cannulated from either the ampulla of Vater, by making a choledochotomy, or through the cystic duct [4]. Simple closure of the perforation with drainage, without diverticulum resection, because of close proximity of the bile duct to the diverticulum, was described in one case report [5].

If the perforated duodenal diverticulum is in the fourth portion of the duodenum, partial duodenectomy can be performed and reconstruction with end-to-side doudenojejunostomy [2].

In the presence of significant inflammation, more complex procedures have been described. A Roux-en-Y loop of the jejunum is brought through a rent in the transverse mesocolon, the duodenum is transected, and the duodenal stump is oversewn. The Roux limb of the jejunum was anastomosed end to end to the duodenum. A jejunojejunostomy is created 40 cm distal to the duodenojejunostomy. A drain should be placed. As an alternative, vagotomy, antrectomy closure of duodenal stump, and Billroth 2 reconstruction can be performed. This decreases the risk of duodenal fistula [3]. For large duodenal diverticulum causing dilation and obstruction of the bile duct, choledochoduodenostomy is the best approach and avoids the complications associated with attempts to resect the diverticulum. Sphincteroplasty has been described as well [4]. For duodenal diverticulum causing bleeding, preoperative localization with endoscopy or angiography should be done. Excision of the diverticulum with suture ligation of the bleeding point is essential [6].

4. Conclusion

Duodenal diverticular perforation can be challenging as it is a rare disease and difficult to diagnose. Nonoperative management is only in selected patient's population. CT scan can help diagnose the perforation and require urgent surgical intervention.

Authors' Contributions

Khuram Khan, MD, and Saqib Saeed, MD, helped in writing the abstract, figure collections, writing, and format. Haytham Maria helped in writing and format. Mohammed Sbeih helped in writing and editing. Farhana Iqbal helped in writing, format, and others. Brian Donaldson and Alexius Ramcharan helped in review and final editing.

References

[1] D. Mantas, S. Kykalos, D. Patsouras, and G. Kouraklis, "Small intestine diverticula: Is there anything new?," *World Journal of Gastrointestinal Surgery*, vol. 3, no. 4, pp. 49–53, 2011.

[2] M. Wilson and A. Bradley, "Management of perforated duodenal diverticula," *Canadian Journal of surgery*, vol. 48, no. 1, pp. 79-80, 2005.

[3] V. C. Simões, B. Santos, S. Magalhães, G. Faria, D. S. Silva, and J. Davide, "Perforated duodenal diverticulum: surgical treatment and literature review," *International Journal of Surgery Case Reports*, vol. 5, no. 8, pp. 547–550, 2014.

[4] J. W. Donald, "Major complications of small bowel diverticula," *Annals of Surgery*, vol. 190, no. 2, pp. 183–188, 1979.

[5] T. De Perrot, P. A. Poletti, C. D. Becker, and A. Platon, "The complicated duodenal diverticulum: retrospective analysis of 11 cases," *Clinical Imaging*, vol. 36, no. 4, pp. 287–294, 2012.

[6] S. Yokomuro, E. Uchida, Y. Arima et al., "Simple closure of a perforated duodenal diverticulum: "a case report"," *Journal of Nippon Medical School*, vol. 71, no. 5, pp. 337–339, 2004.

40

Afferent Loop Syndrome after Roux-en-Y Total Gastrectomy Caused by Volvulus of the Roux-Limb

Hideki Katagiri,[1] **Kana Tahara,**[1] **Kentaro Yoshikawa,**[1]
Alan Kawarai Lefor,[2] **Tadao Kubota,**[1] **and Ken Mizokami**[1]

[1]*Department of Surgery, Tokyo Bay Urayasu Ichikawa Medical Center, 3-4-32 Todaijima, Urayasu, Chiba 279-0001, Japan*
[2]*Department of Surgery, Jichi Medical University, 1-3311 Yakushiji, Shimotsuke, Tochigi Prefecture 329-0498, Japan*

Correspondence should be addressed to Hideki Katagiri; x62h20k38@yahoo.co.jp

Academic Editor: Akihiro Nakajo

Afferent loop syndrome is a rare complication of gastric surgery. An obstruction of the afferent limb can present in various ways. A 73-year-old man presented with one day of persistent abdominal pain, gradually radiating to the back. He had a history of total gastrectomy with a Roux-en-Y reconstruction. Abdominal computed tomography scan revealed dilation of the duodenum and small intestine in the left upper quadrant. Exploratory laparotomy showed volvulus of the biliopancreatic limb that caused afferent loop syndrome. In this patient, the 50 cm long limb was the cause of volvulus. It is important to fashion a Roux-limb of appropriate length to prevent this complication.

1. Introduction

Afferent loop syndrome is a rare complication of gastric surgery. In general, afferent loop syndrome develops after distal gastrectomy following a Billroth II reconstruction. However, the same condition can occur after a Roux-en-Y reconstruction by stenosis or obstruction of "biliopancreatic limb" [1–3]. We present a patient who developed afferent loop syndrome after total gastrectomy with a Roux-en-Y reconstruction caused by volvulus of the biliopancreatic limb.

2. Case Report

A 73-year-old man presented with periumbilical abdominal pain. One day prior to admission, he noticed the gradual onset of abdominal pain. The pain was not severe and he did not seek medical attention at that time. He did not have nausea or vomiting. He was able to eat but tolerated a smaller amount than usual. However, the pain persisted and gradually worsened, and he presented to the hospital.

The patient has a past medical history of hyperthyroidism, aortic valve replacement due to aortic insufficiency one month prior to presentation, and total gastrectomy for gastric cancer two years previously. He has had two episodes of adhesive small bowel obstruction, one of which required operative intervention. On admission, his vital signs were within normal limits except for a respiratory rate of 30/min. Physical examination showed tenderness from the left flank to the right upper quadrant with palpable loops of dilated intestine. During the physical examination, he started complaining of back pain. Laboratory data showed slight elevation of lipase and alkaline phosphatase. Abdominal computed tomography scan with intravenous contrast was obtained, which showed dilated duodenum and small intestine in the left upper quadrant (Figure 1). In addition, slight dilation of the main pancreatic duct and the intrahepatic bile duct was seen (Figures 2(a) and 2(b)).

Based on these findings, afferent loop syndrome was highly suspected, and we performed exploratory laparotomy urgently. On exploration, there were dilated loops of small intestine without adhesions in the left upper quadrant. The jejunum, from the ligament of Treitz to the site of the jejunojejunal anastomosis, was twisted 360 degrees counterclockwise (Figure 3). We reduced the volvulus manually without difficulty and the dilation of the bowel rapidly resolved. There was no evidence of intestinal necrosis.

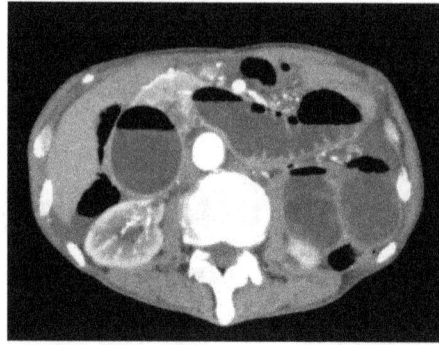

FIGURE 1: Abdominal computed tomography scan revealed dilation of the duodenum and small intestine in the left upper quadrant.

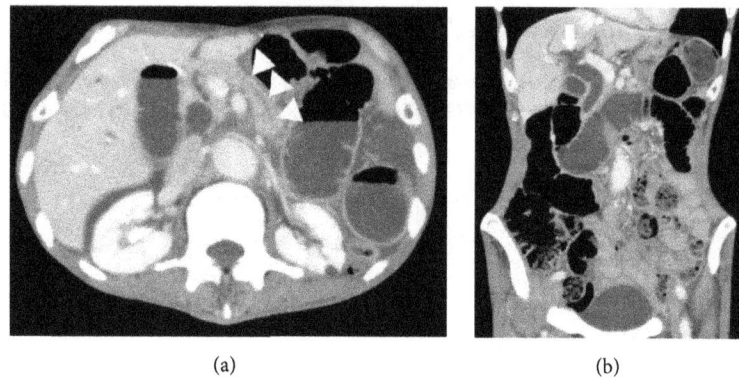

(a)   (b)

FIGURE 2: Computed tomography scan images with axial and coronal views showing slight dilation of the main pancreatic duct (arrow heads) and the intrahepatic bile duct (arrow).

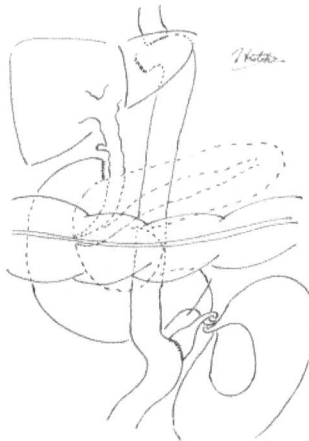

FIGURE 3: Schematic diagram of intraoperative findings. The patient previously underwent total gastrectomy and cholecystectomy. The afferent (biliopancreatic) limb was twisted 360 degrees.

The postoperative course was uneventful and the patient was discharged from hospital.

3. Discussion

Afferent loop syndrome is a rare complication that occurs in 0.2 to 1.0% of patients after gastrectomy with a Billroth

II or Roux-en-Y reconstruction [1, 2, 4, 5]. To be accurate, the afferent limb is not only the afferent limb in patients following a Billroth II reconstruction but also refers to the biliopancreatic limb in patients following a Roux-en-Y reconstruction, in this discussion. Afferent loop syndrome can be caused by internal herniation, kinking at the anastomotic site, adhesions, stomal stenosis, a gastrointestinal stone, recurrent malignancy, and volvulus [1–5]. An obstruction of the afferent limb disrupts the flow of bile and pancreatic juice, resulting in acute pancreatitis or obstructive jaundice [4]. In some patients, afferent loop syndrome can rapidly develop, followed by perforation or peritonitis [1]. In the present patient, the volvulus resulted in complete obstruction of the afferent limb and the patient's condition worsened rapidly.

The diagnosis of afferent loop syndrome is challenging because the symptoms are generally nonspecific [1]. Abdominal pain is one of the common symptoms. Vomiting may occur in patients with afferent loop syndrome; however, it is very difficult to assess. In patients with incomplete obstruction, patients may vomit and the vomitus can contain bile. However, in patients with complete obstruction, patients do not vomit (as in the present patient), because the afferent limb is completely obstructed. As the condition worsens, patients may develop acute pancreatitis or obstructive jaundice, which also makes establishing the diagnosis challenging. Early diagnosis and intervention is important to decrease the mortality rate, especially when the condition develops acutely [1].

In the present patient, slight elevation of lipase and alkaline phosphatase, slight dilation of the common pancreatic duct and the bile duct, and the onset of back pain all suggested high intraluminal pressure and reflux of intestinal fluid to the ducts. Prolonged high intraluminal pressure can result in intestinal necrosis, making early diagnosis and intervention essential.

In the present patient, volvulus of the afferent limb caused afferent loop syndrome. In general, the length of jejunum between the ligament of Treitz and the jejunojejunal anastomosis is typically 20 to 30 cm. However, in the present patient, it was longer than 50 cm. This is longer than usual and may have facilitated the development of volvulus. This patient emphasizes the importance of the length of the afferent limb in gastric surgery. As it is easy to shorten the afferent limb, especially for a Roux-en-Y reconstruction, fashioning an appropriate length for the afferent limb can potentially prevent this complication.

Treatment of afferent loop syndrome depends on the etiology. In the present patient, reduction of the volvulus resolved the condition. In patients with benign etiologies, surgical management including adhesiolysis, bypass, or reconstruction of the limb can generally resolve the cause [2]. In patients with afferent loop syndrome caused by recurrent tumor, the goal of the treatment changes to palliation. In some settings, drainage by percutaneous or endoscopic stent placement has been reported to achieve palliation in patients with cancer [4, 6].

In conclusion, afferent loop syndrome is a rare complication after gastric surgery. Although rare, it is important for surgeons to fashion an afferent limb of appropriate length to prevent this complication.

Competing Interests

The authors declare that there is no conflict of interests regarding the publication of this paper.

References

[1] M. Aoki, M. Saka, S. Morita, T. Fukagawa, and H. Katai, "Afferent loop obstruction after distal gastrectomy with Roux-en-Y reconstruction," *World Journal of Surgery*, vol. 34, no. 10, pp. 2389–2392, 2010.

[2] H.-C. Kim, J. K. Han, K. W. Kim et al., "Afferent loop obstruction after gastric cancer surgery: helical CT findings," *Abdominal Imaging*, vol. 28, no. 5, pp. 624–630, 2003.

[3] P. S. Fleser and M. Villalba, "Afferent limb volvulus and perforation of the bypassed stomach as a complication of Roux-en-Y gastric bypass," *Obesity Surgery*, vol. 13, no. 3, pp. 453–456, 2003.

[4] K. Han, H.-Y. Song, J. H. Kim et al., "Afferent loop syndrome: treatment by means of the placement of dual stents," *American Journal of Roentgenology*, vol. 199, no. 6, pp. W761–W766, 2012.

[5] Y. S. Cho, T. H. Lee, S. O. Hwang et al., "Electrohydraulic lithotripsy of an impacted enterolith causing acute afferent loop syndrome," *Clinical Endoscopy*, vol. 47, no. 4, pp. 367–370, 2014.

[6] P. Taunk, N. Cosgrove, D. E. Loren, T. Kowalski, and A. A. Siddiqui, "Endoscopic ultrasound-guided gastroenterostomy using a lumen-apposing self-expanding metal stent for decompression of afferent loop obstruction," *Endoscopy*, vol. 47, pp. E395–E396, 2015.

41

An Exceptional Case of Ileocolic Intussusception Secondary to Burkitt's Lymphoma: What Variations are There in the Presentation and Management of those Patients who Approach Adolescence?

Krish Kulendran (D), [1,2] **Kay Tai Choy**, [1,2] **Cian Keogh**, [1,2] and **Dinesh Ratnapala** [1,2]

[1]*Cairns Hospital, Cairns, QLD, Australia*
[2]*Ipswich Hospital, Ipswich, QLD, Australia*

Correspondence should be addressed to Krish Kulendran; krishkulendran@gmail.com

Academic Editor: Paola De Nardi

Intussusception is a common cause of abdominal pain among the paediatric population with up to 10% of cases occurring secondary to a pathological lead point. Burkitt's lymphoma (BL) is a highly malignant and rapidly growing B-cell neoplasm which in extremely rare cases can present as intussusception. We report a case in an otherwise healthy 15-year-old male who presented with atypical abdominal pain. Imaging subsequently indicated an ileocolic intussusception, and given that the suspicion of a pathological lead point mandates a laparotomy and bowel resection, he proceeded to surgery. The histopathology confirmed Burkitt's lymphoma as the aetiology responsible for this intussuscepted mass. A detailed discussion including a systematic review of all previous case reports explore the diagnostic dilemma of intussusceptions secondary to BL. This case report aims to highlight the clinical challenges in establishing such a diagnosis and an appreciation for the subtle variations in clinical features, as well as the differences in management between infants and adolescents.

1. Introduction

In 1958, the surgeon Dennis Burkitt first observed a tumour affecting the jaw of one of the paediatric population of Equatorial Africa. This tumour was initially purported as a sarcoma of the jaw; however, it was promptly reclassified as a distinct form of non-Hodgkin's lymphoma (NHL) based on its histopathological features [1].

BL is a rapidly growing B-cell neoplasm which is highly malignant and aggressive. The variants of BL are illustrated below in Table 1.

BL is now recognized in a variety of extranodal sites, including the ileocaecal region. Here, it may cause either indirect pressure symptoms or via direct luminal involvement, intestinal obstruction, or intussusception. Complete resection of this tumour is required for optimal patient survival [3].

This case details a rare cause of intussusception secondary to Burkitt's lymphoma. In infants this is often treated with air enema reduction, but in adult populations intussusceptions are normally associated with a lead point and so surgical management is essential [4]. Identifying this diagnosis in this intervening age group is clinically challenging and a high index of suspicion is necessary. This report contains interesting diagnostic imaging, operative details, and specimen photographs.

2. Case Report

A healthy 15-year-old male presented with a three-week history of irretractable abdominal pain, vomiting, and anorexia. There was no previous similar history or abdominal surgery. He associated the onset of symptoms with a recent contraction of gastroenteritis within the family. There

TABLE 1: Describing variants of BL [2].

Variants of BL	
Type	Features
Endemic	Largely prevalent in the African continent, develops due to chromosomal translocation between chromosomes 8 and 14 causing tumours of the facial bones.
Sporadic	Nonendemic and primarily affects the abdominal viscera. It is subsequently described outside of Africa. This variant occurs due to chromosome 8 translocation involving the c-myc oncogene. This form tends to present with the lymphoid tissues of the gut. The disease can present as masses affecting the terminal ileum, caecum, and abdominal mesentery.
Immunodeficient	Frequently presents with diffuse lymphadenopathy. The Epstein-Barr and human immunodeficiency viruses are a recognized association with all forms of BL, not just the immunodeficient forms.

was no improvement in his condition despite his family contacts recovering.

On examination, he was afebrile and haemodynamically stable. There was a scaphoid abdomen with maximal tenderness in the right upper quadrant. There was significant guarding. Bowel sounds were audible. His abdominal X-ray and routine blood test results were both unremarkable, other than a raised C-reactive protein of 92.

His high opioid requirement, chronicity of symptoms, and examination findings prompted further evaluation with CT. This revealed right-sided abdominal mass and a layering effect at the caecal pole consistent with an intussusception. The appearance was similar to a "pseudokidney," as shown in Figure 1. There was marked free fluid within the abdominal cavity. After resuscitation, he proceeded to a laparotomy.

A diagnostic laparotomy was performed for the inspection of abdominal contents. It confirmed radiological findings of an intussusception of the terminal ileum within the caecal pole. A hard mass was noted within the hepatic flexure region. There was a dilated terminal ileum and multiple lymph nodes noted within the mesentery.

A right hemicolectomy was performed. Vascular pedicles were taken high for an appropriate oncological resection, given the suspicion. Primary ileocolic stapled side-to-side anastomosis was performed. The recovery was uncomplicated and the patient was discharged home three days postoperatively.

As shown in Figure 2, the histopathology of the excised mass proved to be Burkitt's lymphoma of the terminal ileum causing ileocolic intussusception. It extensively involved the appendiceal serosa, mesentery, and omentum.

The tumour was an ulcerated lesion infiltrating all layers of the bowel wall. As shown in Figure 3 microscopically, the characteristic starry sky growth pattern was visualised, with the cells having round nuclei, finely clumped chromatin, and small basophilic nucleoli.

A panel of immunostains was performed on bowel tumour, the regional lymph nodes, and the omentum. The tumour cells in all three sites are CD20, CD10, BCL6, and C-MYC positive (see Figure 4). The tumour has a very high proliferative index with almost 100% of the tumour expressing Ki67. BCL2, Cyclin D1, TdT, CD3, CD5, CD23, and CD30 are negative. Fluorescence in situ hybridisation (FISH) detected a reciprocal t(8;14) translocation and rearrangement of the C-MYC gene. As only chromosome-specific probes

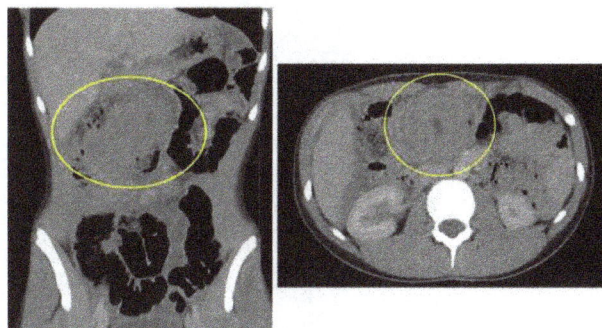

FIGURE 1: CT imaging indicating intussusception.

were used, the presence of other abnormalities cannot be excluded. The above profile supports the original diagnosis of BL.

2.1. Systematic Review of Relevant Literature. The medical literature in the PubMed and Medline/EMBASE databases was reviewed for cases of Burkitt's lymphoma-related intussusception. All publications were scrutinized that contained keywords of "intussusception" and "Burkitt lymphoma." The literature search was limited to paediatric patients under 18 years old, and restricted to papers written in English.

A systematic review of relevant literature was performed to ascertain variance of clinical features in primary presentations of BL-related intussusception. The following information on patient numbers, demographic, main presenting complaint, disease stage, and diagnostic methods were obtained in this meta-analysis.

3. Results

A literature search was performed using the PUBMED medical database. A broad scope of analysis is ensured by including all relevant papers that fulfilled the keyword search, irrespective of age, location, or outcome measurements. Non-English papers were excluded, as time resources could not be allocated for interpretation.

The literature review identified relevant papers when searching for keywords of "Burkitt lymphoma" and "intussusception." This yielded 31 publications reporting on 226 patients in total. However, the majority of these papers reported presentations of intussusception in known BL, rather than primary presentations. These were therefore

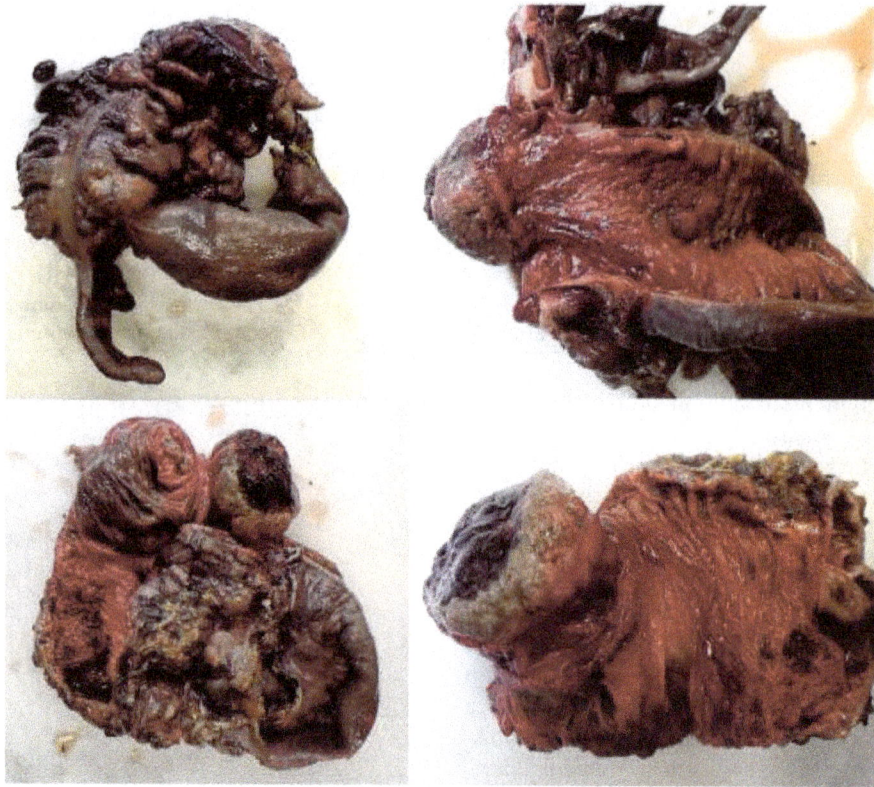

FIGURE 2: Right hemicolectomy specimen demonstrating ileocolic intussusception.

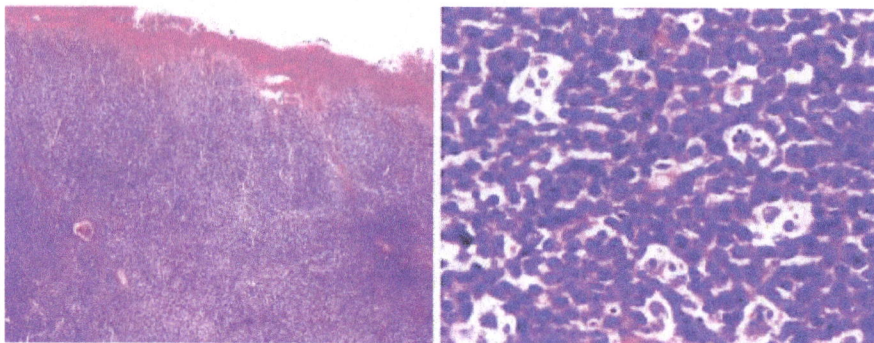

FIGURE 3: Histopathology slides demonstrating characteristic features of BL.

excluded from the analysis, leaving 21 valid publications reporting on 70 paediatric patients.

The mean (s.d.) age was 5.28 (range 2.5–17) years. Sex was recorded in most cases, with a male preponderance of almost 2 : 1 distribution. A solitary case report detailed BL-related intussusception in a patient with Wiskott-Aldrich syndrome, with the remainder of the cases eliciting no significant medical background.

From our cases, the most common presenting complaint was abdominal pain, occurring in 95% of the patients. Importantly, all of these cases mentioned "recurrent" or having painful symptoms lasting >1 week. Other common symptoms included vomiting (28%), altered bowel habits (11%), and bloody stools (13%). Systemic symptoms included weight loss/malaise/fatigue in 7%. Only

13% had a palpable abdominal mass on examination. Only 1 case reported a rectal prolapse as a case of BL-related intussusception.

The investigations that were performed revealed no clear pattern—with nonspecific rises in inflammatory markers described in four cases. Every patient underwent preoperative diagnostic imaging studies—with the majority of them ultrasound/CT, which confirmed the presence of intestinal intussusception. All but one patient had ileocolic intussusception (98%), with the one exception of colocolonic intussusception at the transverse colon.

Regarding outcomes, these results were only available for 54 out of the 70 patients. Using the St. Jude staging system, the stage of disease was determined in these 54 patients. Results show that the 67% of all patients who presented with

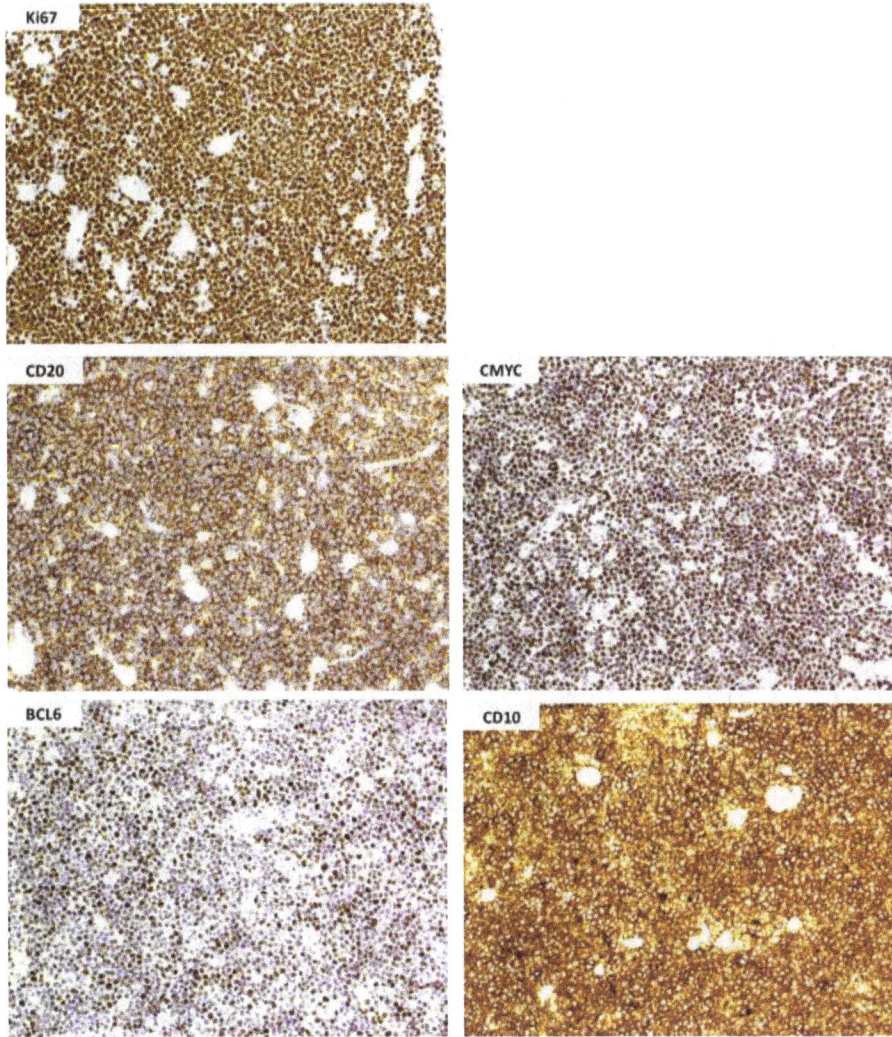

FIGURE 4: Histopathology slides demonstrating positive CD20, CD10, C-MYC, BCL6, and Ki67 immunostains.

intussusception had predominantly Grades I-II disease. 36 out of the 54 patients subsequently received complete tumour resection due to the disease being limited to the area of intussusception. Complete resection was not achieved in the remaining 18 patients, of whom 12 had stage III disease (i.e., ascites, retroperitoneal nodal involvement, and liver involvement) and 6 had stage IV disease (i.e., bone marrow involvement) (Table 2).

4. Discussion

Primary gastrointestinal lymphoma represents 1–4% of all gastrointestinal malignancies [5], with Burkitt's lymphoma accounting for 0.3–1.3% of all non-Hodgkin's lymphomas. While BL accounts for only 1% of all adult lymphomas, it constitutes ~30% of all paediatric NHL, hence representing a significant burden of disease in this age group. As most reported cases in children affect the distal ileum/ileocaecal region, intussusception has been identified as a common presentation [5].

While the classical triad for diagnosis of intussusception comprises of abdominal colic, "red-currant jelly stools,"

TABLE 2: Clinical manifestations of BL-related intussusception.

Trait	No. of patients (%)
Sex	
Male	46 (65)
Female	10 (15)
Unspecified	14 (20)
Stage of disease at diagnosis	
I	1 (2)
II	35 (65)
III	12 (22)
IV	6 (11)
Symptoms/signs	
Abdominal pain	67 (95)
Nausea/vomiting	20 (28)
Altered bowel habits	8 (11)
Blood in stools	9 (13)
Fatigue/malaise/wt. loss	5 (7)
Abdominal mass	9 (13)
Duration > 1 weeks	67 (95)

and palpable abdominal mass, there remains a diagnostic dilemma due to the subtler presentation of intussusception in postinfancy children older than 2-3 years where the classic triad of symptoms may not be present, such as in our case (1, 3). Among the 70 cases analysed above, only 12.8% satisfied the classical triad of intussusception at time of presentation, with the majority of cases just presenting with abdominal pain alone. However, 95% had recurrent symptoms lasting greater than a week, which highlights the importance of recognizing these atypical symptoms for intussusception.

In terms of history, previous literature have described predisposing factors for lymphoma of the small intestine including prior malabsorption syndromes, inflammatory bowel disease, and an immune-deficient state [6]. Our patient's EBV and HIV serology was checked postoperatively and found to be undetected.

Common investigations used today to workup a paediatric patient with concerning abdominal symptoms include blood tests and imaging. Common blood tests associated with an intra-abdominal neoplastic event—such as LDH, was only reported to be elevated in a small number of cases. While not elaborated in detail, most cases reported a fairly unremarkable blood panel in their patients with BL-associated intussusceptions.

Many previous case reports have described misdiagnosis at presentation with differential diagnoses including appendicitis, inflamed Meckel's diverticulum, intestinal infections, and ischaemic gut. In child-bearing females, it is essential to rule out catastrophic causes of ovarian torsion and ectopic pregnancies.

Ultrasonography has a false-negative rate approaching zero and is a reliable screening tool for children at low risk for intussusceptions. Almost 95% of the previously reported cases utilised ultrasound or computer tomography to confirm the presence of intussusception. Some consequently received a contrast enema, which is both diagnostic (the gold standard in the diagnosis of intussusception) and therapeutic [7]. Our patient's presentation and demographic was atypical of idiopathic intussusception and thus a CT was more appropriate to investigate his inexplicable pain, and identify any pathological lead point. This case highlights the importance of being aware of the differing aetiology and consequent management between young infants and adolescents.

In summary, BL-related intussusception is often challenging to diagnose, but must be considered even when facing a child who does not present with the classical triad. The suspicion of intestinal intussusception at a lead point necessitates a laparotomy. Laparotomy remains the gold standard in both diagnosis and treatment, ensuring the excision of the entire tumour with appropriate margins [8]. A multidisciplinary approach is mandatory to ensure that appropriate therapeutic management, as well as necessary follow-up, occurs [9].

This case serves as a reminder to clinicians to maintain vigilance regarding this diagnosis and the subtle variations in its presentations and management among the adolescent/paediatric population.

References

[1] D. Burkitt, "A sarcoma involving the jaws in African children," *British Journal of Surgery*, vol. 46, no. 197, pp. 218–223, 1958.

[2] S. Cogliatti, U. Novak, S. Henz, U. Schmid, P. Möller, and T. Barth, "Diagnosis of Burkitt's lymphoma in due time: a practical approach," *Diagnostic Pathology*, vol. 2, Supplement 1, p. S6, 2007.

[3] F. T. Hoxha, S. I. Hashani, A. S. Krasniqi et al., "Intussusceptions as acute abdomen caused by Burkitt lymphoma: a case report," *Cases Journal*, vol. 2, no. 1, p. 9322, 2009.

[4] A. Attarbaschi, G. Mann, M. Dworzak et al., "The role of surgery in the treatment of pediatric B-cell non-Hodgkin's lymphoma," *Journal of Pediatric Surgery*, vol. 37, no. 10, pp. 1470–1475, 2002.

[5] C. A. I. Bethel, N. Bhattacharyya, C. Hutchinson, F. Ruymann, and D. R. Cooney, "Alimentary tract malignancies in children," *Journal of Pediatric Surgery*, vol. 32, no. 7, pp. 1004–1009, 1997.

[6] D. Bernardi, E. Asti, and L. Bonavina, "Adult ileocolic intussusception caused by Burkitt lymphoma," *BMJ Case Reports*, 2016.

[7] F. Lindbichler and E. Sorantin, "Management of intussusception," *European Radiology Supplements*, vol. 14, no. 4, pp. L146–L154, 2004.

[8] S.-M. Wang, F.-C. Huang, C.-H. Wu, S.-F. Ko, S.-Y. Lee, and C.-C. Hsiao, "Ileocecal Burkitt's lymphoma presenting as ileocolic intussusception with appendiceal invagination and acute appendicitis," *Journal of the Formosan Medical Association*, vol. 109, no. 6, pp. 476–479, 2010.

[9] H. Gupta, A. M. Davidoff, C.-H. Pui, S. J. Shochat, and J. T. Sandlund, "Clinical implications and surgical management of intussusception in pediatric patients with Burkitt lymphoma," *Journal of Pediatric Surgery*, vol. 42, no. 6, pp. 998–1001, 2007.

42

Intestinal Obstruction caused by Ileocolic and Colocolic Intussusception in an Adult Patient with Cecal Lipoma

Tiziana Casiraghi,[1] **Alessandro Masetto,**[2] **Massimo Beltramo,**[3]
Mauro Girlando,[3] **and Camillo Di Bella**[3]

[1] *Azienda Socio-Sanitaria di Vimercate, Presidio di Carate, Via Mosè Bianchi 9, 20841 Carate Brianza, Italy*
[2] *Azienda Socio-Sanitaria di Vimercate, Presidio di Vimercate, Via Santi Cosma e Damiano 10, 20871 Vimercate, Italy*
[3] *Azienda Ospedaliera di Desio e Vimercate, Presidio di Carate, Via Mosè Bianchi 9, 20841 Carate Brianza, Italy*

Correspondence should be addressed to Tiziana Casiraghi; tiziana.casiraghi@asst-vimercate.it

Academic Editor: Paola De Nardi

Introduction. Intussusception is a rare clinical entity in adults (<1% of intestinal obstructions). Colonic intussusception is even rarer, particularly when caused by lipomas. *Case Presentation.* A 47-year-old woman presented to our emergency department complaining of abdominal pain with vomiting and diarrhoea. X-ray and CT showed bowel obstruction due to ileocolonic and colocolonic intussusception; a giant colonic lipoma ($9 \times 4 \times 4$ cm) was recognizable immediately distally to the splenic flexure of the colon. The patient underwent emergency laparotomy and right hemicolectomy. Assessment of the resected specimen confirmed the diagnosis of giant colonic polypoid lesion near to the ileocecal valve, causing a 12 cm long intussusception with moderate ischemic damage. *Conclusion.* Colonic obstruction due to intussusception caused by lipomas is a very rare condition that needs urgent treatment. CT is the radiologic modality of choice for diagnosis (sensitivity 80%, specificity near 100%); since the majority of colonic intussusceptions are caused by primary adenocarcinoma, if the etiology is uncertain, the lesion must be interpreted as malignant and extensive resection is recommended. At present, surgery is the treatment of choice and determines an excellent outcome.

1. Introduction

Lipoma of the gastrointestinal tract is a rare condition described for the first time in 1757 by Baurer and reported in only 0.2%–4.4% of large autopsy series since 1955 [1].

Intussusception was first described by Barbette of Amsterdam in 1674 [2]. It is relatively frequent in children but rare in adults, representing 5% of all bowel intussusceptions and 1% of all bowel obstruction [2, 3].

Colic intussusception is even rarer, above all when caused by lipomas: thirty-seven definite cases have been reported in the English-language literature over the past 45 years [4].

2. Case Report

A 47-year-old woman presented to our emergency department with abdominal pain associated to vomiting and diarrhoea for one week. She was known for a suspicious history of Crohn.

In the emergency department laboratory tests showed PCR 5.89 mg/dl and Hb 10.3 g/dl; an X-ray showed signs of bowel subocclusion. The patient was admitted to the hospital and a CT scan revealed the bowel obstruction with ileocolonic and colocolonic intussusception as far as splenic flexure of the colon; on the left side there was a formation characterised by fat-equivalent density and intralesional septa. CT findings were suggestive of giant lipoma ($9 \times 4 \times 4$ cm). Moderate free fluid was also present (Figures 1, 2, and 3).

The patient underwent emergency laparotomy. Surgical exploration confirmed the colocolonic intussusception; the last ileal loops migrated in the colon, too. The condition appeared to be due to an intraluminal colonic polypoid lesion, appreciable at the level of the splenic flexure at palpation.

Conservative treatment was not possible due to ischemia of involved segments, and right hemicolectomy was performed. The resection was extended from the last ileal loop

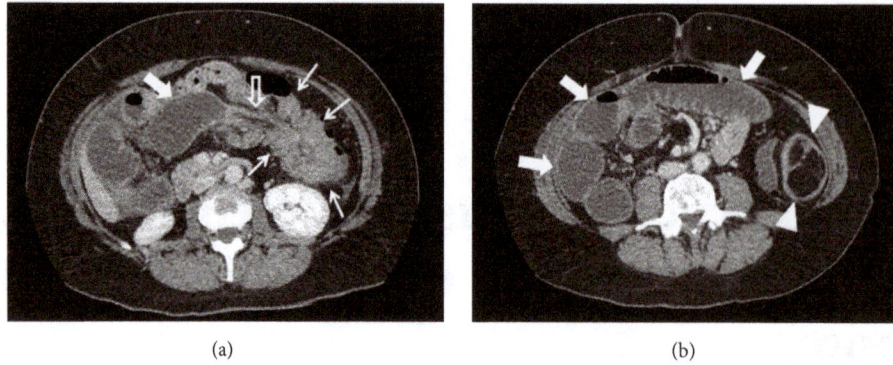

(a)   (b)

FIGURE 1: Contrast-enhanced CT, portal venous phase, axial images. In (a) the last ileal loop is dilated (full arrow); a part of the right colon and its mesentery (empty arrow) are recognizable inside the left colon (thin arrows). In (b) the section is at a lower level; on the left side, the colonic lipoma (arrowheads) is recognizable as a lobulated lesion with fat-equivalent density and with inner septa. On the right side notice dilated small bowel loops (full arrows) and absence of the right colon.

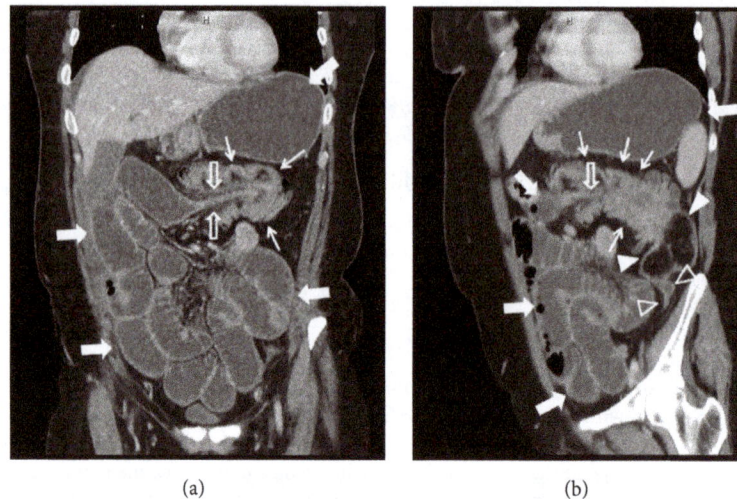

(a)   (b)

FIGURE 2: Contrast-enhanced CT, portal venous phase, multiplanar reconstructions (coronal plane, (a), and paracoronal plane, (b)). The same features described in (a) can be appreciated: the dilated stomach and small bowel loops (full arrows), the right colon, intussusceptum (empty arrows), the left colon, intussuscipiens (thin arrows), the colonic lipoma (full arrowheads), and the collapsed left colon distal to the lipoma (empty arrowheads).

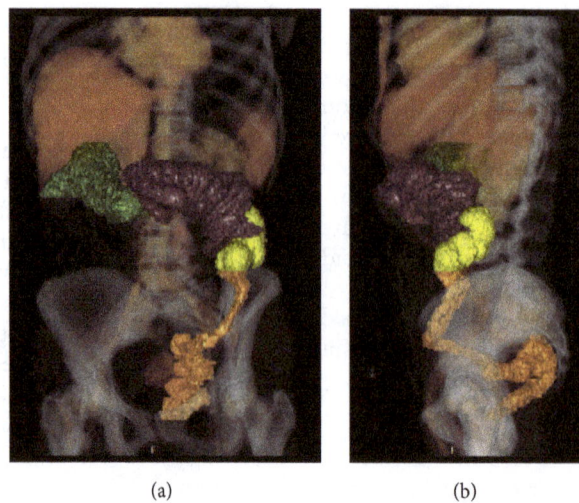

(a)   (b)

FIGURE 3: Contrast-enhanced CT, portal venous phase, 3D volume rendering reconstructions. The anatomical structures of interest were segmented for a panoramic view: the dilated last ileal loop (green), the intussuscepted colonic segments (purple-brown), the lipoma (yellow), the collapsed distal third of the left colon, and the sigmoid and rectum (orange). The skeletal structures and the parenchymatous organs were left in transparency.

to the right colon as far as the big polypoid lesion. An ileotransverse colon manual anastomosis was performed.

The postoperative course was uneventful and the patient was discharged on the seventh postoperative day.

Macroscopic assessment of the resected specimen showed the presence of a giant (8.5 × 5 × 3 cm) colic polypoid lesion near the ileocecal valve, causing intussusception of a 12 cm long intestinal segment.

After the cut the polyp showed a yellow homogeneous nodule with well demarcated margins.

The final result was polypoid colonic lipoma causing intussusception and moderate ischemic damage with reactive lymphadenitis.

3. Discussion

Intussusception is a rare condition in adults (1% of bowel obstructions). 90% of cases have an organic cause, 60% due to neoplasm (60% malign and 40% benign) [2]; in particular 65–70% of adult colonic intussusceptions are caused by carcinomas [3]. Colonic lipoma is the most common benign tumor which causes colonic intussusception in adults, but very rarely [5].

Colonic lipomas are more common in women with a peak incidence between 50 and 60 years of age [6, 7]. They are mostly located in the right colon: 19% in cecum, 38% in ascending colon, 22% in transverse colon, 13% in the descending colon, and 8% into the sigma [4].

They arise from the submucosa in approximately 90% of cases, occasionally extending into the muscularis propria, and up to 10% are subserosal [8]. The size described in the literature ranges from 2 mm to 30 cm. They are multiple in 10–20% of cases and infrequently are pedunculated [4, 9, 10].

In general colonic lipomas are silent. Only 25% of patients develop symptoms: history of abdominal pain from mild to severe cramping followed by spontaneous improvement and recurrent episodes of constipation, nausea, and vomiting. Size of the lipoma is a predictor of symptomatology: lipomas larger than 4 cm cause symptoms in 75% of cases.

After intussusception abdominal pain is associated with vomiting, palpable mass, and bloody stool, presenting for many days or even weeks [3, 4, 7].

For the diagnosis, colonoscopy allows direct visualization of the submucosal lipoma, which appears as a mass covered by normal mucosa, but it can also show ulcerated or necrotic overlying mucosa [4, 8, 11]. Colonoscopic biopsy confirms the nature, but inadequate tissue samples often indicate nonspecific colitis with mucosal inflammation [12].

In case of intussusception, abdominal CT scanning is the radiologic modality of choice, above all when giant lipomas are present, with a 70–80% sensitivity and near 100% specificity [3, 13]. Lipoma appears with fat-equivalent density, near ovoidal shape, and smooth margins. However, intussuscepted lipomas may have a heterogeneous appearance reflecting the degree of infarction and fat necrosis [3, 14].

There are different options for treatment.

Small lipomas, less than 2 cm, can be endoscopically removed. Since lipomas show no malignant degeneration, if the biopsy is unequivocal, they may not need treatment and can be observed [4].

Some authors have reported that large pedunculated lesions can be removed without perforation using clipping or endoloop ligation [13, 15], but in most series endoscopic removal of lipomas larger than 2 cm is associated with a greater risk of perforation [4, 13].

It is therefore recommended that tumors larger than 2 cm must be resected surgically [13].

Moreover, the size of the lipoma is an essential factor leading to colonic intussusception, particularly when main axis of the lesion is over 4 cm. This is the reason why colonic lipomas of 4 cm or more must be resected before intussusception occurs [4].

The presence of intussusception leads to an emergency operation [3, 4].

Chiang recommended operative reduction for small bowel intussusceptions, but not for colonic ones [15].

If a colonic lipoma is diagnosed before surgery, segmental resection is an adequate treatment [4].

Since the majority of colonic intussusceptions are caused by primary adenocarcinoma, in view of the uncertain etiology, nondiagnosed lipoma before operation must be interpreted as for cancer, and a more or less extensive resection of the colon is recommended, depending on the location of the tumor. Patients must undergo more or less extensive resection of the colon also depending on the length of the intussusception segment [4, 15].

Even if additional cases are needed to optimize the standard management, surgery is always the treatment of choice and produces an excellent prognosis.

Competing Interests

The authors declare that there is no conflict of interests regarding the publication of this paper.

References

[1] E. Grasso and T. Guastella, "Giant submucosal lipoma cause colo-colonic intussusception. A case report and review of literature," *Annali Italiani di Chirurgia*, vol. 83, no. 6, pp. 559–562, 2012.

[2] A. S. Krasniqi, A. R. Hamza, L. M. Salihu et al., "Compound double ileoileal and ileocecocolic intussusception caused by lipoma of the ileum in an adult patient. A case report," *Journal of Medical Case Reports*, vol. 5, article 452, 2011.

[3] O. Mouaqit, H. Hasnai, L. Chbani et al., "Pedunculated lipoma causing colo-colonic intussusception: a rare case report," *BMC Surgery*, vol. 13, no. 1, article 51, 2013.

[4] S. Paškauskas, T. Latkauskas, G. Valeikaite et al., "Colonic intussusception caused by colonic lipoma: a case report," *Medicina*, vol. 46, no. 7, pp. 477–481, 2010.

[5] G. Ghidirim, I. Mishin, E. Gutsu, I. Gagauz, A. Danch, and S. Russu, "Giant submucosal lipoma of the cecum. Report of a case and review of literature," *Romanian Journal of Gastroenterology*, vol. 14, no. 4, pp. 393–396, 2005.

[6] R. A. De Beer and H. Shinya, "Colonic lipomas: an endoscopic analysis," *Gastrointestinal Endoscopy*, vol. 22, no. 2, pp. 90–91, 1975.

[7]   B. A. Taylor and B. G. Wolff, "Colonic lipomas - Report of two unusual cases and review of the mayo clinic experience, 1976-1985," *Diseases of the Colon & Rectum*, vol. 30, no. 11, pp. 888–893, 1987.

[8]   M. Michowitz, N. Lazebnik, S. Noy, and R. Lazebnik, "Lipoma of the colon. A report of 22 cases," *American Surgeon*, vol. 51, no. 8, pp. 449–454, 1985.

[9]   H. Zhang, J.-C. Cong, C.-S. Chen, L. Qiao, and E.-Q. Liu, "Submucous colon lipoma: a case report and review of the literature," *World Journal of Gastroenterology*, vol. 11, no. 20, pp. 3167–3169, 2005.

[10] C. Triantopoulou, A. Vassilaki, D. Filippou, S. Velonakis, C. Dervenis, and E. Koulentianos, "Adult ileocolic intussusception secondary to a submucosal cecal lipoma," *Abdominal Imaging*, vol. 29, no. 4, pp. 426–428, 2004.

[11] P. C. Buetow, J. L. Buck, N. J. Carr, L. Pantongrag-Brown, P. R. Ros, and D. F. Cruess, "Intussuscepted colonic lipomas: loss of fat attenuation on CT with pathologic correlation in 10 cases," *Abdominal Imaging*, vol. 21, no. 2, pp. 153–156, 1996.

[12] P. Katsinelos, G. Chatzimavroudis, C. Zavos, G. Paroutoglou, B. Papaziogas, and J. Kountouras, "A novel technique for the treatment of a symptomatic giant colonic lipoma," *Journal of Laparoendoscopic and Advanced Surgical Techniques*, vol. 17, no. 4, pp. 467–469, 2007.

[13] G. S. Raju and G. Gomez, "Endoloop ligation of a large colonic lipoma: a novel technique," *Gastrointestinal Endoscopy*, vol. 62, no. 6, pp. 988–990, 2005.

[14] S. Tamura, Y. Yokoyama, T. Morita, T. Tadokoro, Y. Higashidani, and S. Onishi, "'Giant' colon lipoma: what kind of findings are necessary for the indication of endoscopic resection?" *American Journal of Gastroenterology*, vol. 96, no. 6, pp. 1944–1946, 2001.

[15] J. Y.-M. Chiang and Y.-S. Lin, "Tumor spectrum of adult intussusception," *Journal of Surgical Oncology*, vol. 98, no. 6, pp. 444–447, 2008.

43

Case Report of Foreign Body Stuck in Esophagus with Failure of Endoscopic Management in a Man with a History of Pica

Holly Mulinder, Allison Ammann, Yana Puckett, and Sharmila Dissanaike

Department of General Surgery, School of Medicine, Texas Tech University, Lubbock, TX 79409, USA

Correspondence should be addressed to Holly Mulinder; holly.mulinder@ttuhsc.edu

Academic Editor: Serge Landen

This is a case report of foreign body ingestion in a 55-year-old intellectually disabled man with a history of pica and previous removal of ten plastic gloves from his rectum four months prior to this presentation. The patient presented after ingesting plastic gloves which formed large, rigid esophageal and gastric bezoars that were not amenable to endoscopic removal. An exploratory laparotomy and gastrostomy was performed, and a $10 \times 4.5 \times 2$ cm gastric bezoar consisting of rigid plastic gloves was removed without complication. Special considerations must be taken when considering the ingestion of nonfood items in the intellectually disabled population as these cases may not present classically with symptoms of a gastric bezoar.

1. Introduction

Pica is the compulsive ingestion of food and nonfood items. It is a relatively common disorder in institutionalized patients with severe intellectual disability [1]. Prevalence of pica in this population has been reported as high as 25.8% [2]. Nonfood items ingested include dirt, paper, metal objects, and vinyl or latex gloves.

Complications of pica include malabsorption, constipation, vomiting, intestinal obstruction, lead and nicotine toxicity, parasitic infection, hepatitis, and requirement of surgical intervention [3]. Pica can result in the formation of a bezoar which untreated can result in bleeding, gastric ulcer due to pressure necrosis, perforation of intestine, and death.

Bezoars are most commonly formed in the stomach but may be formed in any part of the gastrointestinal tract. They are typically classified by their composition into four types: phytobezoars (vegetable matter), trichobezoars (hair), pharmacobezoars, and lactobezoars [4]. Bezoars composed of other materials such as vinyl or latex gloves, parasitic worms, and metals are less common.

Diagnosis of a bezoar can be made with computed tomography (CT) scans and esophagogastroduodenoscopy. Imaging can identify that a foreign body or bezoar is present but is unable to determine the material of the object. Gastric bezoars can often be diagnosed via endoscopy. A CT scan is most useful in patients presenting with small bowel bezoars as the site of obstruction within the small bowel can be visualized [4].

Chemical dissolution is an option for phytobezoars, but more invasive techniques are required for bezoars composed of other materials. While some gastric bezoars can be removed endoscopically, surgical removal with laparoscopy and gastrostomy may be required for definitive treatment of other cases [4]. Surgical removal is typically required for bezoars in the small bowel due to obstruction [5].

We present a case of a digestive tract bezoar composed of gloves that failed endoscopic treatment and required surgical management.

2. Case Presentation

The patient was a nonverbal 55-year-old male with a past medical history of severe intellectual disability, cerebral palsy, epilepsy, right eye impairment due to enucleation, severe chronic gastritis, grade B esophagitis, dysphagia, and pica behavior who presented with vinyl glove ingestion resulting in esophageal and gastric bezoars.

The previous year, the patient was placed on pica precautions with continued surveillance abdominal X-rays after

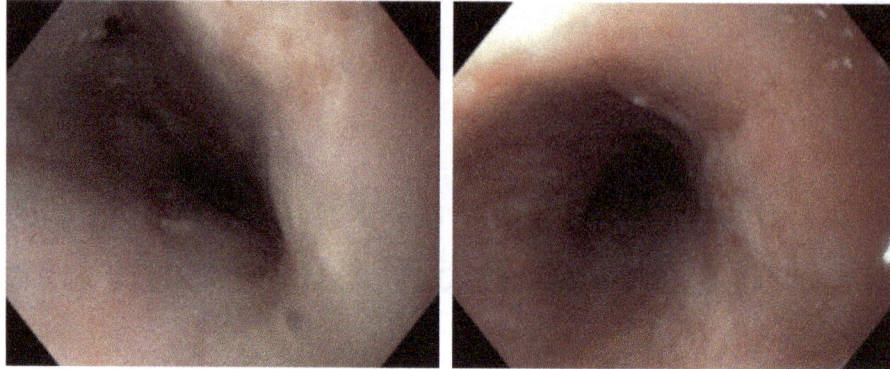

FIGURE 1: Images of esophagogastroduodenoscopy performed just prior to exploratory laparotomy and gastrostomy for evaluation of complete evacuation of foreign bodies in esophagus depicting irritation of the esophagus.

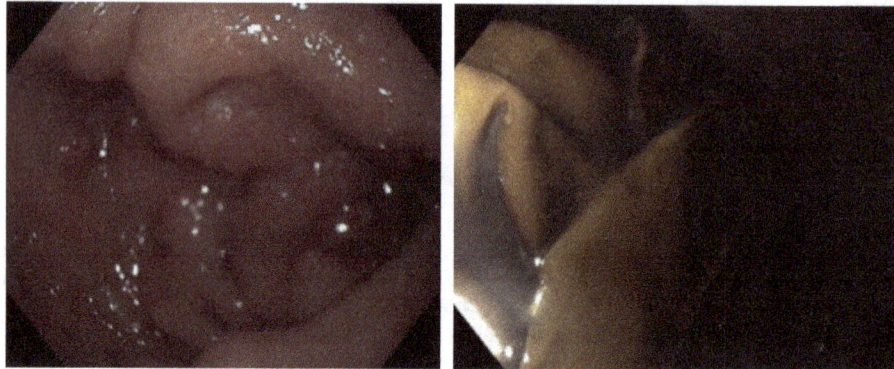

FIGURE 2: Esophagogastroduodenoscopy images of the antrum of the stomach depicting gastric hyperplasia and gastric bezoar composed of gloves.

three documented cases of pica activity in six months. The most recent pica-related event was four months prior to this admission when the patient presented with a rectal mass. At that time, ten plastic gloves were removed from the rectum via colonoscopy. Due to the patient's status, no verbal complaints were noted.

For this case, the patient presented to the gastroenterology clinic after an abdominal X-ray obtained for surveillance showed an esophageal bezoar of unknown etiology. At this time, no nausea, vomiting, constipation, or diarrhea was documented. After a period of observation, a flexible upper GI endoscopy was performed on hospital day 1 and showed a foreign body thought to be ingested vinyl gloves in the lower portion of the esophagus as well as in the gastric fundus. An endoscopic removal was attempted but due to the large size and stiffness of the bezoar, an endoscopic snare became entangled and the removal was abandoned. At this time, a decision was made to leave the patient's endotracheal tube in place due to the fear that removal could result in inhalation of the gloves into the patient's airway. The surgical team was consulted, and the patient was admitted to the surgical intensive care unit (SICU).

A direct laryngoscopy was then performed bedside with failure to visualize the bezoar. A CT chest/abdomen/pelvis was performed, and it showed a bezoar within the proximal esophagus at level of thyroid cartilage extending inferiorly to level of carina, measuring approximately 10 cm in craniocaudal length (Figure 1). It also showed an additional bezoar within the stomach measuring about 6 cm in transverse diameter and 6 cm in craniocaudal diameter.

Out of concern for esophageal damage, the esophageal bezoar was pushed into the stomach via rigid EGD. On hospital day 2, the patient underwent a repeat EGD (Figure 2) and exploratory laparotomy with gastrostomy and evacuation of gastric contents where a $10 \times 4.5 \times 2$ cm bezoar of the plastic glove material was removed from the stomach (Figure 3). An open approach was used instead of a minimally invasive approach due to the nonpliable nature of the partially digested gloves, in order to extract the specimen it would require our incision to be approximately the same size as the open approach. The open approach also decreased contamination and infection risk because it allowed for the stomach contents to be removed outside the peritoneal cavity. The gastrostomy layer and fascia layer were closed, and the skin was left open with iodine-soaked kerlix. The patient was extubated in the operating room and transferred to the floor on postop day 1.

Postoperatively, the patient's course was uneventful. The patient received wound care in the hospital until the abdominal wound was closed on postop day 6. The following

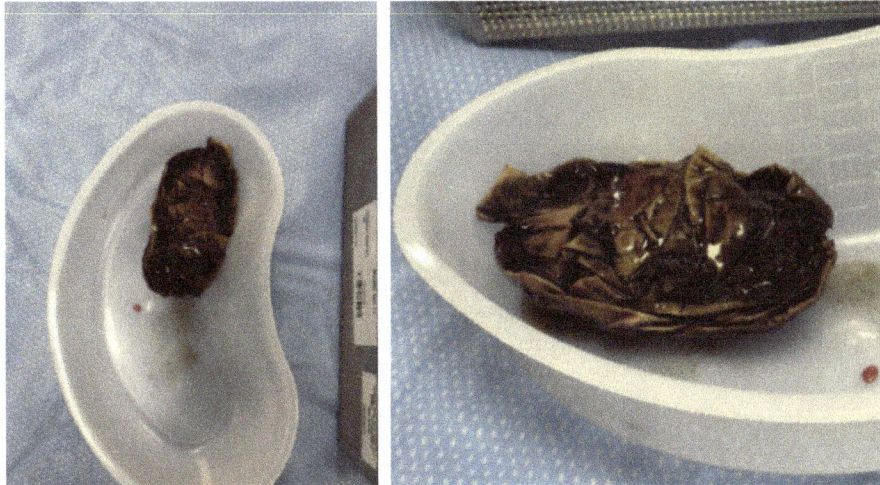

FIGURE 3: Images depicting the gastric bezoar composed of rigid plastic gloves that has just been removed via anterior gastrostomy.

day, the patient was discharged to the state institution where he was previously residing.

3. Discussion

Bezoars composed of usual materials are seen more common in patients with severe intellectual disability than in the general population [1]. Diagnosing a bezoar in adults with severe intellectual disability is often challenging due to the lack of verbal complaints from the patients and unclear physical exam findings. Therefore, when these patients present with anorexia, constipation, vomiting, or change in behavior, it is important to have a high degree of suspicion for a bezoar. This is especially true in patients with a known history of pica. It is also important to note that some patients, such as the one presented in this case, may show no symptoms of a bezoar. Therefore, these patients with a known history of pica behavior should be considered for periodic surveillance with abdominal X-rays [3].

One retrospective study of five adult cases of ingested vinyl gloves found that when ingested, the gloves became stiff and nonpliable [5]. When multiple gloves were ingested together, the bezoar they formed was bulky and rigid resulting in increased risk of bleeding and perforation. A second study reviewing four cases of children ingesting vinyl gloves also reported hardening of the gloves upon ingestion [6].

Due to the unique composition of glove bezoars, treatment with endoscopic fragmentation and removal is not recommended. In these cases, there is an increased risk of snare entrapment and esophageal bleeding [5]. The optimal treatment for these patients is surgical laparotomy and gastrostomy. The postoperative complication rate of these procedures is low and is typically minor such as wound infection [7].

Prevention is an important component of the care of these patients. The institutions that care for these patients must strictly monitor the availability of materials such as gloves.

4. Conclusion

In conclusion, this case examined the ingestion of vinyl gloves in a 55-year-old severely intellectually disabled man with resultant formation of an esophageal and gastric bezoar. After endoscopic management failed, the bezoar was removed via exploratory laparotomy and gastrostomy. This case was unique because the patient had a history of intellectual disability with limited speech, pica, and previous removal of vinyl gloves from the rectum, and the bezoar removed was only discovered due to the implementation of surveillance abdominal X-rays. It is important to consider the material ingested when approaching removal of bezoars. In the case of vinyl glove ingestion, endoscopy has a limited role in the treatment of the resultant bezoar due to the rigid nature of the mass. A more invasive technique such as gastrostomy may be necessary if the mass created is too large to pass through the stomach or causes obstructive symptoms. Lastly, special considerations should be taken in the intellectually disabled population with a history of foreign body ingestion to monitor access to materials as well as symptoms of ingestion. In this population, some form of monitoring such as a KUB used in this case may be necessary to rule out foreign body ingestion when speech is limited.

References

[1] Z. Ali, "Pica in people with intellectual disability: a literature review of aetiology, epidemiology and complications," *Journal of Intellectual and Developmental Disability*, vol. 26, no. 3, pp. 205–215, 2001.

[2] D. E. Danford and A. M. Huber, "Pica among mentally retarded adults," *American Journal of Mental Deficiency*, vol. 87, no. 2, pp. 141–146, 1982.

[3] S. Gravestock, "Eating disorders in adults with intellectual disability," *Journal of Intellectual Disability Research*, vol. 44, no. 6, pp. 625–637, 2000.

[4] M. Iwamuro, H. Okada, K. Matsueda et al., "Review of the diagnosis and management of gastrointestinal bezoars," *World Journal of Gastrointestinal Endoscopy*, vol. 7, no. 4, pp. 336–345, 2015.

[5] I. Kamal, J. Thompson, and D. M. Paquette, "The hazards of vinyl glove ingestion in the mentally retarded patient with pica: new implications for surgical management," *Canadian Journal of Surgery*, vol. 42, no. 3, pp. 201–204, 1999.

[6] G. Stringel, M. Parker, and E. McCoy, "Vinyl glove ingestion in children: a word of caution," *Journal of Pediatric Surgery*, vol. 47, no. 5, pp. 996–998, 2012.

[7] S. L. Castle, O. Zmora, S. Papillon, D. Levin, and J. E. Stein, "Management of complicated gastric bezoars in children and adolescents," *Israel Medical Association Journal*, vol. 17, no. 9, pp. 541–544, 2015.

44

Asymptomatic Gastric Giant Polyp in a Boy with Peutz-Jeghers Syndrome Presented with Multiple Café Au Lait Traits

Christos Plataras ⓘ,[1] Efstratios Christianakis,[1] Florentia Fostira ⓘ,[2] George Bourikis,[3] Maria Chorti,[4] Dimitrios Bourikas,[1] Nikolaos Fotopoulos,[5] Konstantinos Damalas,[6] and Khalil Eirekat[1]

[1]*Pediatric Surgery Department, Penteli Children's Hospital, Ippokratous 8, Penteli 15236, Greece*
[2]*Department of Genetics, Demokritos Research Center, Neapoleos 10, Agia Paraskevi 153 10, Greece*
[3]*General Surgery Department, Tzanio General Hospital, Leoforos Afentouli ke Zanni, Piraeus 185 36, Greece*
[4]*Histopathology Department, Sismanoglio General Hospital, Sismanogliou 37, Marousi 151 26, Greece*
[5]*General Surgery Department, Sismanoglio General Hospital, Sismanogliou 37, Marousi 15126, Greece*
[6]*General Surgery Department, Agios Savvas Regional Cancer Hospital, Leof. Alexandras 171, Athens 11522, Greece*

Correspondence should be addressed to Christos Plataras; christosplataras@yahoo.gr

Academic Editor: Carmela De Crea

We describe an asymptomatic case of PJS in a six-year-old boy with café au lait spots in several parts of his body, a large gastroduodenal polyp, two polyps near the ampulla of Vater, and another in the jejunum. This patient shows some unique aspects of PJS. No other such large gastric polyp in a Peutz-Jeghers child is reported in the literature. The large size of the gastric polyp with lack of symptoms is unusual and poses a unique challenge in terms of management and surgical resection.

1. Introduction

Peutz-Jeghers syndrome (PJS) is an autosomal dominant disorder distinguished by hamartomatous polyps in the gastrointestinal tract and pigmented mucocutaneous lesions. Coexistence of multiple café au lait spots is rare [1, 2].

We describe an asymptomatic case of PJS in a six-year-old boy with café au lait spots in several parts of his body, a large gastroduodenal polyp, two polyps near the ampulla of Vater, and another in the jejunum.

2. Case Presentation

An asymptomatic 6-year-old boy was referred by a dermatologist because of lesions on the inner side of his lower lip that firstly appeared 4 years ago.

He was a skinny boy, light-coloured skin, blond, and green-eyed that was always eating small meals. He had no previous family history of PJS. On clinical examination, we found seventeen café au lait spots ranging from 0.3–3 cm on the anterior and posterior body surface and extremities (Figure 1).

Blood tests showed mild anemia. Abdominal ultrasound and computed tomography showed a large polypoid gastric mass in the antrum and the beginning of the duodenum (Figure 2).

A large, 8 × 5 cm in size, multilobed polypoid gastric mass situated in the antrum was found in gastroscopy. The mass was hemorrhagic, wide-based, and seemed to enter duodenum but moved back to the antrum with peristaltic movements. Two smaller polyps, 0.5 cm in size, were found at the 2nd part of the duodenum near the ampulla of Vater.

The operation was scheduled for polyp removal. Under general anesthesia, a hard epigastric mass was palpated. We made a midline supraumbilical incision. The hard mass could be palpated at the lower third of the stomach. Palpation

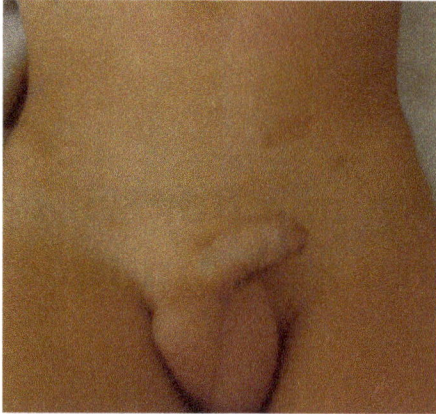

FIGURE 1: Skin lesions resembling café au lait spots.

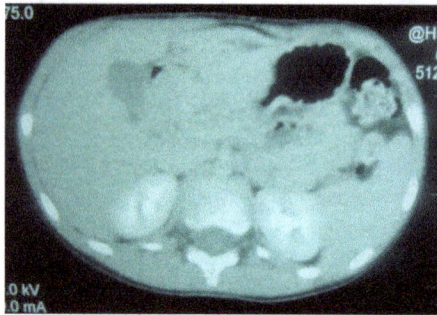

FIGURE 2: Abdominal CT scan. A large polypoid gastric mass in the antrum and the beginning of the duodenum.

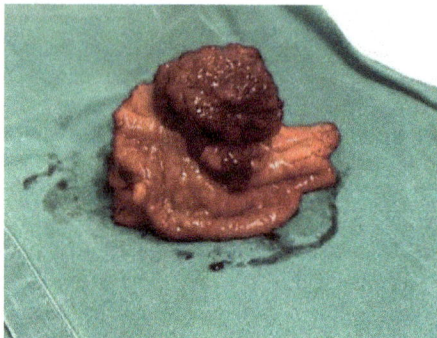

FIGURE 3: Macroscopic appearance of the polyp after surgical removal.

also revealed one lesion at the second part of the duodenum and another in the jejunum. We did a gastrotomy on the anterior surface of the pyloric antrum. The polyp was wide-based (Figure 3), occluding almost completely the pylorus and the duodenum only leaving a space for a hand's little finger to pass. We proceeded to a lower third gastrectomy involving the duodenal bulb, pylorus, and antrum and performed a Billroth I anastomosis. We also did a longitudinal incision of the jejunum 15 cm away from the ligament of Treitz and managed to remove one wide-based polyp, which is 1.5 cm in length. His postoperative course was uneventful.

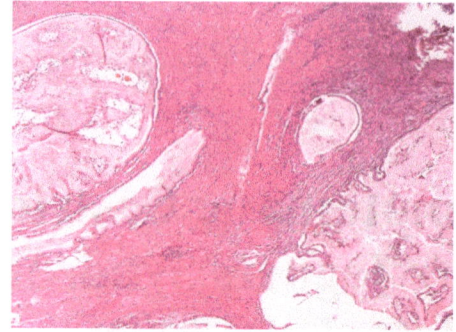

FIGURE 4: Histological appearance of the gastric polyp.

STK11/LKB1 gene identification (a gene encoding a serine/threonine kinase that is responsible for the appearance of the syndrome) (1, 2) showed the splicing mutation: c290 + 1 G > A, in intron 1, which results in aberrant splicing. No family history was reported, so it is highly likely that this mutation was a de novo event. This could not be confirmed, as the patient's parents did not consent to genetic testing.

Postoperative results were excellent. We advised for clinical examination and ultrasound of testis yearly and capsule endoscopy, colonoscopy, and gastroscopy biannually.

At a second look gastroscopy, six months later, we managed to endoscopically remove two smaller polyps near the ampulla of Vater. Colonoscopy was clear. Histology verified the diagnosis of PJS. All 4 polyps showed findings suggestive of hamartomas (Figure 4).

So far, one polyp was detected in the duodenum and another in the sigmoid colon. Polyps were removed by gastroscopy and colonoscopy, respectively. The duodenal polyp was found to be histologically a Peutz-Jeghers polyp, whereas sigmoid polyp was found to be of a hyperplastic type. The gastric polyp was also found to have abnormal (resembling neoplastic) growth in muscularis mucosae where smooth muscle fibers followed the growth of exophytic gastric pits. Biopsies of the esophagus were normal, and gastric biopsies revealed only signs of mild chronic gastritis.

3. Discussion

Primary tumors of the gastrointestinal tract in children are estimated at 1.2% of all pediatric malignancies. They are usually benign. The literature is mainly limited to case studies [3, 4].

The prevalence of gastric polyps in the pediatric population is low compared with that in adults (0.7% vs. 6.35%). The most common pathological types in children are hyperplastic polyps, and most are asymptomatic and do not require removal. Gastric polyps are being encountered in less than 1% of upper gastrointestinal endoscopies performed in children [5, 6].

PJS is an autosomal dominant disease characterized by mucocutaneous pigmentation and hamartomatous polyps of the gastrointestinal tract. The most common location of these polyps is in the small intestine, colon, and stomach, respectively [1, 2].

Our patient shows some unique aspects of PJS. At first, the large size of the gastric polyp with lack of symptoms is unusual and poses a unique challenge in terms of management and surgical resection. No other such large gastric polyp in a Peutz-Jeghers child is reported in the literature. Polypectomy or partial resection was impossible due to its size. The polyp obstructed the view and precluded initial endoscopy of the duodenum. Resection was the only way to inspect the duodenum and first part of the jejunum. Moreover, a Billroth I anastomosis was deemed preferable so that future endoscopies may be facilitated.

Multiple café au lait spots on his body in addition to the classic mucocutaneous macules around the mouth and the buccal mucosa was another unusual finding. Café au lait spots are more often associated with syndromes such as neurofibromatosis type 1 and McCune-Albright syndrome [1, 2]. Unfortunately, skin lesions on our patient were not given attention from his parents and community pediatrician. He was referred for dermatology evaluation many years after the first appearance. So it is important to stress that both unusual and classic hyperpigmentation in children could be the sign of a syndrome that may be "clinically silent" and may have important clinical implications (e.g., in terms of screening). Clinicians should be aware and refer in time.

Surveillance of PJS patients is of critical importance because of the increased risk for malignancies [7, 8]. We advised for clinical examination of testis yearly and capsule endoscopy, colonoscopy, and gastroscopy every three years.

Polyps beyond the reach of conventional endoscopy have been difficult to manage. Until recently, barium contrast upper-gastrointestinal series with a small-bowel follow-through has been recommended. However, recent advances allow better diagnosis and eradication of small-bowel polyps. Video capsule endoscopy (VCE), magnetic resonance enterography (MRE), and double balloon enteroscopy (DBE) are the modern ways of small bowel surveillance [8]. In our patient, we chose VCE due to its availability in our hospital. So far, no malignancy has been found, and the patient remains in excellent clinical condition.

3.1. Summary Box

(i) PJS can present with café au lait traits and hyperpigmented macules of lips

(ii) Unusual and classic hyperpigmentation in children may indicate a "clinically silent" syndrome

(iii) Peutz-Jeghers gastric polyps in children are very rare

(iv) They may become very large in size in small children but still be asymptomatic

(v) Prompt diagnosis may avoid complicated operations and prevent any possibility for malignant transformation

(vi) Follow-up of children with PJS is necessary for early diagnosis and management of possible tumors

Authors' Contributions

Dr. Plataras and Dr. Christianakis wrote the Abstract, Introduction, and Case Presentation and are responsible for the final submission. Dr. Chorti made the histology slides, chose the ones to be published, and edited the pictures. Dr. Fostira made all the gene exams and wrote all the relevant parts of this paper. Mr. Bourikis and Mr. Bourikas wrote the Discussion and collected references. Dr. Eirekat supervised the English language and did the final corrections.

References

[1] S. Brito, M. Póvoas, J. Dupont, and A. I. Lopes, "Peutz-Jeghers syndrome: early clinical expression of a new STK11 gene variant," *BMJ Case Reports*, 2015.

[2] A. Dutta, S. K. Ghosh, and S. K. Kundu, "Peutz-Jegher syndrome," *Indian Pediatrics*, vol. 52, no. 2, pp. 176-177, 2015.

[3] N. Zheng, X. M. Xiao, K. R. Dong, L. Chen, Y. Y. Ma, and K. Li, "Primary gastric tumors in infants and children: 15 cases of 20-year report," *Journal of Cancer Research and Clinical Oncology*, vol. 142, no. 5, pp. 1061–1067, 2016.

[4] S. C. Kim, J. W. Hwang, M. K. Lee, and P. H. Hwang, "Rare case of primary gastric Burkitt lymphoma in a child," *The Korean Journal of Gastroenterology*, vol. 68, no. 2, pp. 87–92, 2016.

[5] S. Diaconescu, I. Miron, N. Gimiga et al., "Unusual endoscopic findings in children: esophageal and gastric polyps: three cases report," *Medicine*, vol. 95, no. 3, article e2539, 2016.

[6] E. Y. Jung, S. O. Choi, K. B. Cho, E. S. Kim, K. S. Park, and J. B. Hwang, "Successful endoscopic submucosal dissection of a giant polyp in a 21-month-old female," *World Journal of Gastroenterology*, vol. 20, no. 1, pp. 323–325, 2014.

[7] M. G. F. van Lier, A. M. Westerman, A. Wagner et al., "High cancer risk and increased mortality in patients with Peutz-Jeghers syndrome," *Gut*, vol. 60, no. 2, pp. 141–147, 2011.

[8] A. Goverde, S. E. Korsse, A. Wagner et al., "Small-bowel surveillance in patients with Peutz-Jeghers syndrome: comparing magnetic resonance enteroclysis and double balloon enteroscopy," *Journal of Clinical Gastroenterology*, vol. 51, no. 4, pp. e27–e33, 2017.

45

Mesh Migration into the J-Pouch in a Patient with Post-Ulcerative Colitis Colectomy

Asem Ghanim,[1] **Benjamin Smood,**[2] **Joseph Martinez,**[1]
Melanie S. Morris,[1] **and John R. Porterfield**[1]

[1]*Department of Surgery, University of Alabama at Birmingham, Birmingham, AL, USA*
[2]*School of Medicine, University of Alabama at Birmingham, Birmingham, AL, USA*

Correspondence should be addressed to John R. Porterfield; jporterfield@uabmc.edu

Academic Editor: Christophoros Foroulis

Mesh repair offers advantages like lower postsurgical pain and earlier return to work. Thus, it has become a widely used treatment option. Here, we present the first case report of a mesh migration into a J-pouch in a patient with history of ulcerative colitis who underwent total abdominal colectomy with J-pouch and ileoanal anastomosis and a subsequent laparoscopic ventral hernia repair with mesh.

1. Introduction

Incisional ventral hernia remains a common complication of abdominal surgery [1, 2]; its incidence is estimated at 10–15% with a recurrence of 20–45% [1, 2]. As such, patients undergoing J-pouch construction are at risk for hernia development and complications of the subsequent repair.

Complications often include infection, seroma, recurrence, or rejection but can include fistulas, erosions, and rarely mesh migration [3–5]. However, the low incidence of serious complications is likely underestimated due to the lack of long-term studies [6]. Several cases have reported bowel obstruction as a result of mesh migration [7, 8]. Although mesh migration to the colon has been reported [9, 10], to our knowledge, this is the first documented patient presentation with mesh migration into a J-pouch following incisional ventral hernia repair.

2. Case Report

A 43-year-old Hispanic male patient presented to the emergency department with intermittent lower abdominal pain and diarrhea. The patient had a previous history of ulcerative colitis and total abdominal colectomy with J-pouch and ileoanal anastomosis (2012) and a laparoscopic incisional ventral hernia repair with mesh (2015) in another institution.

The patient described his pain as intermittent and vague in nature, starting from the suprapubic area and spreading all over his abdomen, rated 6/10. The pain was not associated with fever, nausea, or vomiting. The patient had been having such episodes since his hernia repair but they increased in intensity over the past three weeks. He also had chronic diarrhea with a small amount of blood when he wipes. Physical exam showed a midline incision scar with bulging when coughing and diffuse tenderness all over the abdomen most prominently over the suprapubic/lower abdominal area. The patient looked ill in mild distress and had positive bowel sounds and tachycardia. Initial lab results showed mild normocytic anemia (HGB: 10.5, WBC: 9800, PLT: 579, HCT: 32, and MCV: 70). CT scan (Figure 1) showed thickening and stranding of the J-pouch and rectum, with obliteration of the rectal fat planes, along with mesenteric lymphadenopathy. There was proximal dilatation with partial air-fluid levels within the small bowel, concerning for partial obstruction. A flexible sigmoidoscopy (Figure 2) showed inflamed mucosa with ulceration and adherent mucus. Multiple biopsies were obtained. A large foreign object was visualized in the pouch. It had a rope-like lattice appearance on its outside; the inner

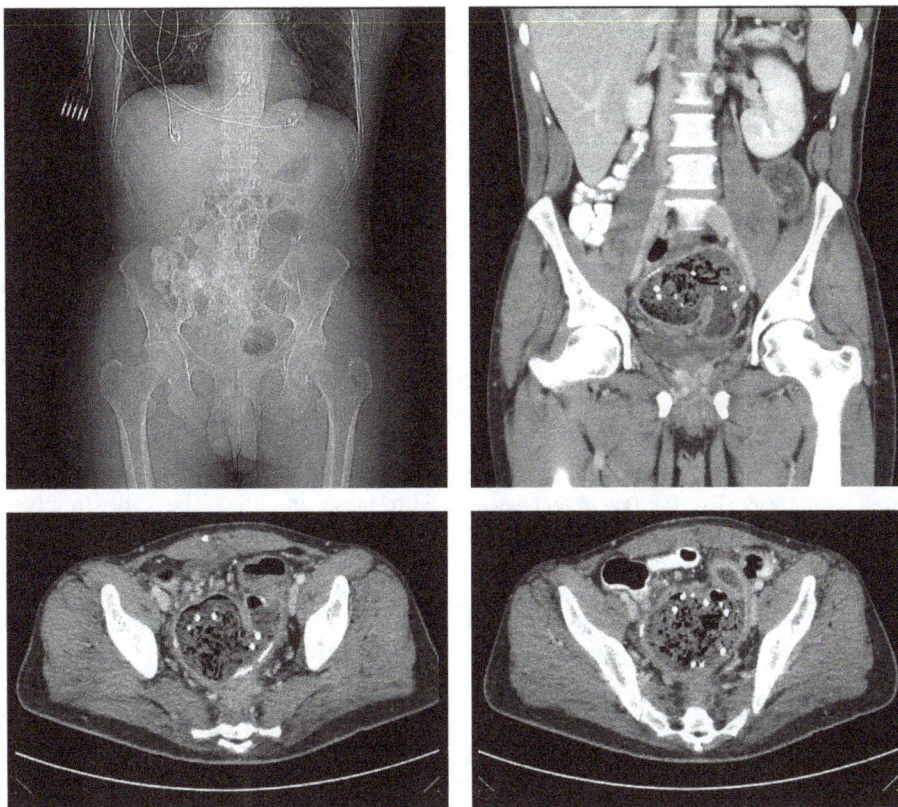

FIGURE 1: CT scan showing thickening and stranding of the J-pouch and rectum, with obliteration of the rectal fat planes, along with mesenteric lymphadenopathy. There was proximal dilatation with partial air-fluid levels within the small bowel, concerning for partial obstruction.

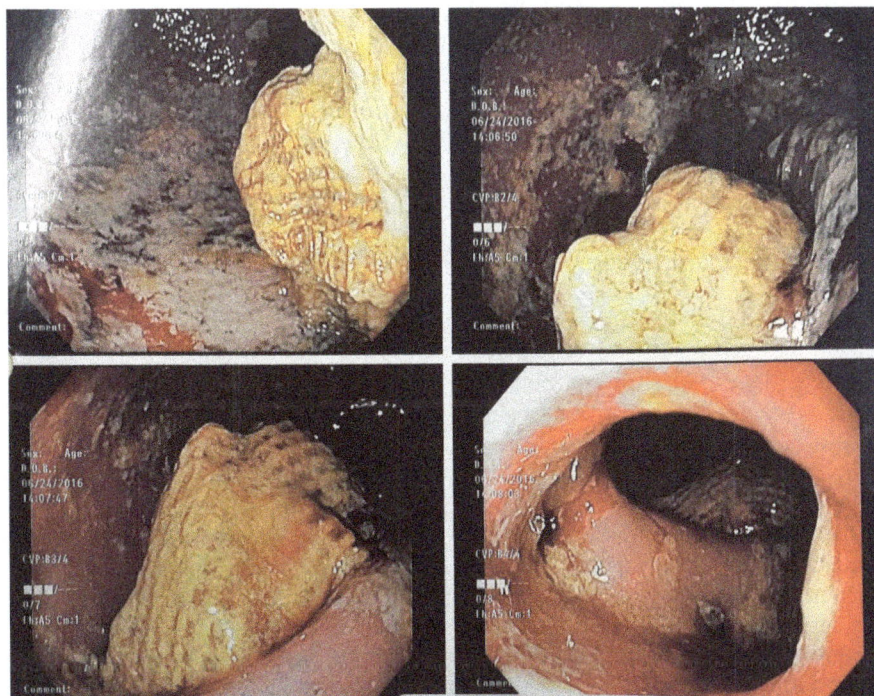

FIGURE 2: A flexible sigmoidoscopy shows inflamed mucosa with ulceration and adherent mucus. A large foreign object was visualized in the pouch.

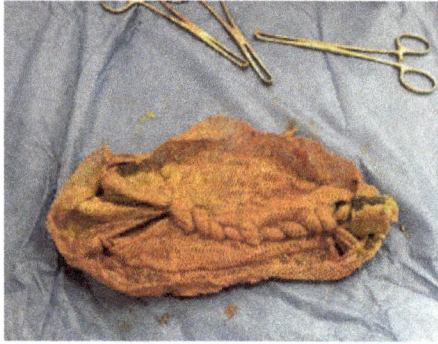

FIGURE 3: The mesh extracted from the J-pouch retaining tacks and sutures attached from the original placement one year previously.

contents were not well visualized. The foreign object was not removed then due to the uncertainty of its origin and extent. The patient was then taken to the operating room for pouch exam under anesthesia where the foreign body was removed in its entirety (Figure 3). The object turned out to be a mesh with tacks and sutures from the original placement one year before. The patient's pain resolved immediately after the procedure and his bowel function returned to normal. The remainder of his postoperative course was unremarkable. He was discharged 2 days after his procedure.

3. Discussion

Review of the literature for mesh migration/erosion case reports showed 86 cases in 79 reports published between 1990 and 2015. There were 23 reported cases of erosions, 24 cases of fistulas, 38 cases of migrations, and one case of coincidental fistula and mesh migration. Destinations for migration/erosion included bowel (30), bladder (14), peritoneum/peritoneal cavity (8), stomach (7), esophagus (3), right lower bronchus (1), scrotum (2), and adnexa (1). Fistulas reported were found between bowel and skin (15), bowel and bladder (2), bowel and another segment of bowel (1), bowel and scrotum (1), and bladder and skin (2). The median time calculated between hernia repair and presentation was 48 months (range: 2–360 months).

Mesh migration is defined as the whole mesh displacing into the organ. Mesh erosion is defined as partial mesh perforation into the organ while a portion is still outside. Mesh fistulation is defined as erosion into two organs causing a tract formation between them or abscess formation that erodes to another organ.

Mesh complication presentations vary drastically from incidental findings to mimicking cancer. Still, common themes are shared, including abdominal pain, gastrointestinal bleeding, bowel obstruction, and diarrhea.

The most common complication for all reported hiatal hernias ($n = 10$) was displacement to the stomach (70%, 7/10) with symptoms of dysphagia. Inguinal hernia mesh repairs ($n = 41$) are most frequently displaced to the bladder (27%, 11/41) while presenting with urinary tract infections or hematuria. Ventral/incisional hernias ($n = 24$) routinely displaced to the bowel (92%, 22/24), presenting with bowel

obstruction or abdominal pain. The median time to presentation was 24, 48, and 60 months for hiatal, inguinal, and ventral/incisional hernias, respectively. As such, despite erosion, fistula, and migration being rare complications, healthcare providers must remain vigilant of the unpredictability of mesh displacement and other serious complications after hernia repair with seemingly unrelated symptoms.

Table 1 in Supplementary Material available online at https://doi.org/10.1155/2017/3617476 reviews the 86 cases of mesh displacement reported between 1990 and 2015. Mesh and procedure types, the various destinations, the main symptoms, and time of presentations are made accessible for future investigators.

The patient in this case presented to the emergency department with nonspecific symptoms following an ileoanal anastomosis in 2012 and an incisional ventral hernia repair with mesh in 2015. The time to presentation for mesh migration (<12 months) was shorter than the median in our review of the literature (48 months). Interestingly, the mesh migration occurred within 1 year of operation, which is a common time frame for pouchitis to develop after ileoanal anastomosis construction (15–18% within 1 postoperative year) [11, 12]. It is worth noting that both pouchitis and mesh migration are associated with postoperative inflammation.

Despite unclear pathophysiology, mesh migration is presumed to be due to inflammation caused by the foreign body, combined with rejection or displacing forces leading to slow erosion of tissue from the prosthesis [5, 13, 14]. It is unclear whether the history of an abdominal surgery with high incidence of pouchitis is related to the unusual presentation of mesh migration to the J-pouch, but similarities in pathophysiology warrant further investigation into operative procedures, materials, and postoperative prevention that may optimize outcomes for patients with specific surgical morbidities [15, 16]. Improvements remain to be made in the balance between durability, foreign body reaction, amount of material, chronic pain, and time to recovery [17].

Disclosure

Dr. John R. Porterfield is a consultant of Intuitive Surgical.

References

[1] O. Bostanci, U. O. Idiz, M. Yazar, and M. Mihmanli, "A rare complication of composite dual mesh: migration and enterocutaneous fistula formation," *Case Reports in Surgery*, vol. 2015, Article ID 293659, 3 pages, 2015.

[2] A. Kingsnorth and K. LeBlanc, "Hernias: inguinal and incisional," *The Lancet*, vol. 362, no. 9395, pp. 1561–1571, 2003.

[3] M. T. Nguyen, R. L. Berger, S. C. Hicks et al., "Comparison of outcomes of synthetic mesh vs suture repair of elective primary ventral herniorrhaphy: a systematic review and meta-analysis," *JAMA Surgery*, vol. 149, no. 5, pp. 415–421, 2014.

[4] F. Aziz and M. Zaeemb, "Chronic abdominal pain secondary to mesh erosion into ceacum following incisional hernia repair: a

case report and literature review," *Journal of Clinical Medicine Research*, vol. 6, no. 2, pp. 153–155, 2014.

[5] A. Agrawal and R. Avill, "Mesh migration following repair of inguinal hernia: a case report and review of literature," *Hernia*, vol. 10, no. 1, pp. 79–82, 2006.

[6] J. W. A. Burger, R. W. Luijendijk, W. C. J. Hop et al., "Long-term follow-up of a randomized controlled trial of suture versus mesh repair of incisional hernia," *Annals of Surgery*, vol. 240, no. 4, pp. 578–585, 2004.

[7] I. Yilmaz, D. O. Karakaş, I. Sucullu, Y. Ozdemir, and E. Yucel, "A rare cause of mechanical bowel obstruction: mesh migration," *Hernia*, vol. 17, no. 2, pp. 267–269, 2013.

[8] M.-J. Chen and Y.-F. Tian, "Intraperitoneal migration of a mesh plug with a small intestinal perforation: report of a case," *Surgery Today*, vol. 40, no. 6, pp. 566–568, 2010.

[9] E. C. Nelson and T. J. Vidovszky, "Composite mesh migration into the sigmoid colon following ventral hernia repair," *Hernia*, vol. 15, no. 1, pp. 101–103, 2011.

[10] S. Al-Subaie, M. Al-Haddad, W. Al-Yaqout, M. Al-Hajeri, and C. Claus, "A case of a colocutaneous fistula: a rare complication of mesh migration into the sigmoid colon after open tension-free hernia repair," *International Journal of Surgery Case Reports*, vol. 14, pp. 26–29, 2015.

[11] G. Cárdenas, R. Bravo, S. Delgado et al., "Recurrent volvular herniation of the ileal pouch: a case report and literature review," *International Journal of Colorectal Disease*, vol. 31, no. 3, pp. 749-750, 2016.

[12] E. Gorgun and F. H. Remzi, "Complications of Ileoanal Pouches," *Clinics in Colon and Rectal Surgery*, vol. 17, no. 1, pp. 43–55, 2004.

[13] A. Celik, S. Kutun, C. Kockar, N. Mengi, H. Ulucanlar, and A. Cetin, "Colonoscopic removal of inguinal hernia mesh: report of a case and literature review," *Journal of Laparoendoscopic and Advanced Surgical Techniques - Part A*, vol. 15, no. 4, pp. 408–410, 2005.

[14] S. R. Yolen and E. T. Grossman, "Colonoscopic removal of a postoperative foreign body," *Journal of Clinical Gastroenterology*, vol. 11, no. 4, article 483, 1989.

[15] E. P. Misiakos, P. Patapis, N. Zavras, P. Tzanetis, and A. Machairas, "Current trends in laparoscopic ventral hernia repair," *Journal of the Society of Laparoendoscopic Surgeons*, vol. 19, no. 3, Article ID e2015.00048, 2015.

[16] M. Śmietański, K. Bury, A. Tomaszewska, I. Lubowiecka, and C. Szymczak, "Biomechanics of the front abdominal wall as a potential factor leading to recurrence with laparoscopic ventral hernia repair," *Surgical Endoscopy and Other Interventional Techniques*, vol. 26, no. 5, pp. 1461–1467, 2012.

[17] A. L. Vorst, "Evolution and advances in laparoscopic ventral and incisional hernia repair," *World Journal of Gastrointestinal Surgery*, vol. 7, no. 11, pp. 293–305, 2015.

46

Management of Small Bowel Perforation by a Bizarre Foreign Body in a 55-Year-Old Woman

Francesca D'Auria,[1] **Vincenzo Consalvo** (ID)**,**[1,2] **Antonio Canero,**[3] **Maria Russo,**[3] **Carmela Rescigno,**[3] **and Domenico Lombardi**[3]

[1]*General Surgery, Università degli Studi di Salerno, Via Giovanni Paolo II, 132, 84084 Fisciano, Italy*
[2]*Clinique Clementville, rue de Clementville, Montpellier, France*
[3]*Azienda Ospedaliera Universitaria San Giovanni di Dio e Ruggi d'Aragona, Via San Leonardo, 1, Salerno, Italy*

Correspondence should be addressed to Vincenzo Consalvo; vincenzoconsa@gmail.com

Academic Editor: Gabriel Sandblom

Introduction. Ingestion of foreign bodies including dentures, fishbone, screw, and/or surgical devices can be a cause of morbidity, and it rarely could be fatal. *Presentation of Case.* We present the first hitherto reported case of mussel shell ingestion, which caused acute abdominal pain in a 55-year-old woman. The shell pierced ileal loops, and it was found in the abdominal cavity. *Discussion.* The accidental or voluntary ingestion of a foreign body is an uncommon event compared to the other causes of bowel perforation. It is fundamental to immediately remove the intestinal fluid, repair the tear, and prevent sepsis, because each delay in diagnosis can lead to a worst outcome. *Conclusion.* In case of bowel perforation, it important for surgeons, who are dealing with these acute care patients, to be aware of different designs and constructions of possible foreign bodies, in order to be prepared to deal with different possible scenarios and be able to manage them properly.

1. Introduction

Foreign body ingestion is a commonly seen accident in emergencies [1–3]. It may accidentally occur in children or intentionally in psychiatric patients. In the 90% of ingested foreign bodies, they pass through the gastrointestinal tract without complications as punching or obstruction, but in the 10% of the case, they required a surgical removal [4]. Ingestion of foreign bodies including dentures, fishbone, screw, and/or surgical devices can be a cause of morbidity and mortality [5–7]. We report the first case of mussel shell ingestion which caused acute abdomen.

2. Ethical and Administrative Information

The patients gave her consent to the publication of scientific data. The authors declare that there will not be any communication to the third party for the respect of her privacy. This study was written respecting the ethical principles for medical research involving human subjects (Declaration of Helsinki). This article was written according to SCARE 2016 guidelines on case report writing. Since other few cases have been reported, it was not necessary to publish on a public registry.

3. Case Report

A 55-year-old Caucasian obese woman (body mass index = 35) was admitted to Surgical Department of our institution for acute abdominal pain. Her past medical history was negative for previous gastrointestinal disease or surgery. She was on medical therapy for hypertension, type II diabetes, and minor depression. Glasgow coma scale was 15. She referred an increasing acute abdominal pain risen 5 hours ago after a fish-based dinner. She has showed an acute diffuse peritonitis. White blood cell count was 32.000 U/μL, with neutrophilia (90%); other blood tests were in normal range. Body temperature was 39.2°C. Electrocardiogram showed sinus rhythm with 92 heart rate. Chest X-ray was normal. Abdominal X-ray showed free subdiaphragmatic

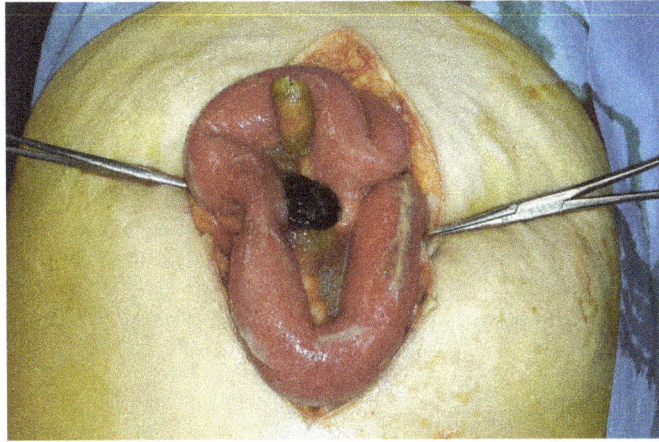

FIGURE 1: View of the abdomen at the opening of the peritoneum.

air. CT scan confirmed the suspicion of small bowel perforation because of the finding of free fluid in the abdomen and an inhomogeneous mass in the small bowel. A nasogastric tube was placed, and it drained 50 mL of biliogastric material. Because of her status, she was immediately ran to the theater for exploratory laparotomy under general anesthesia and oral intubation. Although each clinical finding suggested a colonic or caecum perforation, during the systematic exploration of the bowel loops, surgeons found free intestinal fluid in the abdomen, fecal peritonitis, and (at 60–70 from ileocaecal valve) a 3 cm linear tear of the ileum which was caused by the curve edge of a shell mussel (Figure 1). The foreign body was completely extracted from the lumen through the hole (Figure 2), and the breach was sutured with simple double-strand stitches of polyglactin 3/0 parallel to the bowel tearing. Abdominal cavity washing was carried out with 2 liters of saline. Two drains were placed on suction for 24 hours. Antibiotic therapy (ciprofloxacin, meropenem, and metronidazole) and nil by mouth regimen were started. Patient was admitted in Intensive Care Unit for 12 hours, the weaning from the ventilator, and she was discharged at home in healthy status from the ward on the sixth postoperative day. At the 30-day follow-up, the patient was in good clinical condition, surgical wounds were completely sealed, blood tests were normal, and bowel function was recovered.

4. Discussion

The accidental or intentional ingestion of foreign bodies including dentures, fishbone, screw, magnets, lithium batteries, and/or surgical devices can be a cause of morbidity, but mortality rates have been extremely low. As a matter of facts, a compilation of multiple studies including 2 large series report no deaths in 852 adults and 1 death in 2206 children; mortality rate is extremely low [1, 2]. In the 90% of ingested foreign bodies, they pass through the gastrointestinal tract without complications as punching or obstruction, but in the up to 10% of the case, they required an endoscopic or open/laparoscopic surgical removal [4, 5]. The foreign body ingestion is a commonly seen in emergency setting

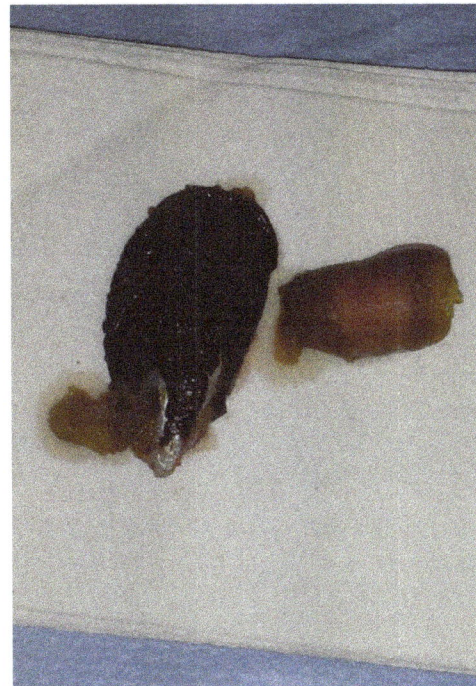

FIGURE 2: Complete extraction of the foreign body.

[7, 8]. It may accidentally occur in children, elderly, edentulous patients, patients with neurological disorders, and addicted patients or intentionally in psychiatric patients or prisoners. A slight prevalence in male is documented [1–3]. Any foreign body that remains in the tract may cause obstruction, perforation or hemorrhage, and fistula formation. The most common sites of perforation are the ileocaecal junction and sigmoid colon. Other potential sites are the duodenojejunal flexure, appendix, colonic flexure, diverticula, and the anal sphincter [8]. Exploratory laparotomy has been the main treatment for patients requiring surgery. However, surgeons are trying to routinely use laparoscopy in the emergency setting aiming reduction in the length of stay and for esthetical purpose [5]. In the diagnosis management, CT scan is a mandatory requirement to orient the endoscopic

or surgical management. In case of bowel perforation, the correct management should be the precocious removal of the foreign body, the suture of the breach, and the toilette of the abdominal cavity in order to reduce the septic risk and restore bowel function [8, 9].

5. Conclusion

Inflammatory bowel disease, appendicitis, diverticula, gallstone migration, cancer, endometriosis, trauma, infection, autoimmune disease, drugs, vasculopathy [10–13], and foreign bodies can cause an acute bowel perforation. It is fundamental to immediately remove the intestinal fluid, repair the tear, and prevent sepsis. Each delay in diagnosis can lead to a worst outcome. Because the accidental or voluntary ingestion of a foreign body is uncommon compared to the other causes of bowel perforation, it is important to remember that it is a possible event which deserves to be contemplated in the list of causes to be investigated in case of free air in abdomen.

Additional Points

Highlights. A foreign body ingestion is an uncommon cause of bowel perforation. It may accidentally occur in children or intentionally in psychiatric patients. Differential diagnosis is mandatory, i.e., IBD, diverticula, vasculopathy, etc. It is fundamental to remove intestinal fluid, repair bowel tear, and prevent sepsis. Each delay in diagnosis can lead to a worst outcome.

Authors' Contributions

Vincenzo Consalvo and Francesca D'Auria wrote the case. The surgeons Domenico Lombardi, Carmela Rescigno, and Antonio Canero reviewed the care. Maria Russo also reviewed the care.

References

[1] N. G. Velitchkov, G. I. Grigorov, J. E. Losanoff, and K. T. Kjossev, "Ingested foreign bodies of the gastrointestinal tract: retrospective analysis of 542 cases," *World Journal of Surgery*, vol. 20, no. 8, pp. 1001–1005, 1996.

[2] E. Panieri and D. H. Bass, "The management of ingested foreign bodies in children—a review of 663 cases," *European Journal of Emergency Medicine*, vol. 2, no. 2, pp. 83–87, 1995.

[3] A. Gałczyński, E. Cieplińska, and A. Konturek, "Habitual intentional foreign body ingestion - a literature review," *Polski Przeglad Chirurgiczny*, vol. 88, no. 5, pp. 290–297, 2016.

[4] M. Bekkerman, A. H. Sachdev, J. Andrade, Y. Twersky, and S. Iqbal, "Endoscopic management of foreign bodies in the gastrointestinal tract: a review of the literature," *Gastroenterology Research and Practice*, vol. 2016, Article ID 8520767, 6 pages, 2016.

[5] B. Mohamed Aboulkacem, M. Ghalleb, A. Khemir et al., "Laparoscopic assisted foreign body extraction from the small bowel: a case report," *International Journal of Surgery Case Reports*, vol. 41, pp. 283–286, 2017.

[6] M. A. Memon and R. J. Fitztgibbons Jr., "The role of minimal access surgery in the acute abdomen," *The Surgical Clinics of North America*, vol. 77, no. 6, pp. 1333–1353, 1997.

[7] V. Papastergiou, N. Mathou, K. Manes et al., "When perforation is not the culprit: case report and systematic review of mechanical small-bowel obstruction complicating colonoscopy," *Acta Gastroenterologica Belgica*, vol. 81, no. 1, pp. 89–92, 2018.

[8] M. A. Revell, M. A. Pugh, and M. McGhee, "Gastrointestinal traumatic injuries: gastrointestinal perforation," *Critical Care Nursing Clinics of North America*, vol. 30, no. 1, pp. 157–166, 2018.

[9] S. R. Rami Reddy and M. S. Cappell, "A systematic review of the clinical presentation, diagnosis, and treatment of small bowel obstruction," *Current Gastroenterology Reports*, vol. 19, no. 6, p. 28, 2017.

[10] A. A. Mohamed, C. J. Richards, K. Boyle, and G. Faust, "Severe inflammatory ileitis resulting in ileal perforation in association with combination immune checkpoint blockade for metastatic malignant melanoma," *BMJ Case Reports*, vol. 2018, p. 5, 2018.

[11] P. Lebert, I. Millet, O. Ernst et al., "Acute jejunoileal diverticulitis: multicenter descriptive study of 33 patients," *American Journal of Roentgenology*, vol. 210, no. 6, pp. 1245–1251, 2018.

[12] C. Y. Louie, M. A. DiMaio, G. W. Charville, G. J. Berry, and T. A. Longacre, "Gastrointestinal tract vasculopathy: clinicopathology and description of a possible "new entity" with protean features," *The American Journal of Surgical Pathology*, vol. 42, no. 7, pp. 866–876, 2018.

[13] M. T. Glavind, M. V. Møllgaard, M. L. Iversen, L. H. Arendt, and A. Forman, "Obstetrical outcome in women with endometriosis including spontaneous hemoperitoneum and bowel perforation: a systematic review," *Best Practice & Research. Clinical Obstetrics & Gynaecology*, vol. 21, 2018.

47

Management and Reconstruction of a Gastroesophageal Junction Adenocarcinoma Patient Three Years after Pancreaticoduodenectomy: A Surgical Puzzle

Dionysios Dellaportas, James A. Gossage, and Andrew R. Davies

Department of Oesophagogastric Surgery, St Thomas' Hospital, King's College London, London, UK

Correspondence should be addressed to Dionysios Dellaportas; dellapdio@gmail.com

Academic Editor: Alexander R. Novotny

Introduction. With the improving survival of cancer patients, the development of a secondary primary cancer is an increasingly common phenomenon. Extensive surgery during initial treatment may pose significant challenges to surgeons managing the second primary cancer. *Case Presentation.* A 69-year-old male, who had a pancreaticoduodenectomy three years ago for pancreatic head adenocarcinoma, underwent an uneventful extended total gastrectomy for gastroesophageal junctional adenocarcinoma. The reconstruction controversies and considerations are highlighted. *Discussion.* Genetic, environmental, and lifestyle factors are common for several gastrointestinal malignancies. However, the occurrence of a second unfavorable cancer such as gastroesophageal adenocarcinoma after pancreatic head cancer treatment is extremely uncommon. This clinical scenario possesses numerous difficulties for the surgeon, since surgical resection is the mainstay of treatment for both malignancies. Gastrointestinal reconstruction becomes challenging and requires careful planning and meticulous surgical technique along with sound intraoperative judgement.

1. Introduction

Improvement of management for cancer patients, increased overall survival, and identification of the disease in early stages have led to the rare event of patients developing a second primary cancer later in their lives. In various studies the incidence of second primary cancer is 6.6–9% [1]. Complex surgery during initial cancer treatment can limit surgical options during management plan of the secondary malignancy. We present an interesting case of a 69-year-old male treated successfully in our institution, who developed gastroesophageal junction adenocarcinoma three years after pancreaticoduodenectomy for pancreatic head adenocarcinoma and finally underwent an extended total gastrectomy. The aim of our study is to highlight the treatment options, the controversies, and the challenging surgical reconstructive options in such a clinical scenario.

2. Case Presentation

A 69-year-old white male patient was investigated for dysphagia and vomiting associated with weight loss. The patient had a medical history of hypertension and hyperlipidemia and a surgical history of pylorus-preserving pancreaticoduodenectomy three years ago for pancreatic head adenocarcinoma. The latter's histopathological stage was pT1N0 (TNM 7th Edition AJCC classification) and the patient received no adjuvant treatment. Upper gastrointestinal endoscopy revealed an ulcerated, friable tumour of the gastroesophageal junction (GOJ) and histopathology confirmed the presence of poorly differentiated adenocarcinoma. Formal staging of the disease was performed with computed tomography (CT) scan, followed by positron emission tomography (PET/CT) scan and endoscopic ultrasound (EUS) and after multidisciplinary team (MDT) discussion the patient was staged as Siewert type II cT2N1M0 GOJ adenocarcinoma [2]. No evidence of distant disease from either malignancy was revealed and the patient was considered for radical treatment. According to usual management [3] he received three cycles of neoadjuvant chemotherapy with epirubicin, cisplatin, and capecitabine (ECX protocol), which was well tolerated and with good radiological and clinical response. Restaging CT scan demonstrated regression of the two enlarged left-gastric lymph nodes. The patient was offered either surgery or definite chemoradiotherapy for locoregional control of the disease and chose the former option after extensive counselling as to the associated risks and benefits.

Surgical planning raised some anatomical challenges. Reviewing the pancreaticoduodenectomy reconstruction method from his operative note three years ago, the patient had a pylorus-preserving pancreaticoduodenectomy (PPPD) with an isolated Roux-en-Y reconstruction for the pancreaticojejunal anastomosis. Ligation of the gastroduodenal artery (GDA) was done during PPPD, which gives rise to the right gastroepiploic artery precluding the use of the stomach as conduit for any kind of oesophagogastrectomy. Moreover, the use of colon as a conduit is appealing, but the use of either the left or the right colon involves dissection of the middle colic vessels and meticulous preservation of anastomotic arcades, in an area where the isolated jejunal Roux limb may ascend, retrocolic, and to the left of the above vessels for the pancreaticojejunal anastomosis. Extensive adhesiolysis may be anticipated since the superior mesenteric vessels, which give rise to the middle colic vessels, were dissected during the PPPD.

With all the above in mind, surgical exploration was decided and performed through the old bilateral subcostal incision. The primary tumour involved the GOJ, but after transhiatal mobilization and intraoperative upper gastrointestinal endoscopy it became feasible to get to macroscopically clear margins to the thoracic oesophagus without the need of thoracotomy. In addition, duodenojejunostomy was antecolic and performed on the long blind ended jejunal loop that originated just below the duodenojejunal flexure from the previous Whipple procedure. After division of the jejunum, an extended total gastrectomy was performed. Oesophagojejunal anastomosis was the only reconstructive anastomosis needed in this complex case to reestablish gastrointestinal continuity. Total operative time was 170 minutes. Final histopathology showed a complete resection (R0) of a ypT1bN0 GOJ poorly differentiated adenocarcinoma, with negative lymph nodes (0/29). The patient had an uneventful postoperative course and was discharged on the 10th postoperative day, while MDT decision was for no adjuvant treatment. He remains well on postoperative surveillance.

3. Discussion

The development of a second malignancy as mentioned above is an unusual event, which is increasingly common in an era of improved survival for cancer patients. Particularly for patients with unfavorable malignancies, like pancreatic, oesophageal, or gastric cancer, the incidence of second primary cancer is less than 5% [1]. Simultaneous

or metachronous occurrence of gastroesophageal adenocarcinoma with periampullary tumours is extremely unusual. In an interesting review of more than 10.000 gastric cancer patients [4], 96 of them had a second primary malignancy and only 5 of them had pancreatic adenocarcinoma. For oesophageal adenocarcinoma patients, the most common second primary malignancies are gastric, oropharyngeal, and lung cancer, while pancreatic cancer is extremely rare [5]. Obviously, common risk factors such as genetic, lifestyle, or dietary factors can give rise to gastrointestinal malignancies of different sites, and if the patient survives long enough after an initial treatment, a second primary gastrointestinal cancer may develop. Surgical resection remains the mainstay of treatment for pancreatic, gastric, and oesophageal cancer.

Technically, surgical strategies have been described in the setting of previous oesophagogastrectomy for the performance of pancreaticoduodenectomy [6], mostly involving the use of colon as conduit, and in the form of case reports. Other challenging options when the right gastroepiploic vessels are compromised include the use of supercharged jejunal interposition conduits [7] or microvascular reconstruction methods for the right gastroepiploic vessels [8, 9]. Oesophagogastrectomy and pancreaticoduodenectomy are individually extensive operations, and their combination either simultaneously or metachronously poses unique challenges. In a recent review of such cases, only three cases involved oesophageal resection after pancreaticoduodenectomy [10]. Our case involved an extended total gastrectomy and intrathoracic oesophagojejunal anastomosis, and to the best of our knowledge it is the first case reporting such a reconstruction configuration.

We suggest careful preoperative planning which includes understanding the method of reconstruction following the previous Whipple procedure and endoscopic assessment of the oesophagogastric primary by the surgical team themselves to establish its exact location. Having at one's disposal, a variety of surgical strategies for junctional tumours (e.g., extended total gastrectomy, left thoracoabdominal oesophagogastrectomy, substernal colonic interposition, and supercharged jejunal reconstruction methods) afford flexibility that may be crucial in determining success. Furthermore, it is probably unnecessary to dissect all of the jejununa to the pancreas and bile duct in these cases, which may lead to complications. The simplest option remains to use the loop of small bowel previously anastomosed to the stomach/duodenum and (staying close to the bowel wall during its division) mobilize this to reach the oesophagus. Failing this, the jejunum can simply be stapled off and either a Roux loop created distally (beyond the pancreatico- and hepaticojejunostomies) or a colon interposition is used. Postoperatively, nutritional monitoring plays a key role as these patients are at higher risk of the many side effects of complex gastrointestinal surgery such as pancreatic insufficiency, small intestinal bacterial overgrowth, and vitamin/mineral deficiencies.

The use of complex surgery in treatment of cancer patients has made reoperations challenging; however reconstruction options exist and meticulous preoperative planning, imaging tests, and intraoperative judgement help the surgeon to perform extensive and successful oncologically sound procedures.

Abbreviations

GOJ: Gastroesophageal junction
CT: Computed tomography
PET/CT: Positron emission tomography/computed tomography
EUS: Endoscopic ultrasound
MDT: Multidisciplinary team
PPPD: Pylorus-preserving pancreaticoduodenectomy
GDA: Gastroduodenal artery
R0:   Complete macroscopic/microscopic resection in clear margins.

Competing Interests

The authors declare that there is no conflict of interests regarding the publication of this paper.

References

[1] R. T. Grundmann and F. Meyer, "Second primary malignancy among cancer survivors—epidemiology, prognosis and clinical relevance," *Zentralblatt für Chirurgie*, vol. 137, pp. 565–574, 2012.

[2] J. R. Siewert and H. J. Stein, "Classification of adenocarcinoma of the oesophagogastric junction," *British Journal of Surgery*, vol. 85, no. 11, pp. 1457–1459, 1998.

[3] D. Cunningham, W. H. Allum, S. P. Stenning et al., "Perioperative chemotherapy versus surgery alone for resectable gastroesophageal cancer," *The New England Journal of Medicine*, vol. 355, no. 1, pp. 11–20, 2006.

[4] T. K. Ha, J. Y. An, H. G. Youn, J. H. Noh, T. S. Sohn, and S. Kim, "Surgical outcome of synchronous second primary cancer in patients with gastric cancer," *Yonsei Medical Journal*, vol. 48, no. 6, pp. 981–987, 2007.

[5] N. Nandy and C. A. Dasanu, "Incidence of second primary malignancies in patients with esophageal cancer: a comprehensive review," *Current Medical Research and Opinion*, vol. 29, no. 9, pp. 1055–1065, 2013.

[6] D. E. Gyorki, N. E. Clarke, M. W. Hii, S. W. Banting, and R. J. Cade, "Management of synchronous tumours of the oesophagus and pancreatic head: a novel approach," *Annals of the Royal College of Surgeons of England*, vol. 93, no. 6, pp. e111–e113, 2011.

[7] J. Y. Kim, M. M. Hanasono, J. B. Fleming, M. D. Berry, and W. L. Hofstetter, "Combined esophagectomy and pancreaticoduodenectomy: expanded indication for supercharged jejunal interposition," *Journal of Gastrointestinal Surgery*, vol. 15, no. 10, pp. 1893–1895, 2011.

[8] A. Inoue, H. Akita, H. Eguchi et al., "Gastric conduit-preserving, radical pancreaticoduodenectomy with microvascular reconstruction for pancreatic head cancer after esophagectomy: report of a case," *Surgery Today*, vol. 44, no. 4, pp. 786–791, 2014.

[9] S. Pagkratis, D. Virvilis, B. T. Phillips et al., "Creation of gastric conduit free-graft with intraoperative perfusion imaging during pancreaticoduodenectomy in a patient post esophagectomy," *International Journal of Surgery Case Reports*, vol. 9, pp. 39–43, 2015.

[10] Y. N. Shiryajev, I. Kurosaki, Y. V. Radionov, A. A. Kashintsev, and N. Y. Kokhanenko, "Esophagectomy and pancreatoduodenectomy in the same patient: tactical and technical considerations," *Hepato-Gastroenterology*, vol. 61, no. 133, pp. 1246–1252, 2014.

48

Subcutaneous Emphysema caused by an Extraperitoneal Diverticulum Perforation: Description of Two Rare Cases

Gael Kuhn, Jean Bruno Lekeufack, Michael Chilcott, and Zacharia Mbaidjol ⓘ

Hôpital Fribourgeois Riaz, Rue de l'Hôpital 9, Case Postale 70, Riaz, 1632 Fribourg, Switzerland

Correspondence should be addressed to Zacharia Mbaidjol; zahqaria@gmail.com

Academic Editor: Christophoros Foroulis

The onset of colon diverticular disease is a frequent event, with a prevalence that increases with age. Amongst possible complications, free peritoneal perforation with abscess formation may occur. We herein describe two rare presentations of an extraperitoneal sigmoid diverticulum perforation. Our first patient, an 89-year-old female with no signs of distress, developed a subcutaneous abscess and emphysema in an incisional hernia following an appendectomy through a McBurney incision. The second patient, an 82-year-old female, was in general distress at the time of her admission and had a more advanced infection following the occurrence of a sigmoid perforation in a hernial sac. Complicated diverticulitis has a known course and evolution, but with an extraperitoneal presentation, this etiology is not expected. A computed tomography (CT) scan should be completed if the patient is hemodynamically stable, and wide debridement should be performed. Subcutaneous emphysema with an acute abdomen may be a sign of sigmoid perforation. Clinicians should keep this etiology in mind, regardless of the initial presentation.

1. Introduction

Diverticular disease is a "Western" disease with a prevalence increasing with age, with 50% to 60% of people over the age of 80 being affected. The distal colon is mostly impacted, with 10% to 20% of patients afflicted with diverticular disease presenting with diverticulitis [1–4]. Perforation of the diverticulum may occur, causing a wide range of complications that are mainly intraperitoneal in nature, such as abscessation, fistulization, and hemorrhage. In rare cases, the diverticulum can perforate in an extraperitoneal manner. In 1853, the first case of a subcutaneous emphysema secondary to the perforation of a hallow viscous was described [5]. Herein, we report two unusual presentations of the extraperitoneal manifestation of a perforated diverticulitis.

1.1. Case 1 Presentation. An 89-year-old fit female with a history of chronic back pain and an appendectomy during her youth completed using a McBurney incision presented with a one-day history of spontaneous pain in her right flank without any fever, chills, or other symptoms. At the time of

her admission, she was not in distress, she was not febrile, and her vital signs were within normal values. On clinical examination, there was swelling with a red area measuring 12 cm × 4 cm and tenderness of the right flank around her appendectomy scar. Crepitus could be felt diffusely on her right and left flanks and the periumbilical and epigastric regions upon palpation. Blood test showed the presence of mild inflammation, with a CRP value of 7 mg/l (within normal values) and an elevated white blood cell count of 18 G/l. The rest of the laboratory results were normal. Emergency ultrasonography was unhelpful because of air interference. An abdominal CT scan (Figure 1) showed diffuse subcutaneous abdominal emphysema extending to the pelvis on the left side that was more pronounced on the right inguinal fossa with a bowel loop in contact with the abdominal wall. An emergency laparotomy centered on the McBurney incision showed feces and pus within the subcutaneous compartment. Furthermore, at the level of the aponeurosis of the external oblique muscle, an inflammatory diverticulum could be seen fistulizing between the lumen of the sigmoid colon loop and the necrotic

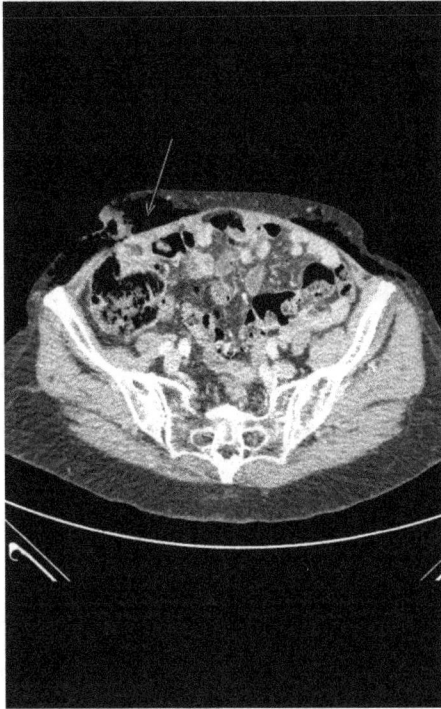

FIGURE 1: CT findings of the first case. The arrow indicates the extraperitoneal perforation.

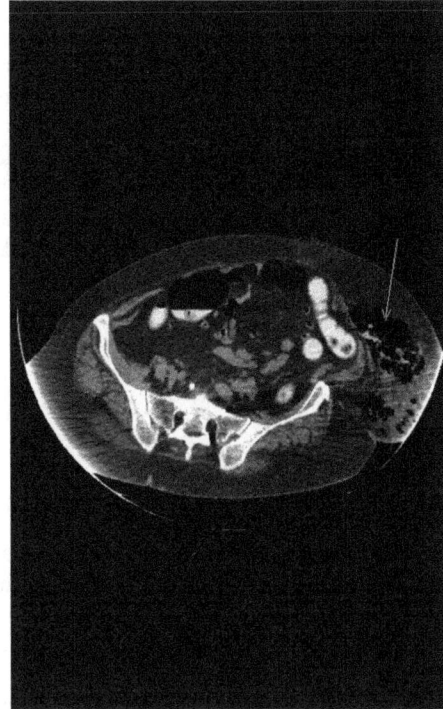

FIGURE 2: CT findings of the second case. The arrow represents once again the extraperitoneal perforation.

subcutaneous tissue. We subsequently diagnosed intraoperatively a subcutaneous abscess and emphysema with an enteroparietal fistula caused by a ruptured sigmoid diverticulum in an incisional hernia. The necrotic tissues were excised, and the punctiform sigmoid colon fistula was closed. Revision of the rest of the sigmoid showed important adhesions between the sigmoid colon and the parietal peritoneum of the right flank and between the caecum and the sigmoid colon, respectively. The sigmoid colon also showed diffused diverticulosis with no inflammation. The cutaneous and subcutaneous tissues were left open and dressed with a negative pressure-assisted closure device on postoperative day 1. The patient received intravenous antibiotherapy for two weeks with quinolones and a third-generation cephalosporin at first which was then switched to aztreonam due to an allergic reaction. Bacteriological studies showed polymicrobial digestive bacteria (i.e., *Escherichia coli*, *Streptococcus equinus*, and *Enterococcus*). Subsequently, there was good clinical and biological evolution. At two weeks postoperation, she was reoperated on for closure of the wound. She was discharged from the hospital three weeks after her initial surgical intervention with the indication to continue antibiotics for a total of four weeks.

1.2. Case 2 Presentation. An 82-year-old patient with a history of diverticular disease, a hysterectomy 20 years ago, and a gastric ulcer who had experienced a digestive hemorrhage 18 years ago was admitted to the emergency room with a one-week history of diminished general health associated with abdominal pain, diarrhea, and fever. Her general practitioner reported that she had sustained many falls during the

past week and had felt sleepy since the previous day. At the time of her admission, the patient was very weak but had a normal state of consciousness. She had no fever (36.8°), a blood pressure of 80/40 mmHg, a pulse rate of 100 beats/minute, and a room air saturation at 80%. The physical examination showed a woman in general distress with a diffusely sensitive lower abdomen. Her left inguinal fossa demonstrated an important hematoma extending to the left flank (resulting from the various falls) that was in the process of abscessation with phlyctena and a local smell of necrosis. The rest of her abdomen was nontender. A blood test revealed a marked inflammation with a CRP value of 440 mg/l and a white blood cell count of 22 G/l, with a left shift. Her creatinine clearance value was 25 ml/mn. The abdominal X-ray gave an impression of subcutaneous feces on the left flank. An abdominal CT confirmed the presence of a sigmoid perforation, with liquid extending from a suprapubic hernial sac all the way to the subcutaneous tissue on the left abdominal wall, which contained free air and feces (Figure 2).

The diagnosis of septic shock with subcutaneous emphysema caused by a sigmoid perforation was retained, and an emergency surgical laparotomy was suggested. The patient received wide-spectrum antibiotics, and a segmental sigmoid resection was performed with creation of a Hartmann terminal colostomy. Culture swab and biopsies yielded a mixed flora (e.g., *Streptococcus dysgalactiae*, *Klebsiella oxytoca*, *Proteus mirabilis*, *Morganella morganii*, and *Enterococcus*). The necrotic cutaneous and subcutaneous tissues on the left abdominal wall were widely excised, all the way to the muscular fascia from the left flank to the left inguinal fossa. The wound was then partially closed on multiple drains. Twenty-four hours later, she was reoperated upon for more extensive debridement of the soft tissues and the abdominal fascia on the right and left inguinal fossa and the supra pubic region. The wound was then dressed with a negative pressure-assisted closure device and closed on drains located near each parietal colic space. Pathology findings confirmed the diagnosis of severe and perforated diverticulitis with necrosis of the abdominal wall. In the postoperative course, her general status degraded with the development of a cardiorespiratory distress condition requiring intubation and amines. The patient died 12 days later from complications of her disease.

2. Discussion

Diverticular disease of the colon is a multifactorial disease influenced by ethnicity, diet, and possibly genetics [2]. It is also an age-related disease affecting less than 10% of people younger than the age of 40 to two-thirds (67%) of the population older than 80 [2–4]. In one study, diverticulum of the descending colon and sigmoid was recorded in more than 5% of postmortem examinations performed in persons aged 40 and older at the Mayo Clinic [1]. The disease has a high prevalence in Western countries. It affects mostly the distal colon, with 90% of cases having a sigmoid involvement and 15% having a right-sided diverticulum [4]. Between 10% and 20% of patients affected with diverticular disease present with diverticulitis [2–4]. Perforation can be localized and cause an abscess, which may be drained under CT guidance or it may perforate into the free peritoneal cavity and cause extensive peritonitis [1]. To our knowledge, there have been only three descriptions of a sigmoid diverticulitis perforation into an inguinal hernia [6–8] and only one previous case of a subcutaneous emphysema with necrotizing fasciitis caused by a sigmoid diverticulitis perforation reported in the literature [9]. Furthermore, we believe that this present case report is the first description of subcutaneous emphysema caused by a diverticulum perforating into an incisional hernia following an appendectomy. In both of our cases, perforation of the diverticulum into the extraperitoneal space occurred via a point of weakness in the abdominal wall. In the first case, it was through an incisional hernia. By definition, these hernias develop at the site at which an incision has been made for a previous surgery, complicate 5% to 11% of wound closures [10], and carry a relatively high mortality rate (5.3%) with complications such as an enterocutaneous fistula, adhesions, and strangulation [10]. In the second case, the sigmoid diverticulum perforated into an inguinal hernia. Salemis et al. described a case of an incarceration of Meckel's diverticulum through a ventral incisional defect [11], while Alvarez-Zepeda et al. reported a case of perforated sigmoid diverticulum in a Spigelian hernia causing a necrotizing fasciitis [12]. Both of these cases are already very rare presentations of diverticulum perforation. Diverticula most commonly form due to a rise in intraabdominal pressure, such as that caused by muscle contractions during straining for defecation. They usually occur on the antimesenteric border, at a point of weakness on the musculature wall of the bowel, mostly

between the taeniae coli around the point of entry of the vasa recta [3, 4, 13]. Patients in Western nations mostly present with left-sided involvement of the colon (90%), whereas, in contrast, those in Asian nations show right-sided involvement [3, 4]. Painter and Burkitt suggested that a poor-fiber diet predisposes individuals to diverticular disease by increasing transit time and decreasing stool volume [4, 14] and therefore, diverticular disease is a preventable condition. One feared complication of diverticular disease is perforation with abscess formation. In very rare instances, gas cracklings under the skin can be felt following perforation. Subcutaneous emphysema can be a nonspecific sign of rupture of a hollow organ [5, 13, 15]. Air formation can occur by way of two different mechanisms, either (1) due to the air gradient between the perforated organ with the persistent peristalsis and the subcutaneous tissues or (2) secondary to an infection by gas-forming bacteria, mainly *Escherichia coli*, *Clostridium sporogenes*, *Enterobacter aerogenes*, *Klebsiella*, and *Proteus* [5, 16, 17]. In some cases, perforation of the gastrointestinal tract may drain to the buttock, hip, thigh, or lower extremities or into the retroperitoneal space of the abdomen by dissecting along the anatomical planes [18]. Morton reported a case of a sigmoid diverticulitis perforating into the right buttock, the left buttock, and the hips [1]. In gas gangrene, due to the above-cited microorganisms, the air lies within the muscles, as opposed to that in the case of subcutaneous emphysema, where it lies in between the muscles and interstitial tissues [16]. In our first case, the gas had spread via a complicated diverticulitis, which had caused a colocutaneous fistula and the perforation of a diverticulum in the abdominal wall, possibly secondary to a weakened abdominal wall and previous surgery. During her physical examination, the crackling was extending diffusely on her abdomen, but there were no signs of peritonitis or widespread cellulitis, suggesting a direct spread of gas into the subcutaneous tissues. Furthermore, the bacteria found with the culture swab were organisms that were part of the endogenous flora. The perforation was localized and occurred on the opposite side due to a redundant sigmoid loop. In our second case, which had a fatal outcome, the patient first presented with a cellulitis that evolved into a necrotizing fasciitis of the anterior lateral wall, requiring another surgery. There was also no gas gangrene, but, with the infection being more advanced, the case required a sigmoid resection, extensive necrosectomy, and a Hartmann terminal colectomy. Neither of the two patients were diabetics, but the second patient was obese and had hypertension, chronic renal insufficiency, and chronic venous lower extremity insufficiency, whereas the first patient was in good general heath otherwise. Fecal peritonitis, which has a high mortality rate (46%) [9], was not present in both of the cases we have described, as the feces had accumulated in the extraperitoneal space. CT scanning, which was necessary in both cases to determine the nature of the disease and the extent of the perforation, is the best imaging modality available to clinicians at this time and permits the elucidation of characteristic features for detecting the site of perforation, free gas, or fluid accumulation, allowing for an easier differentiation between air and fatty tissues. The findings can be wall thickening, pericolonic stranding, or a massive pneumoperitoneum [19]. An emergency surgery with extensive debridement and necrosectomy is the usual outcome of such findings, as simple percutaneous drainage is rarely enough and a second operation is often needed. Agaba et al. reported a case of subcutaneous emphysema with muscular necrosis and necrotizing fasciitis from a perforated sigmoid diverticulitis that required two consecutive surgeries [9]. During the operation, it is important for the surgeon to differentiate between a subcutaneous tissue infection with emphysema caused by free air drained in the subcutaneous tissue and necrotizing fasciitis and gas gangrene, as the latter two carry much higher rates of mortality and morbidity. This diagnosis should be considered in patient experiencing exquisite pain with a systemic toxicity, extensive cellulitis, crepitus, and/or hyponatremia [20, 21]. In both of our current cases, the wounds were then closed with a vacuum-assisted closure device very early on, which helps with wound healing by stimulating blood flow, decreasing local tissue edema, and removing excess fluid. Its use also increases cell division, tissue granulation, and bacterial clearance [9, 22]. Notably, despite the administration of prompt and appropriate treatment, the outcome of our second case was fatal. This outlines the difficulty that persists in handling such infections.

3. Conclusion

Diverticular disease is a frequent disease with known evolutions and complications. In some rare instances, which we have illustrated herein, complications may occur in a setting that renders the diagnosis more complicated. Extraperitoneal sigmoid diverticulum perforation is an unusual occurrence. Furthermore, crepitus and abdominal subcutaneous emphysema on imagery represent a high index of suspicion and warrant a search for the cause. Aggressive surgical debridement should immediately be performed. A better prognostic outcome can be expected with a prompt diagnosis and when the fascia is not affected, but, ultimately, the end result depends on the patient's comorbidities.

References

[1] J. J. Morton, "Diverticulitis of the colon," Annals of Surgery, vol. 124, no. 4, pp. 725–745, 1946.

[2] J. M. Radhi, J. A. Ramsay, and O. Boutross-Tadross, "Diverticular disease of the right colon," BMC Research Notes, vol. 4, no. 1, p. 383, 2011.

[3] D. M. Commane, R. P. Arasaradnam, S. Mills, J. C. Mathers, and M. Bradburn, "Diet, ageing and genetic factors in the pathogenesis of diverticular disease," World Journal of Gastroenterology, vol. 15, no. 20, pp. 2479–2488, 2009.

[4] N. Stollman and J. B. Raskin, "Diverticular disease of the colon," Lancet, vol. 363, no. 9409, pp. 631–639, 2004.

[5] T. W. Fiss Jr., O. S. Cigtay, A. J. Miele, and H. L. Twigg, "Perforated viscus presenting with gas in the soft tissues (subcutaneous emphysema)," The American Journal of Roent-

genology, Radium Therapy, and Nuclear Medicine, vol. 125, no. 1, pp. 226–233, 1975.

[6] B. P. Colcock and J. E. Hull, "Diverticulitis with perforation into hernial sac," The Lahey Clinic Bulletin, vol. 9, no. 2, pp. 46-47, 1954.

[7] N. Tanner, "Strangulated femoral hernia appendix with perforated sigmoid diverticulitis," Proceedings of the Royal Society of Medicine, vol. 56, pp. 1105-1106, 1963.

[8] M. L. A. Tufnell and C. Abraham-Igwe, "A perforated diverticulum of the sigmoid colon found within a strangulated inguinal hernia," Hernia, vol. 12, no. 4, pp. 421–423, 2008.

[9] E. A. Agaba, A. R. Kandel, P. O. Agaba, and L. S. Wong, "Subcutaneous emphysema, muscular necrosis, and necrotizing fasciitis: an unusual presentation of perforated sigmoid diverticulitis," Southern Medical Journal, vol. 103, no. 4, pp. 350–352, 2010.

[10] C. D. George and H. Ellis, "The results of incisional hernia repair: a twelve year review," Annals of the Royal College of Surgeons of England, vol. 68, no. 4, pp. 185–187, 1986.

[11] N. S. Salemis, "Incarceration of Meckel's diverticulum through a ventral incisional defect: a rare presentation of Littre's hernia," Hernia, vol. 13, no. 4, pp. 443–445, 2009.

[12] C. Alvarez-Zepeda, C. Hermansen-Truan, O. Valencia-Lazo, R. Azolas-Marcos, F. Gatica-Jimenez, and J. Castillo-Avendano, "Necrotizing fasciitis of the abdominal wall secondary to a perforated sigmoid diverticulum in a Spiegel's hernia. A case report," Cirugia y Cirujanos, vol. 73, no. 2, pp. 133–136, 2005.

[13] T. Ashizawa, K. Hama, H. Tanaka, and M. Ando, "Intramesocolic diverticular perforation of the sigmoid colon diagnosed by detecting air collection in anterior pararenal space on computed tomography: report of a case," Acta Medica Okayama, vol. 61, no. 5, pp. 299–303, 2007.

[14] N. S. Painter and D. P. Burkitt, "Diverticular disease of the colon: a deficiency disease of western civilization," British Medical Journal, vol. 2, no. 5759, pp. 450–454, 1971.

[15] L. R. H. Stahlgren and G. Thabit Jr., "Subcutaneous emphysema: an important sign of intra-abdominal abscess," Annals of Surgery, vol. 153, no. 1, pp. 126–133, 1961.

[16] C. H. Tan, R. Vikram, P. Boonsirikamchai, S. C. Faria, C. Charnsangavej, and P. R. Bhosale, "Pathways of extrapelvic spread of pelvic disease: imaging findings," Radiographics, vol. 31, no. 1, pp. 117–133, 2011.

[17] T. Brightmore, "Non-clostridial gas infection," Proceedings of the Royal Society of Medicine, vol. 64, no. 10, pp. 1084-1085, 1971.

[18] B. Ravo, S. A. Khan, R. Ger, A. Mishrick, and H. S. Soroff, "Unusual extraperitoneal presentations of diverticulitis," The American Journal of Gastroenterology, vol. 80, no. 5, pp. 346–351, 1985.

[19] J. P. Singh, M. J. Steward, T. C. Booth, H. Mukhtar, and D. Murray, "Evolution of imaging for abdominal perforation," Annals of the Royal College of Surgeons of England, vol. 92, no. 3, pp. 182–188, 2010.

[20] C. D. Marron, M. Khadim, D. McKay, E. J. Mackle, and J. W. R. Peyton, "Amyand's hernia causing necrotising fasciitis of the anterior abdominal wall," Hernia, vol. 9, no. 4, pp. 381–383, 2005.

[21] R. J. Green, D. C. Dafoe, and T. A. Rajfin, "Necrotizing fasciitis," Chest, vol. 110, no. 1, pp. 219–229, 1996.

49

Managing a Colonoscopic Perforation in a Patient with No Abdominal Wall

Jayan George⑩, Michael Peirson, Samuel Birks, and Paul Skinner

Department of General Surgery, Northern General Hospital, Herries Road, Sheffield S5 7AU, UK

Correspondence should be addressed to Jayan George; jayan.george@aol.com

Academic Editor: Tahsin Colak

We describe the case of a 37-year-old gentleman with Crohn's disease and a complex surgical history including a giant incisional hernia with no abdominal wall. He presented on a Sunday to the general surgical on-call with a four-day history of generalised abdominal pain, nausea, and decreased stoma output following colonoscopy. After CT imaging, he was diagnosed with a large colonic perforation. Initially, he was worked up for theatre but following early senior input, a conservative approach with antibiotics was adopted. The patient improved significantly and is currently awaiting plastic surgery input for the management of his abdominal wall defect.

1. Introduction

Crohn's disease is a condition affecting approximately 145/100,000 people [1]. Within this population, 70% will undergo surgery and of that number 30–70% will require repeat or multiple procedures[2]. The management of these patients can be quite complex. Surgical intervention is normally reserved for when medical therapy has failed [3].

Colonoscopy is a common procedure performed for diagnostic and therapeutic purposes. It is estimated that up to fifteen million colonoscopies were performed in the United States in 2012 [4, 5]. Colonoscopic perforation is a serious complication and can occur at rates ranging from 0.016 to 0.8% [6–11].

We describe the case of a patient with a background of Crohn's disease resulting in multiple operations leading to loss of his abdominal wall (and a subsequent giant incisional hernia) presenting with colonic perforation. The patient presented on a Sunday to the general surgical on-call. Experienced registrars were present and the patient could have been taken to theatre. This case is unique, and many experienced clinicians are not likely to have encountered an abdomen such as this. To our knowledge, this is the first case of its kind.

2. Case Report

We report the case of a 37-year-old gentleman who presented on a Sunday to the general surgical on-call with a four-day history of generalised abdominal pain postcolonoscopy. He had associated nausea and slightly reduced stoma output.

Past medical history includes asthma and Crohn's disease which had settled at the time leading up to the colonoscopy. There were no known drug allergies, and the patient takes azathioprine, salbutamol, and beclometasone. He is a nonsmoker and drinks minimal alcohol.

Past surgical history includes a complicated appendicectomy in 2007 resulting in a colostomy; a colonic perforation and retroperitoneal abscess secondary to Crohn's disease led to an ileostomy in 2010, and the ileostomy was reversed with an ileocolonic anastomosis formed in 2012. Anastomotic dehiscence occurred leading to major sepsis with abdominal wall breakdown and abdominal compartment syndrome. A debridement of the area was performed and left as a laparostomy, and an ileostomy was reformed. The area was later covered by a large skin graft in 2012. His colonoscopy was part of a preoperative workup for a procedure in a quaternary centre to assess his viability to repair his complex hernia.

On examination, his heart rate was 117 beats per minute (bpm), blood pressure 128/81 mmHg, respiratory rate 15, and oxygen saturation 98% on air. There was a large mass overlying the hernia to the left of the midline and on abdominal palpation; the mass was ballotable with crepitus, was slightly tender, and had a cough impulse (Figures 1–3). In addition, a stoma was present. The chest was clear to auscultation, and GCS was 15/15.

Bloods on admission revealed a C-reactive protein of 219 mg/L (0–5 mg/L) and were otherwise unremarkable.

2.1. Computed Tomography Scan of the Abdomen and Pelvis with Contrast (Day of Admission). There is a huge amount of free air, which is most likely secondary to a recent colonoscopy that has probably blown off the ascending colon stump. The colon cannot be traced beyond the midtransverse colon in the current scan (Figure 4). A large midline abdominal wall hernia containing several bowel loops with most of the gas seeping into the mesentery within the hernia can be seen. Part of the gas is also seen in the intrahepatic and right perinephric space.

The patient was managed with an ABCDE approach. Tazobactam with piperacillin (Tazocin) was administered as per local guidelines. Intravenous fluids, analgesia, and monitoring of output were commenced.

Given the result of the computed tomography scan, the surgical registrars had consented the patient for a laparotomy plus proceed as necessary. This was halted when the consultant on-call reviewed the patient an hour later.

A conservative approach was adopted, and the patient was discharged just days following admission. He did very well and is currently undergoing review at one of our quaternary centres for his abdominal wall reconstruction.

Following his admission and conservative management, contact was made with the quaternary centre and they reported that the colonoscopy had gone to plan and was carried out meticulously and there was no evidence of a perforation; it was noted that there was evidence of inflammation macroscopically and microscopically and this was determined to be nonspecific.

3. Discussion

Colonic perforations are a rare complication, but when they occur, they can be quite significant with morbidity rates of up to 55% [12]. Mortality can range from 0 to 20% [13, 14]. A systematic review examining imaging techniques to diagnose colonic perforation suggests CT in the first instance unless the patient is haemodynamically unstable, where a decubitus or upright abdominal film could be used instead [6]. Our patient was haemodynamically stable and was referred to us having had a CT scan confirming perforation, and prompt action was taken (Figures 3 and 4).

A recent systematic review indicated that the management of the stable colonic perforation is to observe and treat conservatively unless any of the following findings are present: diffuse peritonitis on examination, heart rate > 100 bpm, temperature > 38°C or < 36°C, respiratory rate > 20 breaths per minute, PaCO2 < 2.7 kPa, white blood

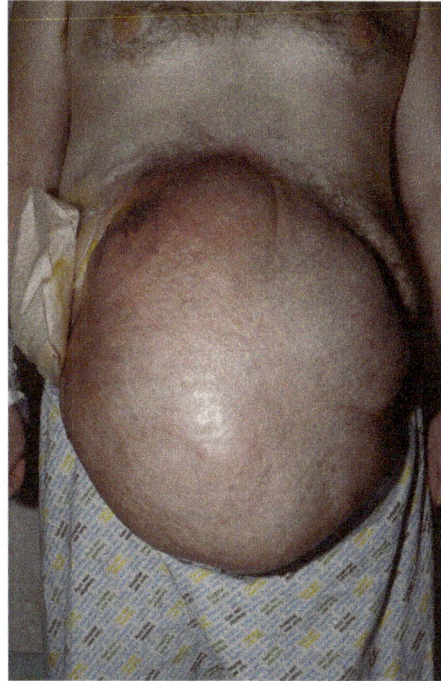

Figure 1: Anterior view of large abdominal hernia.

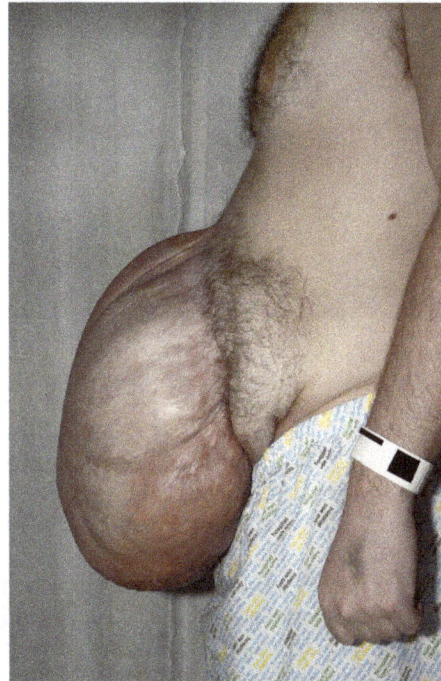

Figure 2: Lateral view of large abdominal hernia.

cell count > 12×10^9/L or < 4×10^9/L or > 10% immature (band) forms, mean arterial pressure < 65 mmHg or relative hypotension, or altered mental status [6]. Our patient was haemodynamically stable with raised inflammatory markers and a very pronounced abdominal hernia; given the fact that he had little abdominal wall, he would not present as a typical peritonitic abdomen (Figures 1 and 2). This

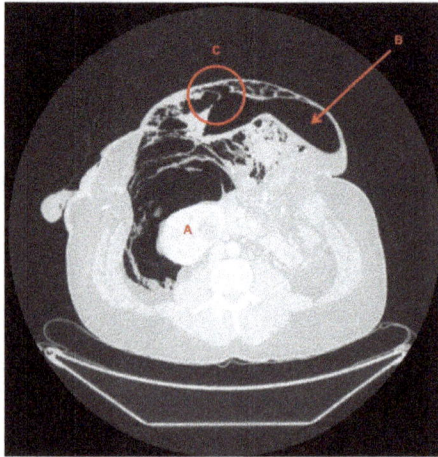

FIGURE 3: Axial CT image showing (A) retroperitoneal free gas around the right kidney (not typical with transverse colon perforation), (B) transverse colon, and (C) perforation of the transverse colon.

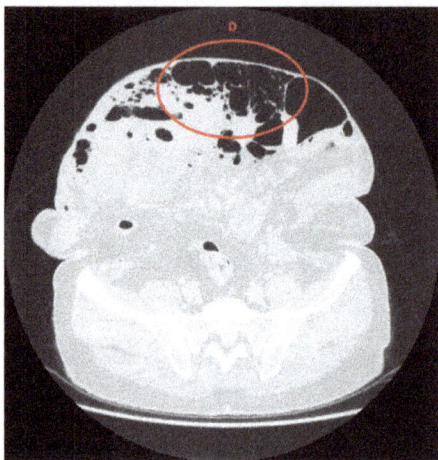

FIGURE 4: Axial CT image showing (D) septated free gas, presumed to be located in the mesentery of the colon.

led to the concern that he needed to go to theatre and the patient was consented and prepped; however, he was clinically stable and following senior input, conservative management continued.

Very few studies have looked at which antibiotic is appropriate, but aerobic and anaerobic cover is suggested [15]. We used Tazocin as per our local guidance for intra-abdominal sepsis, and this has good cover for both types of organisms.

Hawkins et al. have developed an algorithm based on best evidence to manage the patient surgically: for a small perforation, they advocate that surgical repair is preferable but for large perforations, obstruction, malignancy, or inflammatory bowel disease, a surgical resection is more appropriate [6]. In this case, surgery for the patient would be incredibly difficult and would carry a significant risk given his lack of an abdominal wall, especially during postoperative recovery.

The biggest determining factor in this patient's management was early consultant input. Whilst the patient was worked up for theatre, the consultant on-call was informed, and this prompted an early senior review which led to the conservative management approach being followed. This is a reminder for all trainees to focus on the pathology and the patient's clinical status in initiating treatment and not to be distracted by the obvious abdominal wall defect and CT images (Figures 1–4).

Acknowledgments

The authors would like to acknowledge Dr. Catherine Clout, Consultant Radiologist, for her input in attaining the imaging.

References

[1] G. P. Rubin, A. P. Hungin, P. J. Kelly, and J. Ling, "Inflammatory bowel disease: epidemiology and management in an English general practice population," *Alimentary Pharmacology and Therapeutics*, vol. 14, no. 12, pp. 1553–1559, 2000.

[2] H.-J. Duepree, A. J. Senagore, C. P. Delaney, K. M. Brady, and V. W. Fazio, "Advantages of laparoscopic resection for ileocecal Crohn's disease," *Diseases of the Colon & Rectum*, vol. 45, no. 5, pp. 605–610, 2002.

[3] S. A. Patil and R. K. Cross, "Medical versus surgical management of penetrating Crohn's disease: the current situation and future perspectives," *Expert Review of Gastroenterology & Hepatology*, vol. 11, no. 9, pp. 843–848, 2017.

[4] M.-C. Jaberoo, J. Joseph, G. Korgaonkar, K. Mylvaganam, B. Adams, and M. Keene, "Medico-legal and ethical aspects of nasal fractures secondary to assault: do we owe a duty of care to advise patients to have a facial x-ray?," *Journal of Medical Ethics*, vol. 39, no. 2, pp. 125-126, 2013.

[5] D. A. Joseph, R. G. S. Meester, A. G. Zauber et al., "Colorectal cancer screening: estimated future colonoscopy need and current volume and capacity," *Cancer*, vol. 122, no. 16, pp. 2479–2486, 2016.

[6] A. T. Hawkins, K. W. Sharp, M. M. Ford, R. L. Muldoon, M. B. Hopkins, and T. M. Geiger, "Management of colonoscopic perforations: a systematic review," *The American Journal of Surgery*, vol. 215, no. 4, pp. 712–718, 2018.

[7] J. S. Kim, B.-W. Kim, J. I. Kim et al., "Endoscopic clip closure versus surgery for the treatment of iatrogenic colon perforations developed during diagnostic colonoscopy: a review of 115,285 patients," *Surgical Endoscopy*, vol. 27, no. 2, pp. 501–504, 2013.

[8] V. Lohsiriwat, "Colonoscopic perforation: incidence, risk factors, management and outcome," *World Journal of Gastroenterology*, vol. 16, no. 4, pp. 425–430, 2010.

[9] A. C. Silva, M. Pimenta, and L. S. Guimaraes, "Small bowel obstruction: what to look for," *Radio Graphics*, vol. 29, no. 2, pp. 423–439, 2009.

[10] J. W. Scott, O. A. Olufajo, G. A. Brat et al., "Use of national burden to define operative emergency general surgery," *JAMA Surgery*, vol. 151, no. 6, article e160480, 2016.

[11] R. Magdeburg, P. Collet, S. Post, and G. Kaehler, "Endoclipping of iatrogenic colonic perforation to avoid surgery," *Surgical Endoscopy*, vol. 22, no. 6, pp. 1500–1504, 2008.

[12] M. S. Tam and M. A. Abbas, "Perforation following colorectal endoscopy: what happens beyond the endoscopy suite?," *The Permanente Journal*, vol. 17, no. 2, pp. 17–21, 2013.

[13] H.-H. Kim, B.-H. Kye, H.-J. Kim, and H. M. Cho, "Prompt management is most important for colonic perforation after colonoscopy," *Annals of Coloproctology*, vol. 30, no. 5, pp. 228–231, 2014.

[14] A. Y. B. Teoh, C. M. Poon, J. F. Y. Lee et al., "Outcomes and predictors of mortality and stoma formation in surgical management of colonoscopic perforations: a multicenter review," *Archives of Surgery*, vol. 144, no. 1, pp. 9–13, 2009.

[15] R. Magdeburg, M. Sold, S. Post, and G. Kaehler, "Differences in the endoscopic closure of colonic perforation due to diagnostic or therapeutic colonoscopy," *Scandinavian Journal of Gastroenterology*, vol. 48, no. 7, pp. 862–867, 2013.

50

Abdominal Pregnancy in the Small Intestine Presenting as Acute Massive Lower Gastrointestinal Hemorrhage

Apiradee Pichaichanlert,[1] Vor Luvira,[1] and Nakhon Tipsunthonsak[2]

[1]*Department of Surgery, Faculty of Medicine, Khon Kaen University, Khon Kaen, Thailand*
[2]*Surgery Unit, Khon Kaen Hospital, Khon Kaen, Thailand*

Correspondence should be addressed to Vor Luvira; vor_110@yahoo.com

Academic Editor: Dimitrios Mantas

An abdominal pregnancy is an ectopic pregnancy in which the implantation site occurs in the abdominal cavity outside the female reproductive organs. There have been four reported cases that ruptured into the gastrointestinal tract and into the large intestine. We present the first case of an abdominal pregnancy rupturing into the small intestine with a good outcome.

1. Introduction

Acute lower gastrointestinal hemorrhage (LGIH) is defined as the onset of hematochezia, originating from either the colon or rectum. The most common causes of acute severe LGIH include diverticulosis, angioectasia, postpolypectomy bleeding, and ischemic colitis [1]. Ectopic pregnancy refers to the implantation of an embryo outside the uterus and is classified into two major types, according to the location of the implant—viz., a tubal or a nontubal pregnancy. The most common type of ectopic pregnancy (95%) is the tubal, which includes all parts of the fallopian tube (i.e., the fimbria, ampulla, isthmus, and cornual or interstitial part). An abdominal pregnancy is a nontubal pregnancy in which the implantation site occurs in the abdominal cavity and has a very low incidence (1%) [2]. Massive rectal bleeding is an unusual complication of ectopic pregnancy and carries with it a high mortality rate. We reviewed all cases of ectopic pregnancy that presented with LGIH [3–15] (Table 1) and only four of these were abdominal pregnancies.

For all reported cases of abdominal pregnancy presenting with lower GI bleeding, the gestational sac ruptured into the large intestine (colon or rectum). Herein, we present a case of an abdominal pregnancy in which the gestational sac ruptured into the small intestine and presented as severe hematochezia.

2. Case Presentation

A 32-year-old woman sought care at a provincial hospital after passing loose and dark stool about 10 times in a single day. She had been healthy until the diarrhea occurred and was not taking any medications. Her past medical history was unremarkable, except that she had undergone tubal surgery for pelvic inflammatory disease three years priorly. She had one child who was born by vaginal delivery. She had never undergone an instrumental pregnancy termination or intrauterine device insertion, which might lead to uterine perforation. She had no history of amenorrhea or abnormal vaginal discharge. Her initial diagnosis was upper gastrointestinal hemorrhage, but this was changed when bile was observed in the nasogastric tube after which the patient developed exsanguinating hematochezia and severe hypotension requiring 11 units of packed red cell transfusion for stabilization. Soon after, she was transferred to a tertiary care center.

The patient's blood pressure was 70/40 mmHg, and her pulse rate was 120 beats/min. The abdominal examination was unremarkable. The per-rectal examination revealed excessive bleeding without any discernible cause. The laboratory tests showed a hemoglobin level of 6.3 g/dL and a platelet count of $28 \times 10^3/\mu L$. Owing to the unstable condition of the patient, an emergency exploratory laparotomy was conducted in order to localize and control the bleeding. During the laparotomy,

TABLE 1: Reported cases of intestinal hemorrhage associated with ectopic pregnancy.

Author	Reported year	Patient	Site of ectopic pregnancy	Location of placental erosion	Gestational age (weeks)	Maternal outcome	Fetal outcome
Armstrong [3]	1835	NA	NA	NA	24	Dead	NA
Edgar [4]	1901	NA	NA	Sigmoid	NA	Dead	NA
Clark [5]	1932	Female, 25 years	Left interstitial	Sigmoid	6	Alive	Dead
Webster and Kerr [6]	1956	NA	Right interstitial	Appendix and ileum	NA	Dead	NA
Engel [7]	1961	NA	Left interstitial	Ileum	NA	Dead	NA
Shirkey et. al. [8]	1964	Female, 38 years	Left interstitial	Ileum	NA	Alive	Dead
Bigg et al. [9]	1965	Female, 19 years	Right interstitial	Caecum	NA	Alive	Dead
Bornman et al. [10]	1985	Female, 29 years	Abdominal (posterior wall of uterus)	Sigmoid	34	Alive	Alive
Seow et al. [11]	1992	NA	Abdominal	Caecum	NA	NA	NA
Verma et al. [12]	1996	Female, 38 years	Left fallopian tube	Sigmoid	4–8	Alive	Dead
Warshal et al. [13]	1996	Female, 36 years	Right interstitial	Ileum	12–16	Alive	Dead
Saravanane et al. [14]	1997	Female, 30 years	Abdominal (pouch of Douglas)	Rectum	14	Alive	Dead
Ekwaro et al. [15]	2004	Female, 26 years	Abdominal (fundus of uterus)	Sigmoid	NA	Dead	Dead
Present study	2017	Female, 32 years	Abdominal (fundus of uterus)	Ileum	16	Alive	Dead

blood was found in the peritoneal cavity and a segment of the ileum attached to the fundus of uterus (Figure 1(a)). The intraluminal content was palpated in the adhered ileal segment (Figure 1(b)). An enterotomy revealed a fetus 7.5 cm in crown-rump length and fresh blood in the ileal lumen (Figure 1(c)). The placental tissue had implanted at the fundal dome of the uterus and eroded into the small bowel (Figure 1(d)). A segmental small bowel resection was performed along with reanastomosis. The placental tissue was removed by way of a wedge resection of the uterine wall. The patient had an uneventful postoperative course and was discharged on postoperative day 7.

Histologic examination of the resected specimens later confirmed the diagnosis of an abdominal pregnancy which included a male fetus of 4 months' gestational age (Figure 2), normal cord, subserous uterine myoma, and submucosal hemorrhage in the small intestine.

3. Discussion

A case of acute massive lower gastrointestinal hemorrhage, caused by an abdominal pregnancy that ruptured into the small intestine, is discussed. This is a rare gynecologic condition, considered to be an underlying cause of rectal bleeding, and is usually misdiagnosed, resulting in delayed treatment. Due to the rarity of the condition and the associated high mortality of abdominal pregnancy, despite having a high index of suspicion, it is not possible to diagnose the condition before surgery.

Lower gastrointestinal hemorrhage is defined as bleeding originating distal to the ligament of Treitz. Typically, massive bleeding is thought to require more than 3 to 5 units of blood transfused over 24 h. Although LGIH can occur at any age, the disease presentation for adults trends to be diverticular bleeding, inflammatory bowel disease, or neoplasm, and with advancing age, bleeding from an arteriovenous malformation, diverticular bleeding, or neoplasm [16]. The other common causes of LGIH are ischemic colitis, postpolypectomy bleeding, hemorrhoids, and stercoral ulcer.

We searched for reports on intestinal hemorrhage associated with ectopic pregnancy and found only 13 cases (Table 1). The site of the ectopic pregnancy was not identified in the first two reported cases. The first [3] was a case of a syphilitic woman six months pregnant, dying of hemorrhage and suddenly passing bloody stool containing fetal bones, and the second [4] was a case of rectal hemorrhage, proven at autopsy to have arisen from an ectopic gestational sac rupture into the sigmoid colon. The other 11 reports in the literature identified the implantation sites; for most of which (six cases) the implantation site was at the uterine cornu—that is, interstitial pregnancies, accounting for 1% of tubal pregnancies [13]. The literature indicated that the ectopic gestational sac usually ruptured into the ileum in cases of interstitial pregnancy. Four of the 13 cases were abdominal pregnancies, and the implantation site was usually situated at the uterine serosa and typically ruptured into the large intestine. The remaining case was a tubal ectopic pregnancy that ruptured into the sigmoid colon.

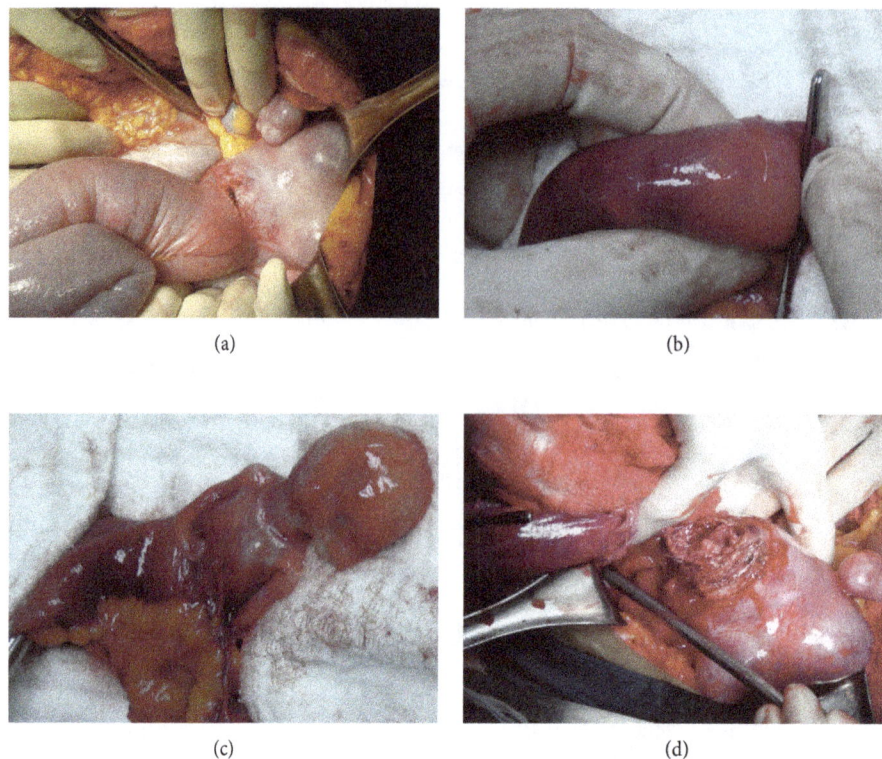

(a)

(b)

(c)

(d)

FIGURE 1: Photographs of intraoperative findings. (a) Exploratory laparotomy showing the adherence between the ileum and uterine fundus. (b) The intraluminal ileal mass palpable near the adherence site. (c) The opened ileum revealing a dead fetus. (d) Photograph showing the placenta in the uterus after detaching the ileum from the uterine fundus.

All types of ectopic pregnancies result in high maternal mortality, caused by delayed treatment of life-threatening hemorrhages. It is estimated that a woman with an abdominal pregnancy is 90 times more likely to die compared to a woman with an intrauterine pregnancy [17]. Historically, lack of knowledge of the condition was associated with mortality of the mother. Even today, the fetus almost always dies in ectopic pregnancies, although we did find one case of an abdominal pregnancy that presented as massive rectal bleeding, where both the mother and neonate survived [10].

The abnormal implantation site of an ectopic pregnancy leads to denigration of the trophoblastic tissue [13], which grows by invading the adjacent structures that are prone to the implantation site where there is greater blood supply. The communication of the intestinal tract with the ectopic gestational sac is called an enteroamniotic fistula, which follows the villous invasion of the bowel wall. When the gestational sac approximates to the intestine, there is an inflammatory reaction and an infection develops, resulting in a fistula. The vascularized gestational structures are aggravated by infection and villous invasion of the adjacent vascular structures, leading to massive hemorrhage [8]. The terminal ileum, sigmoid colon, and caecum are the parts of the gastrointestinal tract that are usually involved [14]. The small intestine is associated with interstitial and not abdominal pregnancies, which are usually associated with invasion of the large intestine. We have thus presented the first case of a ruptured abdominal pregnancy into the small intestine, which caused massive lower gastrointestinal hemorrhage.

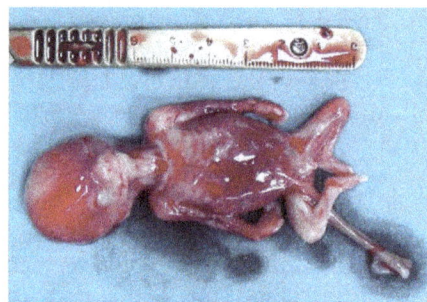

FIGURE 2: Photograph of the dead fetus.

Attending physicians need to be aware of the possibility of a fistula between the ectopic gestational sac and the bowel in any pregnant woman who presents with obscure intestinal hemorrhage, and to initiate prompt surgery. Although women with ectopic pregnancy frequently have no identifiable risk factors, a prospective case-controlled study revealed that increased awareness of ectopic pregnancy and knowledge of the associated risk factors help to identify women at higher risk and early diagnosis. In our case, we did not consider this condition initially but performed an emergency surgery after massive blood transfusions. During laparotomy—in order to control the bleeding and to prevent intraabdominal abscess formation or peritoneal sepsis—we resected the infected fistula, a segment of the small bowel, the wall of the involved uterus, and the ectopic fetus and placental tissue. After recovering from the surgery, the patient was discharged without any major morbidity.

In conclusion, abdominal pregnancy is a rare life-threatening condition requiring prompt treatment. This is the first report of an abdominal pregnancy that ruptured into the small intestine with a good outcome.

Acknowledgments

The authors thank (a) the patient and her family for permission to share the case, (b) the support from the Faculty of Medicine, Khon Kaen University, (c) Mr. Dylan Southard for editing suggestions, and (d) Mr. Bryan Roderick Hamman for assistance with the English-language presentation of the manuscript under the aegis of the KKU Publication Clinic.

References

[1] L. L. Strate and I. M. Gralnek, "ACG clinical guideline: management of patients with acute lower gastrointestinal bleeding," *American Journal of Gastroenterology*, vol. 111, no. 4, pp. 459–474, 2016.

[2] N. Agarwal and F. Odejinmi, "Early abdominal ectopic pregnancy: challenges, update and review of current management," *Obstetrician & Gynaecologist*, vol. 16, no. 3, pp. 193–198, 2014.

[3] J. Armstrong, "Anomalous case of ectopic pregnancy in a syphilitic patient; discharge of fetal bones by the rectum," *London Medical Gazette*, vol. 16, pp. 51-52, 1835.

[4] J. Edgar, "Ectopic gestation with formation of large hematocele and secondary rupture into upper third of sigmoid flexure," *Glasgow Medical Journal*, vol. 56, pp. 143-144, 1901.

[5] S. G. Clark, "Ectopic pregnancy complicated by rupture into the intestine," *Journal of the American Medical Association*, vol. 99, no. 15, pp. 1253-1254, 1932.

[6] A. Webster and C. H. Kerr, "A case of interstitial tubal pregnancy with rupture into the bowel," *American Journal of Obstetrics and Gynecology*, vol. 72, no. 2, pp. 430–432, 1956.

[7] G. Engel, "Verblutungstod durch perforation einer intramuralen graviditat in den dunndarm," *Münchener Medizinische Wochenschrift*, vol. 103, p. 1726, 1961.

[8] A. L. Shirkey, D. C. Wukasch, G. B. Matthews, A. C. Beall Jr., and M. E. DeBakey, "Profuse hemorrhage from ruptured ectopic pregnancy: report of a successfully treated case and review of the literature," *Annals of surgery*, vol. 160, no. 5, pp. 839–843, 1964.

[9] R. L. Bigg, C. Jarolim, D. D. Kram, and H. E. Bessinger, "Ruptured interstitial pregnancy causing massive rectal bleeding," *Archives of Surgery*, vol. 91, no. 6, pp. 1021-1022, 1965.

[10] P. C. Bornman, J. S. Collins, M. J. Abrahamson, and N. H. Gilinsky, "Live abdominal pregnancy presenting as massive rectal bleeding," *Postgraduate Medical Journal*, vol. 61, no. 718, pp. 759-760, 1985.

[11] C. Seow, H. S. Goh, and C. S. Sim, "Massive bleeding per rectum from a caecal pregnancy," *Annals of the Academy of Medicine, Singapore*, vol. 21, no. 6, pp. 818–820, 1992.

[12] G. R. Verma, R. Kochhar, and A. Rajwanshi, "Ectopic pregnancy presenting as lower gastro-intestinal hemorrhage," *Indian Journal of Gastroenterology*, vol. 15, no. 4, p. 151, 1996.

[13] D. P. Warshal, P. J. Fultz, A. E. Dawson, G. Del Priore, and B. DuBeshter, "Interstitial pregnancy complicated by rectal bleeding," *American Journal of Obstetrics and Gynecology*, vol. 175, no. 5, pp. 1373-1375, 1996.

[14] C. Saravanane, S. R. Smile, S. S. Chandra, and S. Habeebullah, "Rectal bleeding: a rare complication of abdominal pregnancy," *Australian and New Zealand Journal of Obstetrics and Gynaecology*, vol. 37, no. 1, pp. 124-125, 1997.

[15] L. Ekwaro, P. M. Kizza, G. Nassdi, and J. Lubega, "Ectopic pregnancy: an unusual cause of lower GIT bleeding. A case report," *East and Central African Journal of Surgery*, vol. 9, no. 1, 2004, http://www.ajol.info/index.php/ecajs/article/view/137205.

[16] T. Raphaeli and R. Menon, "Current treatment of lower gastrointestinal hemorrhage," *Clinics in Colon and Rectal Surgery*, vol. 25, no. 4, pp. 219–227, 2012.

[17] G. Masukume, "Live births resulting from advanced abdominal extrauterine pregnancy, a review of cases reported from 2008 to 2013," *Webmed Central Obstetrics and Gynaecology*, vol. 5, no. 1, p. WMC004510, 2014, http://www.webmedcentral.com/.

51

Biliary Tract Abnormalities as a cause of Distal Bowel Gas in Neonatal Duodenal Atresia

Surasak Puvabanditsin ⓘ, Marissa Botwinick, Charlotte Wang Chen, Aditya Joshi, and Rajeev Mehta

Department of Pediatrics, Rutgers Robert Wood Johnson Medical School, One Robert Wood Johnson Place, New Brunswick, NJ 08903, USA

Correspondence should be addressed to Surasak Puvabanditsin; surasak1@aol.com

Academic Editor: Serge Landen

Background. The presence of distal bowel gas in an infant does not exclude the diagnosis of duodenal atresia. *Case Presentation.* We report a term neonate with Down syndrome. The infant developed vomiting and cyanosis with each feeding soon after birth. Plain film abdominal X-rays showed a nonspecific gas-filled stomach and small bowel. Duodenal atresia and an anomalous common bile were noted on an upper GI study and exploratory laparotomy. *Conclusion.* In the absence of a "double bubble" appearance and intestinal gas distally on a plain radiograph, one must not exclude duodenal atresia as the differential diagnosis.

1. Introduction

In the newborn with duodenal atresia, the hallmark of an abdominal radiograph is the "double bubble" with a gaseous distension of the stomach and proximal duodenum and the total absence of gas in the distal bowel.

Only 23 cases of duodenal atresia with an anomalous common bile duct have been reported in the literature. We present a case of a Down syndrome neonate with duodenal atresia and gas in the distal intestine without a "double bubble" sign.

2. Case Report

A term female was born at 39 weeks of gestation to a 32-year-old G2P1 by spontaneous vaginal delivery. Apgar scores were 9 and 9 at 1 and 5 minutes, respectively. The pregnancy was uncomplicated. Physical examination revealed a weight of 3650 gm (70th centile), length of 51 cm (60th centile), and head circumference of 33 cm (15th centile). The infant had features of Down syndrome: flattened facies, upslanting palpebral fissures, palmar creases, and sandal gap deformities of the great and second toes. Karyotype was obtained on the first day of life. Recurrent vomiting after each feeding was noted since birth. A plain abdominal radiograph showed a nonspecific bowel gas pattern with gas noted in the stomach, duodenum, and distal bowel (Figure 1). An upper gastrointestinal (UGI) series showed a complete obstruction to the flow of barium at the proximal portion of the duodenum. A small amount of contrast was also seen to exit from the proximal duodenal segment into a biliary duct structure with a retrograde filling of the biliary tree into the intrahepatic system as well as into the gallbladder through the cystic duct. The contrast was also seen in the proximal jejunum which was located in the right upper quadrant (Figures 2 and 3). The patient underwent exploratory

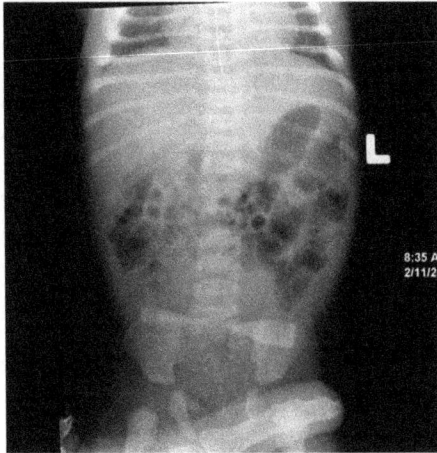

FIGURE 1: Abdominal radiograph showing an air-filled stomach, duodenum, and jejunum.

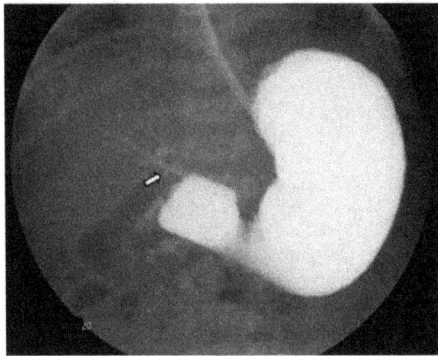

FIGURE 2: Upper gastrointestinal series showing complete obstruction to the flow of contrast at the second portion of the duodenum. There is also contrast filling of the biliary tree above the duodenal bulb noted (arrow).

laparotomy on the 3rd day of life. Duodenal atresia was repaired. Malrotation was identified, and a Ladd procedure and appendectomy were performed. The postoperative course was uneventful, and the infant was discharged home at 35 days of life. Karyotype confirmed the diagnosis of trisomy 21 (Down syndrome).

3. Discussion

Duodenal atresia (DA) occurs in approximately 1 in 2500–7500 live births without a sex-associated difference. Approximately 25–40% of infants with duodenal atresia have trisomy 21 (Down syndrome). Approximately 8% of infants with Down syndrome have duodenal atresia [1–3]. There is also an association of VACTERL anomalies (vertebral, anorectal, cardiac, tracheoesophageal, renal, and limb anomalies). The classic abdominal X-ray depicts the "double bubble" which represents the air-filled stomach and obstructed duodenum and the absence of distal bowel gas [3]. During pregnancy, duodenal atresia can cause an increase of fluid

in the amniotic sac resulting in polyhydramnios; this may be the first sign of a DA. A double bubble can be seen with prenatal ultrasound, in which case the bubbles are filled with fluid. This appearance should be interpreted with caution as transient double bubbles can result from transient duodenal fluid accumulation and slow peristalsis, and these have been observed in fetuses subsequently found to be healthy [3–5]. After delivery, an infant with duodenal atresia generally has a scaphoid abdomen but one may occasionally observe epigastric fullness from dilation of the stomach and proximal duodenum. The passage of meconium within the first 24 hours of life is not usually altered.

Unlike more distal small bowel (jejunal/ileal) atresia which is believed to be caused by an ischemic episode, DA is believed to result from the failure of the recanalization of the bowel lumen following the phase of epithelialization, proliferation, and subsequent vacuolization of the alimentary tract during embryonic development [6–8]. Between the 30th and 60th days of embryonic development, growth and differentiation of the alimentary tract are proceeding at great speed. In a matter of a week or 10 days, its cross-sectional area increases eighty-fold. At the beginning of the sixth week, the duodenum contains a small lumen. From the 7th to 8th weeks, the patency of the duodenal lumen is restored by a coalescence of vacuoles, which produces 2 parallel channels in the duodenum, and at the same time, 2 channels appear in the developing biliary system [7–9]. This is the time when genetic and environmental influences would exert their maximal effect. It is not unreasonable to suppose that during this period, duodenal atresia may develop.

An anomalous bile duct termination may occur when atresia develops between the 2 orifices of the bile ducts. Boyden et al. [10], in discussing the abnormalities which may occur at the entrance of the common bile duct and pancreatic ducts, stated that they were the result of an embryological "traffic jam" [8, 10]. During development, two blindly ending channels appear in the duodenum at the stage of vacuolization and at the same time two channels also appear in the developing biliary system. Each of these joins up separately with the developing duodenal channels. If some accident affected the "embryological events" at this stage of development, aberrations of the lower biliary tract could be expected in association with duodenal atresia. The atretic segment is an abnormally sited bile channel [8, 11]. In the report by Komuro et al. [12], 12 (22.2%) of 54 cases with duodenal atresia and 9 cases with and 3 without distal bowel gas had an anomalous bifurcated bile duct conduit between the proximal and distal segments.

In summary, duodenal atresia with a plain radiograph showing distal bowel gas via anomalies of the bile duct is more common than initially thought. We describe a case with findings that are contradictory to the cardinal sign of duodenal atresia namely the "double bubble" with the absence of gas in the distal intestine. Prenatal sonographic findings suggestive of duodenal atresia should not be dismissed based on plain film findings.

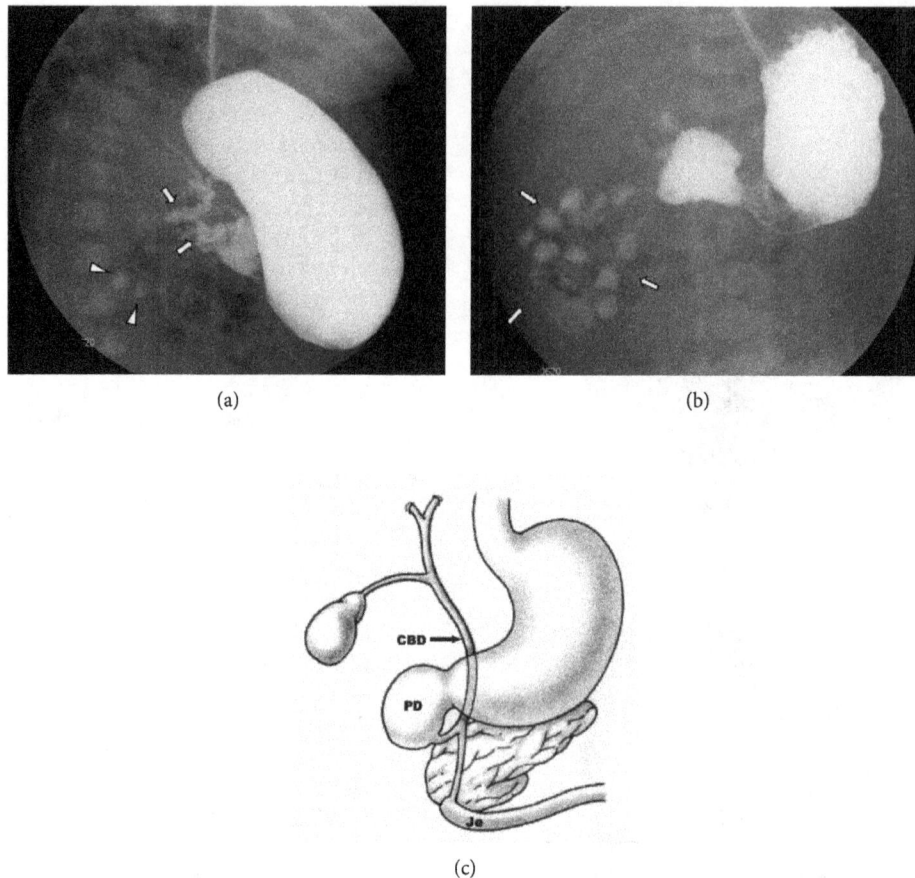

(a)

(b)

(c)

FIGURE 3: (a) Upper gastrointestinal series showing a complete obstruction of the duodenum and contrast filling of anomalous bifurcated bile ducts (arrows). The small contrast was also noted in the distal bowel (arrowheads). (b) Upper gastrointestinal series showing a complete obstruction at the second portion of the duodenum, and contrast was seen in the proximal jejunum which is located in the right upper quadrant. The proximal location of the jejunum indicates a malrotation of the intestine without evidence of a small bowel obstruction. (c) Diagram showing biliary tract abnormality associated with duodenal atresia (PD—proximal duodenum, Je—jejunum, and CBD—common bile duct).

Authors' Contributions

Surasak Puvabanditsin, Charlotte Wang Chen, and Aditya Joshi have analyzed and interpreted the patient data and contributed in writing the manuscript. Rajeev Mehta, Surasak Puvabanditsin, and Marissa Botwinick critically revised the manuscript. All authors read and approved the final manuscript.

Acknowledgments

The authors thank Sylvia Sutton-Thorpe, Chrystal Puvabanditsin, and Christina Puvabanditsin for supporting this effort and preparing the manuscript.

References

[1] S. B. Freeman, C. P. Torfs, P. A. Romitti et al., "Congenital gastrointestinal defects in Down syndrome: a report from the Atlanta and National Down Syndrome Projects," *Clinical Genetics*, vol. 75, no. 2, pp. 180–184, 2009.

[2] F. M. Karrer, "Pediatric duodenal atresia," January 2017, https://emedicine.medscape.com/article/932917.

[3] J. Traubici, "The double bubble sign," *Radiology*, vol. 220, no. 2, pp. 463-464, 2001.

[4] E. Z. Zimmer and M. Bronshtein, "Early diagnosis of duodenal atresia and possible sonographic pitfalls," *Prenatal Diagnosis*, vol. 16, no. 6, pp. 564–566, 1996.

[5] J. L. Grosfeld and F. J. Rescorla, "Duodenal atresia and stenosis: reassessment of treatment and outcome based on antenatal diagnosis, pathologic variance, and long-term follow-up," *World Journal of Surgery*, vol. 17, no. 3, pp. 301–309, 1993.

[6] J. M. Latzman, T. L. Levin, and S. M. Nafday, "Duodenal atresia: not always a double bubble," *Pediatric Radiology*, vol. 44, no. 8, pp. 1031–1034, 2014.

[7] S. J. Knechtle and H. C. Filston, "Anomalous biliary ducts associated with duodenal atresia," *Journal of Pediatric Surgery*, vol. 25, no. 12, pp. 1266–1269, 1990.

[8] D. B. Tashjian and K. P. Moriarty, "Duodenal atresia with an anomalous common bile duct masquerading as a midgut volvulus," *Journal of Pediatric Surgery*, vol. 36, no. 6, pp. 956-957, 2001.

[9] H. Ando, "Embryology of the biliary tract," *Digestive Surgery*, vol. 27, no. 2, pp. 87–89, 2010.

[10] E. A. Boyden, J. G. Cope, and A. H. Bill Jr., "Anatomy and embryology of congenital intrinsic obstruction of the duodenum," *The American Journal of Surgery*, vol. 114, pp. 190–202, 1967.

[11] A. Gourevitch, "Duodenal atresia in the newborn," *Annals of the Royal College of Surgeons of England*, vol. 48, no. 3, pp. 141–158, 1971.

[12] H. Komuro, K. Ono, N. Hoshino et al., "Bile duct duplication as a cause of distal bowel gas in neonatal duodenal obstruction," *Journal of Pediatric Surgery*, vol. 46, no. 12, pp. 2301–2304, 2011.

52

Primarily Proximal Jejunal Stone causing Enterolith Ileus in a Patient without Evidence of Cholecystoenteric Fistula or Jejunal Diverticulosis

Houssam Khodor Abtar,[1] **Mostapha Mneimneh,**[1] **Mazen M. Hammoud,**[1]
Ahmed Zaaroura,[1] **and Yasmina S. Papas**[2]

[1]*Makassed General Hospital, Department of Surgery, Beirut, Lebanon*
[2]*Saint George Hospital University Medical Center, Department of Surgery, Beirut, Lebanon*

Correspondence should be addressed to Houssam Khodor Abtar; dr.houssamabtar@gmail.com

Academic Editor: Boris Kirshtein

Stone formation within the intestinal lumen is called enterolith. This stone can encroach into the lumen causing obstruction and surgical emergency. Jejunal obstruction by an enterolith is a very rare entity and often missed preoperatively. To our knowledge, most cases of jejunal obstruction, secondary to stone, were associated with biliary disease (cholecystoenteric fistula), bezoar, jejunal diverticulosis, or foreign body. Hereby we present a rare case report of small bowel obstruction in an elderly man who was diagnosed lately to have primary proximal jejunal obstruction by an enterolith without evidence of a cholecystoenteric fistula or jejunal diverticulosis. This patient underwent laparotomy, enterotomy with stone extraction, and subsequent primary repair of the bowel.

1. Introduction

The term enterolithiasis defines intestinal intraluminal stone. This pathology can also be described as enterolith ileus or pseudogallstone ileus when it causes small bowel obstruction [1]. Extrinsic, intramural, and intraluminal causes are all possible etiologic factors of small bowel obstruction where postoperative adhesions remain the most common cause and account for 74% of all cases [2]. Gallstone ileus accounts for only 1–4% of cases [3]. Till year 2011 only 39 cases of primary jejunal enterolithiasis resulting in small bowel complication had been reported and the majority of them are related to jejunal diverticulosis [4].

2. Case Report

A 76-year-old male patient presented to our emergency department with a 72-hour history of persistent nausea, vomiting, and generalized fatigue associated with diffuse colicky abdominal pain. He had a long history of intermittent episodes of abdominal pain and distension. He was afebrile and obstipated and did not pass stool for 3 days. His past medical history is significant for hypertension and prostate cancer. He had open prostatectomy 1 year ago. Upon physical exam, the patient was hemodynamically stable and slightly dehydrated. His abdomen was soft with mild diffuse tenderness and distention.

Blood tests revealed a leukocyte count of $11,500 \times 10^9/L$ (neutrophils 92%), C-reactive protein of 36 mg/L, and Cr of 2 mg/dL. The remaining lab studies were within normal limits. We did not order a plain abdominal film as this would not show valuable information regarding the diagnosis.

A computed tomography scan with oral contrast was performed and showed proximal dilated jejunal loop (up to 5 cm in diameter) with a large ring of calcification likely suggestive of ascariasis (Figure 1); the rest of the bowels had a normal caliber. The gall bladder was not distended and there was neither air in the biliary tree (pneumobilia) nor free fluid within the abdominal cavity.

The patient was admitted to the hospital. Conservative management was started with IV hydration, pain management, and a nasogastric tube (drainage of 1.5 L bilious material). He was prepared for exploratory laparotomy through a supraumbilical midline incision.

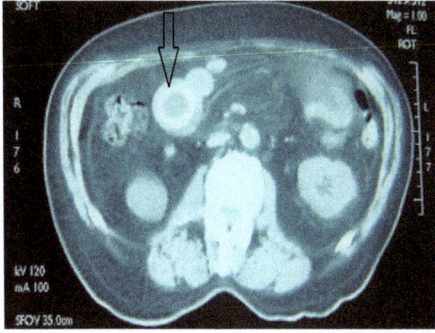

FIGURE 1: Contrast-enhanced computed tomographic image showing dilated jejunal loop (up to 5 cm in diameter) with a large calcified ring (black arrow).

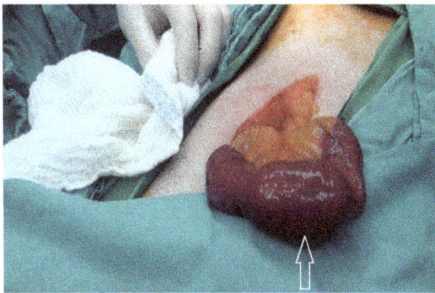

FIGURE 2: Intraoperative findings. Impacted proximal jejunal stone causing obstruction (white arrow).

Upon surgical exploration, the proximal jejunum was found to be dilated, whereas the distal jejunum, ileum, and large bowels were collapsed. A mass about 5.5 cm in size was found to be obstructing the proximal jejunum about 30 cm from the ligament of Treitz (Figure 2). An enterotomy was performed directly over the mass and a large stone was extracted from within the jejunal loop (Figure 3). The opening was closed primarily. The gall bladder appeared normal without evidence of cholecystoenteric fistula. And even so we did not find any jejunal diverticula after complete running of the jejunum. Patient had a smooth postoperative course discharged home without any consequences.

3. Discussion

Proximal jejunal obstructions are typically caused by adhesions or tumors. Less frequently, such cases can be secondary to strictures because of inflammatory bowel disease, gallstone impactions, bezoars, and/or foreign bodies [5]. To our knowledge, most cases of stone-related small bowel obstruction described in the literature were secondary to cholecystoenteric fistulae most commonly located at the level of the terminal ileum [6]. Obstruction at the level of the jejunum by a stone in the absence of a cholecystoenteric fistula, like in the case reported here, has been very rarely reported.

Some authors have found a possible association between primary enteroliths in the jejunum and the presence of small

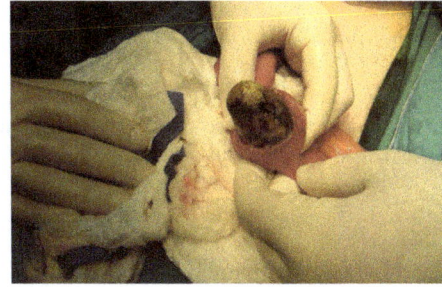

FIGURE 3: Large stone extracted from within the jejunal lumen by enterotomy with subsequent primary closure.

bowel diverticuli. With the usual composition of primary enterolith being choleic acid, an end product of bile salt metabolism, it has been postulated that the formation of these stones is secondary to the acidic pH shift within the small confined bowel diverticulum [7].

Another contributing factor that has been reported is the stasis encountered in patients with bowel hypomotility. Indeed, stasis seems to be necessary to permit the progressive accumulation of particulate matter leading eventually to the formation of a stone [3]. In our case this mechanism played an important role in stone formation.

Other possible causes of enterolith in the small bowel include Meckel's diverticulum, small bowel anastomosis, metabolic diseases, intussusception, intestinal strictures, and inflammatory or infectious enteritis [7]. Congenital defects, such as luminal atresia, stenosis, or intestinal aganglionosis, are of the most common causes of small bowel stone formation in the pediatric population [8].

Concerning the management of such cases crushing the enterolith and milking it distally is the first step to do [7]. If this fails, enterotomy is considered then by most experts to be the standard procedure for the management of mechanical small bowel obstruction by a stone, because conservative management has been found to be frequently unsuccessful [9].

In conclusion, jejunal obstruction by a primary enterolith is a very rare entity. This pathology should be expected when other common pathologies have been excluded for the cause of small bowel obstruction in the elderly population. Hence, diagnosis and management are often delayed. Surgical exploration is often necessary as it can result in serious potential complications.

Competing Interests

The authors declare that there are no competing interests, financial or otherwise, related to the publication of this study or its findings.

References

[1] R. G. K. Watson and T. D. Williams, "Enterolith with pseudo-gallstone ileus and perforation," *Irish Journal of Medical Science*, vol. 150, no. 1, pp. 86–88, 1981.

[2] C. P. Mullan, B. Siewert, and R. L. Eisenberg, "Small bowel obstruction," *American Journal of Roentgenology*, vol. 198, no. 2, pp. W105–W117, 2012.

[3] B. Chaudhery, P. A. Newman, and M. D. Kelly, "Small bowel obstruction and perforation secondary to primary enterolithiasis in a patient with jejunal diverticulosis," *BMJ Case Reports*, vol. 2014, 2014.

[4] R. Nonose, J. S. Valenciano, J. S. de Souza Lima, E. F. Nascimento, C. M. G. Silva, and C. A. R. Martinez, "Jejunal diverticular perforation due to enterolith," *Case Reports in Gastroenterology*, vol. 5, no. 2, pp. 445–451, 2011.

[5] S. Milanchi, C. McVay, and D. E. Fermelia, "Jejunal enterolith causing small-bowel obstruction," *Journal of the American College of Surgeons*, vol. 205, no. 2, p. 377, 2007.

[6] S. Chatterjee, T. Chaudhuri, G. Ghosh, and A. Ganguly, "Gallstone ileus—an atypical presentation and unusual location," *International Journal of Surgery*, vol. 6, no. 6, pp. e55–e56, 2008.

[7] T. Monchal, E. Hornez, S. Bourgouin et al., "Enterolith ileus due to jejunal diverticulosis," *The American Journal of Surgery*, vol. 199, no. 4, pp. e45–e47, 2010.

[8] R. Bergholz and K. Wenke, "Enterolithiasis: a case report and review," *Journal of Pediatric Surgery*, vol. 44, no. 4, pp. 828–830, 2009.

[9] F. Altintoprak, E. Dikicier, U. Deveci et al., "Intestinal obstruction due to bezoars: a retrospective clinical study," *European Journal of Trauma and Emergency Surgery*, vol. 38, no. 5, pp. 569–575, 2012.

53

Metastasis of Hepatocellular Carcinoma to the Esophagus

Jun-ichiro Harada, Takeshi Matsutani ⓘ, Nobutoshi Hagiwara ⓘ, Yoichi Kawano, Akihisa Matsuda, Nobuhiko Taniai, Tsutomu Nomura, and Eiji Uchida ⓘ

Department of Gastrointestinal and Hepato-Biliary-Pancreatic Surgery, Nippon Medical School, 1-1-5 Sendagi, Bunkyo-ku, Tokyo 113-8603, Japan

Correspondence should be addressed to Takeshi Matsutani; matsutani@nms.ac.jp

Academic Editor: Paola De Nardi

A follow-up endoscopy in a 71-year-old Japanese man who had undergone a left lateral segmentectomy for HCC two years ago revealed an approximately 2 cm in diameter pedunculated polypoid mass in the middle part of the thoracic esophagus. Immunohistochemical staining of the endoscopic biopsy revealed a metastatic HCC esophageal tumor. As the patient's disease could be radically removed by preoperative examinations, we resected the metastatic esophageal tumor via right thoracotomy and esophagogastrostomy reconstruction. Histological examination of the resected specimen revealed that the esophageal tumor was compatible with a HCC metastasis. This is an extremely rare case of a solitary metastasis to the esophagus from HCC in the literature.

1. Introduction

Extrahepatic metastasis of hepatocellular carcinoma (HCC) is relatively rare, even in advanced HCC cases that have intrahepatic metastases. The lung, bone, and adrenal gland are the most common sites of distant HCC metastases via hematogenous metastasis through the hepatic artery or portal vessel system [1–3]. The incidence of gastrointestinal tract metastases from HCC is low, with several groups reporting rates between 0.5% and 2%; however, these patients usually have poor outcomes [2, 4, 5]. HCC metastasis to the gastrointestinal tract most commonly involves the duodenum, followed by the stomach and the colon. Esophageal HCC metastases are extremely rare; the reported rates in the literature are less than 0.4% [1–3, 6]. The clinicopathological characteristics of HCC with esophageal involvement remain unknown. Herein, we present a surgically treated case of esophageal metastasis from HCC.

2. Case Report

A 71-year-old Japanese man with a medical history of HCC that resulted from chronic hepatitis B infection underwent a left lateral segmentectomy for HCC at another institute. Pathological findings of the resected specimens were moderately differentiated hepatocellular carcinoma (St-P, 55 × 50 × 38 mm, eg, fc(+), fc-inf(+), sf(−), s0, nx, vp1, vv0, va1, b0, im0, p0, sm(−), and lc lead to pT3 and pStageIII). Two years after surgery, his serum alpha-fetoprotein (AFP) level increased to 1800 ng/ml (normal is 0–10 ng/ml). Physical examination showed no remarkable abnormal findings. Laboratory blood and chemical examination results were also within normal limits. A follow-up examination that included an upper gastrointestinal endoscopy showed a pedunculated polypoid tumor in the middle thoracic esophagus, approximately 2 cm in diameter (Figure 1(a)). Esophageal varices were not seen at the anal side of the tumor. A barium

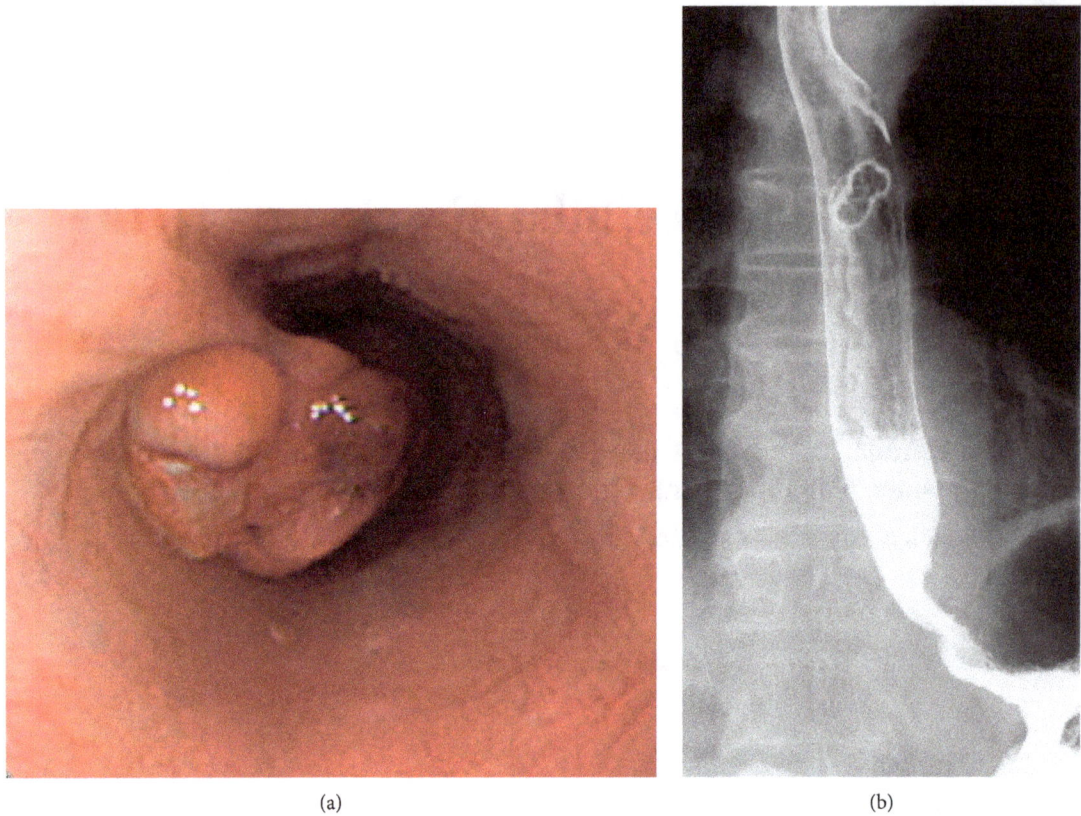

(a)   (b)

FIGURE 1: (a) Upper gastrointestinal endoscopy showing a pedunculated polypoid tumor in the middle thoracic esophagus. (b) Barium esophagography revealing an elevated lesion in the middle thoracic esophagus.

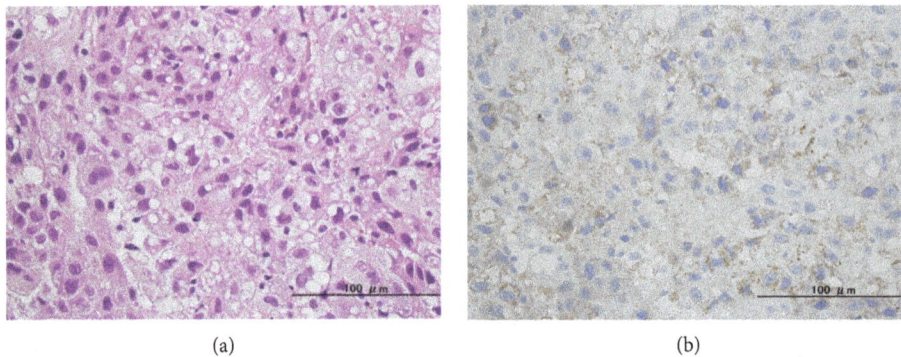

(a)   (b)

FIGURE 2: (a) Pathological findings of biopsy specimens; tumor cells with acidophilic cytoplasm proliferated without a tubular structure. (b) Tumor cells showing immunopositive for hepatocyte stain.

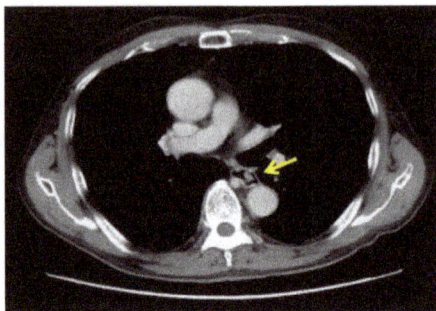

FIGURE 3: Chest computed tomography showing an elevated mass in the esophageal lumen (arrow).

esophagogram showed an elevated mass in the middle thoracic esophagus (Figure 1(b)). The biopsy specimen obtained from the esophageal lesion revealed tumor cells with acidophilic cytoplasm that proliferated without a tubular structure (Figure 2(a)). Tumor cells in the biopsy specimens were positive for hepatocyte stain (monoclonal mouse anti-human hepatocyte antibody) (Figure 2(b)). The esophageal tumor was diagnosed as a metastatic HCC tumor. Chest computed tomography (CT) showed an elevated mass in the esophageal lumen (Figure 3). Abdominal CT detected no evidence of metastasis to the lung or of new HCC lesions in the liver, except for lymph node metastases in the lesser curvature area

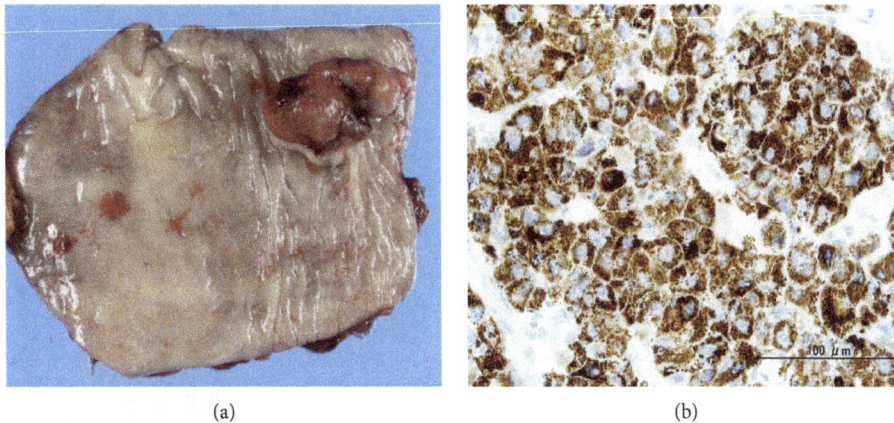

(a)   (b)

FIGURE 4: (a) By gross appearance, the resected specimen shows a reddish polypoid tumor in the middle esophagus. (b) Metastatic hepatocellular carcinoma to the esophagus confirming by positive AFP staining.

of the stomach. However, a portal tumor thrombus was not found. As the patient was in good general condition and preoperative imaging showed resectable disease, we performed surgical resection. Esophageal resection via right thoracotomy was performed with regional lymph node dissection, and the whole stomach for reconstruction was made to provide better protection of the submucosal vessels, compared to gastric tube approach. Esophagogastrostomy was performed at the intrathorax where the gastric tube was lifted up through the posterior mediastinal route. Intraoperative exploration revealed no peritoneal dissemination. The gross appearance of the resected specimen was a reddish polypoid tumor in the middle esophagus (Figure 4(a)). A metastatic esophageal tumor from HCC was confirmed by positive immunohistochemical staining for hepatocyte and AFP (Figure 4(b)). Two months following the operation, a follow-up CT demonstrated multinodular-type HCC in both lobes of the liver. The patient received no additional therapies and died from disease progression two months following the operation.

3. Discussion

Metastatic esophageal tumors are extremely rare in living patients with malignant tumors. A study of 1835 autopsy cases from a variety of malignancies revealed 112 (6.1%) esophageal metastases, and the most common malignancies to produce such metastases were the lung (41/450, 11.3%), breast (14/188, 7.4%), and ovarian cancer (1/40, 2.5%) [7]. In contrast, HCC frequently invades the vascular spaces of the liver; consequently, extrahepatic HCC metastases are rare. The most common extrahepatic HCC metastases diagnosed in autopsy or surgical series were to the lung (18.1%–49.2%) followed by lymph nodes (26.5%–41.7%), bone (4.2%–16.3%), and adrenal glands (8.4%–15.4%) [1, 3, 6]. Incidences of gastrointestinal metastases are infrequent, and metastatic esophageal tumors from HCC are extremely rare, present in less than 0.4% of HCC patients [1–3, 6]. Despite improvements in diagnostic techniques, only 13 cases of esophageal metastasis in living HCC patients have been

reported in the last 20 years on PubMed, including this case (Table 1) [8–18].

The major symptoms of esophageal HCC metastases were gastrointestinal bleeding and dysphagia. Upper gastrointestinal endoscopy is necessary to diagnose esophageal HCC metastases because three previously reported cases, including ours, were asymptomatic [11, 16]. Metastatic esophageal tumors are usually located in the submucosal layer [7]; therefore, esophagography and endoscopy show severe luminal stricture with normal overlying mucosa, which often complicates histological diagnoses. A literature review indicated that the most common endoscopic findings of esophageal HCC metastases were polypoid or submucosal tumors [9, 14, 15]. If an endoscopic biopsy reveals a lack of available tumor cells, several imaging modalities, such as CT, endoscopic ultrasound, or angiography, are necessary to differentiate between primary esophageal cancer and HCC metastases [9]. In this case, the endoscopic and imaging findings were compatible with a metastatic esophageal tumor of HCC origin.

The exact mechanisms involved in esophageal metastasis from HCC are still unknown; however, several possibilities have been proposed. The main possible routes for esophageal involvement are thought to be a direct extension from metastatic mediastinal nodes or spread in the esophageal wall through systemic hematogenous pathways in HCC. The spread of HCC is characterized by disseminating tumor infiltration and the frequent occurrence of tumor thrombi in the portal vein [19]. Moreover, multinodular-type HCC frequently involves portal vein invasion and intrahepatic metastasis [2]. Esophageal metastasis from HCC is presumed to be caused by tumor thrombi invading through the portal system and dissemination from the hepatofugal portal blood flow to the gastrointestinal tract [4, 19]. As HCC frequently invades the portal vein, the involvement of the gastrointestinal tract, including the esophagus, by metastatic HCC via the portal system may not be uncommon. Arakawa et al. [19] found 12 cases (38.7%) that had variceal tumor thrombi among 55 HCC autopsy cases. Thus, esophageal metastasis that is caused by tumor thrombi infiltrating via the portal

TABLE 1: English literature review of esophageal hepatocellular carcinoma metastases.

No.	Author	Year	Age	Sex	Symptoms	Gross type of esophageal tumor	Type of hepatitis	Serum AFP (ng/ml)	Therapy of varices	Therapy for HCC	Therapy for esophageal metastasis	Other metastasis at living	Outcome	Survival time (M)
1	Sohara	2000	54	M	Melena	Submucosal	HCV	4987	Esophageal transection, splenectomy	TAI	–	Lung	Death	3
2			46	M	Hematemesis	Polypoid	NA	990	Esophageal transection, EIS	TACE, radiation	–	–	Death	7
3	Kume	2000	56	M	Dysphagia, tarry stool	Submucosal	HBV	12,200	EIS, EVL	TACE	–	Lung, bone	Death	2
4	Cho	2003	50	M	Dysphagia, hematemesis	Polypoid	NA	Elevated	–	Resection	Radiation, TAI	–	Death	11
5	Tsubouchi	2005	63	M	None	Polypoid	HCV	4130	+	TACE	–	Stomach	Death	7
6	Yan	2007	53	M	Melena	Polypoid	HBV	17,036	–	–	–	–	Death	1
7	Choi	2008	66	M	Melena	Submucosal epolypoid	Non-B, non-C	3.47	EVL	TACE	–	–	Death	7
8	Xie	2008	50	M	Dysphagia, odynophagia	Cauliflower-like	HBV	NA	–	Systemic chemotherapy, OLT, TACE	Radiation	–	Alive	>7
9	Hsu	2009	54	M	Hematemesis, tarry stool	Polypoid	HBV	NA	–	OLT, TACE	–	Stomach	Death	4
10	Kahn	2010	55	M	Dysphagia	Polypoid	HCV	1426	–	OLT, TACE	Hyperthermia, PDT, stent placement	–	Death	10
11	Boonnuch	2011	59	M	Dysphagia	Submucosal	NA	510	–	OLT, TACE	Resection	–	Alive	>2
12	Fukatsu	2012	63	M	None	Polypoid	NA	NA	EVL, EIS	TACE, RFA	–	–	Death	1
13	Our case		71	M	None	Polypoid	HBV	1801	+	Resection	Resection	Lymph node	Death	3

HCV: hepatitis C virus; HBV: hepatitis B virus; NA: not available; EIS: endoscopic injection sclerotherapy; EVL: endoscopic variceal ligation; TAI: transcatheter arterial injection; TACE: transcatheter arterial chemoembolization; OLT: orthotopic liver transplantation; RFA: radiofrequency ablation; PDT: photodynamic therapy.

system and disseminating by hepatofugal portal blood flow might be a route of hematogenous spread. In this case, histological examination of resected specimens did not demonstrate any specific features directly related to these mechanisms, and no existence of portal thrombus was detected on the presurgical abdominal CT scan. Thus, a causative mechanism involved in metastasis to the esophagus from HCC in our case cannot be made at this time. We speculated that this case involved spreading by hepatofugal blood flow because there was no evidence of direct invasion or lymphadenopathy around the esophagus.

Advanced hepatocellular carcinoma (HCC) is one of the most deadly diseases with few systemic therapeutic options. Sorafenib is the first-line molecular target treatment of patients with advanced HCC and increases overall survival by approximately 3 months (10.7 months) compared with placebo (7.7 months). The RESORCE trial demonstrated that regorafenib in the second-line treatment increased from 7.8 months with placebo to 10.6 months with regorafenib after patients experienced disease progression on sorafenib. However, other newer molecular agents have failed to demonstrate significantly improved long survival in clinical trials. The effective systemic, immune, or etiology-specific therapies of patients with advanced HCC have not been established. Despite improvements in therapeutic techniques, a standard treatment for esophageal HCC metastases has not been also established. As the majority of these patients already have terminal disease with distant metastases at multiple sites, palliative chemotherapy or radiation therapy is usually the first treatment choice. The interval between diagnosis of esophageal metastasis and death was short in the 13 reviewed cases, with a mean of only 5.5 months. Thus, esophageal metastasis of HCC has an extremely poor prognosis, and therapy for these HCC cases should be individualized and tailored, whereas HCC is common in Asia. Metastatic HCC generally shows poor responses to chemotherapy and radiation. Several reports have shown that tumor resection can provide excellent palliation and long-term survival in certain cases without metastases to other sites [7, 8]. The resection of metastatic tumors might prolong survival in patients with esophageal metastases from HCC who can tolerate aggressive treatments. If our patient had no lymph node metastases, we could perform an endoscopic submucosal dissection that gives less surgical stress. Our patient had rapid disease progression by two months postsurgery, and it should be discussed with patients whether surgical removal is the optimal treatment.

4. Conclusion

We report a rare case of a preoperatively diagnosed esophageal metastasis from HCC. Specialists in digestive organ diseases should be aware that esophageal metastasis of HCC may exhibit the aforementioned endoscopic characteristics and may cause dysphagia or gastrointestinal bleeding, although this case showed no symptoms from the metastatic esophageal tumor.

References

[1] J. Kaczynski, G. Hansson, and S. Wallerstedt, "Metastases in cases with hepatocellular carcinoma in relation to clinicopathologic features of the tumor. An autopsy study from a low endemic area," *Acta Oncologica*, vol. 34, no. 1, pp. 43–48, 1995.

[2] T. Nakashima, K. Okuda, M. Kojiro et al., "Pathology of hepatocellular carcinoma in Japan. 232 consecutive cases autopsied in ten years," *Cancer*, vol. 51, no. 5, pp. 863–877, 1983.

[3] K. Yuki, S. Hirohashi, M. Sakamoto, T. Kanai, and Y. Shimosato, "Growth and spread of hepatocellular carcinoma. A review of 240 consecutive autopsy cases," *Cancer*, vol. 66, no. 10, pp. 2174–2179, 1990.

[4] L. T. Chen, C. Y. Chen, C. M. Jan et al., "Gastrointestinal tract involvement in hepatocellular carcinoma: clinical, radiological and endoscopic studies," *Endoscopy*, vol. 22, no. 3, pp. 118–123, 1990.

[5] C. P. Lin, J. S. Cheng, K. H. Lai et al., "Gastrointestinal metastasis in hepatocellular carcinoma: radiological and endoscopic studies of 11 cases," *Journal of Gastroenterology and Hepatology*, vol. 15, no. 5, pp. 536–541, 2000.

[6] Liver Cancer Study Group of Japan, "Primary liver cancer in Japan. Clinicopathologic features and results of surgical treatment," *Annals of Surgery*, vol. 211, pp. 277–287, 1990.

[7] S. Mizobuchi, Y. Tachimori, H. Kato, H. Watanabe, Y. Nakanishi, and A. Ochiai, "Metastatic esophageal tumors from distant primary lesions: report of three esophagectomies and study of 1835 autopsy cases," *Japanese Journal of Clinical Oncology*, vol. 27, no. 6, pp. 410–414, 1997.

[8] W. Boonnuch, T. Akaraviputh, C. Nino, A. Yiengpruksawan, and A. A. Christiano, "Successful treatment of esophageal metastasis from hepatocellular carcinoma using the da Vinci robotic surgical system," *World Journal of Gastrointestinal Surgery*, vol. 3, no. 6, pp. 82–85, 2011.

[9] A. Cho, M. Ryu, Y. Yoshinaga et al., "Hepatocellular carcinoma with unusual metastasis to the esophagus," *Hepato-Gastroenterology*, vol. 50, no. 52, pp. 1143–1145, 2003.

[10] C. S. Choi, H. C. Kim, T. H. Kim et al., "Does the endoscopic finding of esophageal metastatic hepatocellular carcinoma progress from submucosal mass to polypoid shape?," *Gastrointestinal Endoscopy*, vol. 68, no. 1, pp. 155–159, 2008.

[11] H. Fukatsu, S. Miura, H. Kishida et al., "Gastrointestinal: esophageal metastasis from hepatocellular carcinoma," *Journal of Gastroenterology and Hepatology*, vol. 27, no. 9, p. 1536, 2012.

[12] K. F. Hsu, T. Y. Hsieh, C. L. Yeh, M. L. Shih, and C. B. Hsieh, "Polypoid esophageal and gastric metastases of recurrent hepatocellular carcinoma after liver transplantation," *Endoscopy*, vol. 41, no. 2, pp. E82–E83, 2009.

[13] J. Kahn, D. Kniepeiss, C. Langner, D. Wagner, F. Iberer, and K. Tscheliessnigg, "Oesophageal metastases of hepatocellular carcinoma after liver transplantation," *Transplant International*, vol. 23, no. 4, pp. 438-439, 2010.

[14] K. Kume, I. Murata, I. Yoshikawa, K. Kanagawa, and M. Otsuki, "Polypoid metastatic hepatocellular carcinoma of the esophagus occurring after endoscopic variceal band ligation," *Endoscopy*, vol. 32, no. 5, pp. 419–421, 2000.

[15] N. Sohara, H. Takagi, T. Yamada et al., "Esophageal metastasis of hepatocellular carcinoma," *Gastrointestinal Endoscopy*, vol. 51, no. 6, pp. 739–741, 2000.

[16] E. Tsubouchi, S. Hirasaki, J. Kataoka et al., "Unusual metasta-sis of hepatocellular carcinoma to the esophagus," *Internal Medicine*, vol. 44, no. 5, pp. 444–447, 2005.

[17] L. Y. Xie, M. Fan, J. Fan, J. Wang, X. L. Xu, and G. L. Jiang, "Metastatic hepatocellular carcinoma in the esophagus follow-ing liver transplantation," *Liver Transplantation*, vol. 14, no. 11, pp. 1680–1682, 2008.

[18] S. L. Yan, Y. H. Hung, and T. H. Yang, "Metastatic hepatocel-lular carcinoma of the esophagus: an unusual cause of upper gastrointestinal bleeding," *Endoscopy*, vol. 39, no. S1, pp. E257–E258, 2007.

[19] M. Arakawa, M. Kage, S. Matsumoto et al., "Frequency and significance of tumor thrombi in esophageal varices in hepato-cellular carcinoma associated with cirrhosis," *Hepatology*, vol. 6, no. 3, pp. 419–422, 1986.

54

Bowel Resection and Ileotransverse Anastomosis as Preferred Therapy for 15 Typhoid Ileal Perforations and Severe Peritoneal Contamination in a very Elderly Patient

Benjamin Momo Kadia,[1,2] **Desmond Aroke,**[3,4] **Martin Hongieh Abanda,**[2,5,6] **Tsi Njim,**[3,7] **and Christian Akem Dimala**[3,8,9]

[1]*Foumbot District Hospital, Foumbot, Cameroon*
[2]*Grace Community Health and Development Association, Kumba, Cameroon*
[3]*Health and Human Development (2HD) Research Network, Douala, Cameroon*
[4]*Mbengwi District Hospital, Mbengwi, Cameroon*
[5]*Non-Communicable Disease Unit, Clinical Research Education, Networking and Consultancy (CRENC), Douala, Cameroon*
[6]*Bafang District Hospital, Bafang, Cameroon*
[7]*Centre for Tropical Medicine and Global Health, Nuffield Department of Medicine, University of Oxford, Oxford, UK*
[8]*Faculty of Epidemiology and Population Health, London School of Hygiene and Tropical Medicine, London, UK*
[9]*Department of Orthopaedics, Southend University Hospital, Essex, UK*

Correspondence should be addressed to Benjamin Momo Kadia; benjaminmomokadia@yahoo.com

Academic Editor: Gaetano La Greca

Typhoid ileal perforation (TIP) is the most lethal complication of typhoid fever. Although TIP is a surgical emergency by consensus, there is still much controversy regarding the most appropriate surgical approach to be used. Bowel exteriorization and secondary closure are usually recommended for patients presenting late with multiple TIPs and heavy peritoneal soiling. We, however, discuss a unique case of an 86-year-old patient with 15 typhoid ileal perforations successfully treated with one-step surgery comprising bowel resection and ileotransverse anastomosis in a resource-constrained setting of Cameroon.

1. Introduction

Typhoid fever is a severe infectious disease caused by the Gram-negative enteric bacillus *Salmonella typhi* [1, 2]. Intestinal perforations are the most frequent cause of typhoid-related morbidity and mortality [2–7]. These lesions commonly occur in the ileum [8]. Typhoid ileal perforation (TIP) is the most lethal complication of typhoid fever [3, 9, 10]. The high case fatality of TIP in low-income countries where typhoid is endemic makes the condition a public health menace in these settings [5, 11]. Mortality rates from TIP vary between 5 and 60% [9, 12]. In Cameroon, a recent cohort study conducted in two regional hospitals revealed that TIP was most frequently associated with peritonitis-related mortality [13].

Although TIP is a surgical emergency by consensus, the most appropriate surgical approach to be used remains controversial [5, 14, 15]. Generally, the appropriate surgical option for managing TIP is contingent on the general state of the patient, the site and number of perforations, and the extent of peritoneal contamination. Closure of the perforation with fresh edges or wedge resection of the ulcer area and closure are recommended for simple perforation with minimal peritoneal soiling. Bowel resection with or without anastomosis and closure of the perforation followed by ileotransverse anastomosis are best reserved for multiple perforations [8]. The recommended options for severely ill patients who present late with heavy peritoneal contamination are ileostomy [6, 15] and laparostomy [8] followed by secondary closure. In low-income countries, however, most severely ill patients are managed in resource-limited hospitals where suboptimal management prevails and TIP is invariably a fatality [5].

The aim of the current paper is to report an unusual case of an 86-year-old patient with 15 typhoid ileal perforations and significant peritoneal soiling successfully managed with one-step surgery comprising bowel resection and ileo-transverse anastomosis in rural Cameroon. The clinical challenges presented by this rare and critical case in a resource-limited setting are also highlighted.

2. Case Presentation

An 86-year-old Cameroonian male was brought to our district hospital with complaints of fever for 4 weeks and abdominal pain and diarrhoea for 2 weeks. The fever was of low grade, intermittent, and without associated symptoms. He automedicated himself with suboptimal doses of amoxicillin, metronidazole, and ibuprofen tablets which were bought over the counter from a drug store. After 2 weeks of continuous use of these drugs, the fever was persistent and became associated with abdominal pain and diarrhoea. The pain was a mild burning intermittent hypogastric pain which was of gradual onset and with no relieving or aggravating factors. The diarrhoea was of gradual onset and started a few hours after the onset of abdominal pain. It was watery and intermittent, and he passed out small quantities of blood-stained yellowish stool about 4 times on average each day. He was taken to a traditional healer who gave him concoctions for 2 weeks during which there was progressive onset of a severe frontal throbbing headache, loss of appetite, and general weakness. The severity of the abdominal pain was increasing. He was then brought to our hospital after 4 weeks of illness.

His past history was significant for moderate arterial hypertension, which was controlled with hydrochlorothiazide. He frequently used nonsteroidal anti-inflammatory drugs for chronic low back pain. His past history was otherwise unremarkable.

On admission, the patient was wasted and prostrated and had sunken eyeballs. His Glasgow coma score was 15/15. His vital signs were: blood pressure 100/60 mm/Hg, pulse 124 beats/minute (regular, rapid, and thready), respiratory rate 29 breaths/min and regular, and temperature 39°C. The capillary refill time was 3 seconds. His conjunctivae were mildly pale, and his sclerae were anicteric. There was no palpable enlarged lymph node. His buccal cavity was dry. The abdomen was symmetrically distended and moved slightly with respiration. There was guarding and rebound tenderness at the hypogastrium. Digital rectal examination was without particularity but for an empty rectum. Bowel sounds were faint and hypoactive. The rest of the physical examination was normal.

In view of these, a diagnosis of localized peritonitis with severe sepsis was made. Aggressive fluid resuscitation with crystalloids was started. The patient was put on nil per os, and a nasogastric tube was inserted. Copious thick greenish fluid was brought out by the nasogastric tube. A urinary catheter was placed, and the urine output was monitored. The patient was placed on intravenous ceftriaxone (1 g, 8 hourly), gentamicin (160 mg daily), metronidazole (500 mg, 8 hourly), and paracetamol (1 g, 8 hourly). The following laboratory investigations were requested:

(1) An erect chest X-ray which revealed air beneath the right hemidiaphragm and distended small-bowel loops.

(2) The Widal test which was positive with a titre of <1/160 for both somatic and flagellar antibodies.

(3) White cell count that showed leucocytosis at 16,000 cells/mm^3 with 72% neutrophils.

(4) Haemoglobin level which was 11.8 g/dL.

Blood cell indices were not fully assessed because our hospital could not do a complete blood count. Based on the historical, clinical, and laboratory data obtained, we considered intestinal perforation due to typhoid fever as the probable aetiology of peritonitis, and the aetiological differentials included perforated peptic ulcer and perforated appendix. However, we could not perform blood or stool culture in our primary care hospital to confirm typhoid fever.

Four hours after admission and continuous resuscitation, the vital signs were blood pressure 120/80 mmHg, pulse 98 beats/min (regular and bounding), respiratory rate 24 breaths/min, and temperature 37.5°C. The patient remained haemodynamically stable the following 3 hours. Urine output was 32 ml/hr. His physical status score at the time of surgery was American Society of Anaesthesiology class IV. Intravenous ceftriaxone alongside other preoperative medication was administered to the patient, and an emergency exploratory laparotomy through a vertical midline incision was performed under general anaesthesia. Intraoperatively, distended small-bowel loops denuded of serosa on multiple spots were observed. Abundant greenish peritoneal fluid mixed with exudate and faecal material was obvious. The operative wound was rated as Altemeier class IV. On further inspection, multiple perforations were observed in the ileum (Figure 1).

A total of 15 perforations scattered over about 26 cm of the distal ileum were found. The perforation closest to the ileocaecal junction was less than 2 cm from the junction. The peritoneal cavity was thoroughly cleaned with warm saline. About 28 cm of the distal ileum including the section with perforations was segmentally resected (Figure 2) to leave clean margins, and then, a manual 2-layer end-to-side anastomosis of the proximal edge of the ileum and the transverse colon was performed.

The distal edge of the ileum was closed as a stump over the caecum, and the ascending colon left as a blind loop. Two abdominal drains were inserted to drain both the paracolic gutters and the rectovesical pouch through the right (Figure 3) and left lower quadrants of the abdomen.

The abdomen was closed layer by layer. Portions of the resected ileum were sent for histopathological analysis in a tertiary hospital. The patient was monitored in the recovery room for 30 minutes during which he remained haemodynamically

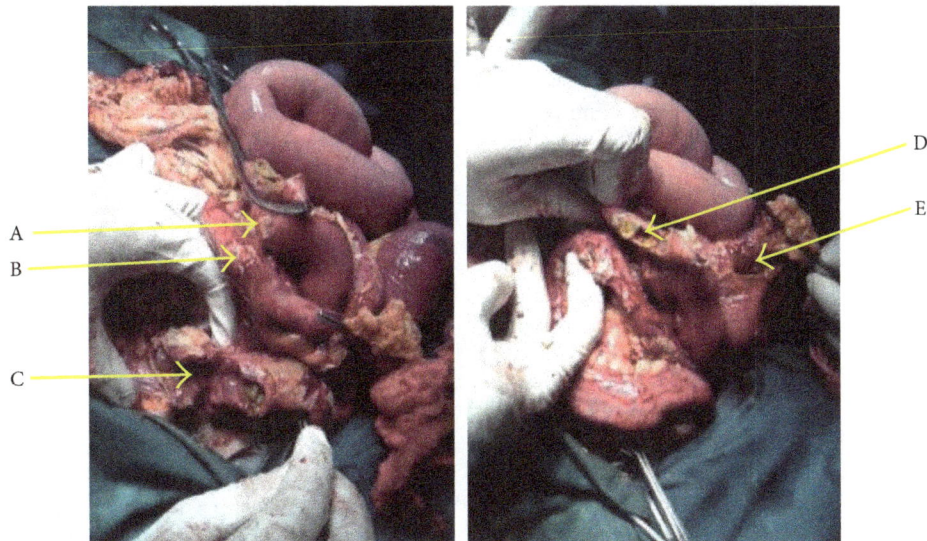

FIGURE 1: Intraoperative view of multiple typhoid ileal perforations (A to E) in the patient.

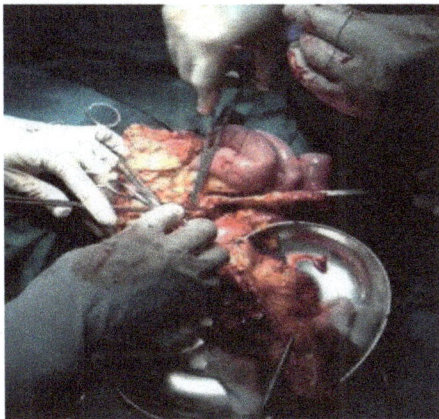

FIGURE 2: Segmental resection of the distal ileum.

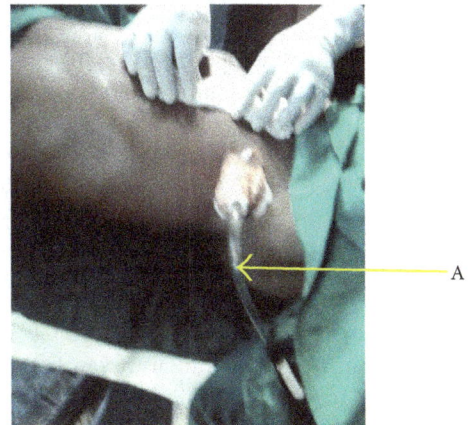

FIGURE 3: Abdominal drain (A).

stable. He was sent to the ward where close monitoring was continued.

Postoperatively, the patient was maintained on intravenous infusions of dextrose-saline, as well as intravenous ciprofloxacin (400 mg, 12 hourly), metronidazole (500 mg, 8 hourly), omeprazole (40 mg, 24 hourly), and intramuscular diclofenac (150 mg daily) for 10 days. Early ambulation was encouraged upon recovery from general anaesthesia. Enteral feeding with fluid diet was started after 26 postoperative hours, and routine postoperative care in the ward was continued. The abdominal drains were removed on the 6th postoperative day. On the 8th postoperative day, bowel sounds could not be perceived. A probable diagnosis of the postoperative paralytic ileus was made. The nasogastric tube was maintained, and enteral feeding halted till the tenth postoperative day when bowel sounds were appreciated. On the tenth postoperative day, suppuration was noticed at the surgical site which necessitated removal of the stitches and opening of the wound at the bedside. The wound was dressed for 3 weeks. Serial (four) Widal tests done at 3 days' interval remained positive with a titre of <1/160 for both somatic and

flagellar antibodies. Histopathology of the resected intestinal tissue revealed diffuse aggregates of enlarged irregular pale cells, with eccentric nuclei, and abundant acidophilic cytoplasm, with phagocytic characteristics. Chronic inflammation of the Peyer patches was also noted. These findings confirmed that the multiple ileal perforations were due to typhoid fever. The patient was discharged home on the thirty-fifth postoperative day and scheduled for regular visits. No other complications were observed after 6 months of follow-up.

3. Discussion

TIP is associated with a characteristic acute abdominal pain which is rather of gradual onset in elderly patients [10]. Furthermore, the severities of the signs and symptoms of TIP do not depend on the multiplicity or sizes of the perforations [14]. These dissociations between TIP and expected clinical features could obscure the sinister course of the illness; delay diagnosis consequently leads to a high degree of peritoneal contamination and mortality in an elderly patient.

A high index of suspicion in elderly patients is therefore imperative.

Delayed presentation of patients is a major hindrance to successful management of TIP in low-income countries. It results in significant changes in the ileum that require extensive surgery which further contributes to high morbidity and mortality [1, 8]. Our report is unique in that it is unusual for a frail and comorbid patient of such advanced age, and invariably depleted physiologic reserves, with multiple negative prognostic factors (including delayed presentation, sepsis, and up to 15 ileal perforations) to have a favourable surgical outcome.

Blood, stool, or bone marrow cultures are the most reliable standards of diagnosing typhoid fever. However, many low-income settings still rely on the Widal test to diagnose typhoid fever [16] which is considered an obsolete approach [8]. This was a major limitation in our preoperative diagnosis of typhoid fever. Diagnosis of intestinal perforation due to typhoid in resource-limited settings like ours is usually on the basis of (i) a history of a febrile illness possibly extending over several weeks, (ii) clinical data suggestive of generalized peritonitis, (iii) radiological data: X-ray showing air under the right hemidiaphragm, and (iv) intraoperative data: visualization of bowel perforations [1].

Generally, perforation occurs after severe inflammation and necrosis of the Peyer patches of the distal ileum [8, 17]. However, the characteristic inflammatory changes and lymphoid tissue involvement typical of typhoid fever require histological confirmation [9, 14], but this is beyond the reach of small hospitals like ours. Another possible aetiology of ileal perforation worth mentioning is frequent use of nonsteroidal anti-inflammatories. Multiple ileal perforations secondary to repeated parenteral diclofenac administration in an elderly patient have been reported [18] although the type of nonsteroidal anti-inflammatory drug and the route and frequency of drug administration differed from our case. Our initiative in sending out a specimen for histological analysis at a tertiary hospital permitted us to definitively confirm typhoid fever as the aetiology of ileal perforations in our patient.

From a treatment perspective, the need for enterostomy ought to be judiciously assessed in spite of clear indications as in our case. Our choice of operative procedure was justified by the known risk of morbidity of bowel exteriorization which is greatest in elderly patients, patients who present late, and patients undergoing emergency surgery. Furthermore, sepsis at presentation and the comorbid state of our patient further increased the risk of complications of bowel exteriorization [19]. Finally, the negative impact of poor stoma care in resource-limited settings cannot be overemphasized. Considering the likelihood of a damaged ileocaecal junction in our case, the option of ileocaecal anastomosis was dismissed since it would have been later on complicated by buildup of the colonic faecal material and toxins into the remaining ileum [20]. Also, primary closure was not a plausible option since most perforations in our case were large. However, considerable ileal resection as in our patient heralds potential complications like malabsorption, osmotic diarrhoea, and derangements in the bile salt metabolism [21]. The ascending colon had no perforations and was salvaged. Resecting this portion of the bowel in order not to leave a blind loop would have rendered the surgical procedure longer and increased the risk of morbidity and mortality in such a critical setting.

Previous case reports indicating more typhoid ileal perforations, albeit in relatively younger patients, indicate different surgical approaches: a case of 25 perforations involving the distal jejunum and entire ileum successfully treated with single-layer closure [22]; a patient with 24 ileal and caecal perforations treated with bowel resection and ileotransverse side-to-side anastomosis with proximal ileostomy [23]; and a child with 27 ileal and colonic perforations necessitating hemicolectomy [24]. From these reports and ours, it is noted that even though the surgical procedures were individualized, optimal perioperative management was common to all the cases. Ameh et al. compared 3 operative procedures in Nigeria (although amongst children) and proposed that although mortality was high following all the types of surgery, bowel resection and anastomosis was a preferred surgical treatment for typhoid perforation in low-income settings [25]. However, a recent study by Caronna et al. in Benin discourages bowel resection and anastomosis. It is, nonetheless, worth noting that Caronna et al. hugely attributed the high morbidity associated with resection and anastomosis to anastomotic complications [15], which based on our assessment did not occur in our patient and explains in part the good outcome. Whichever the surgical approach used, it is recommended to thoroughly search for other sites of perforation or necrosis that might imminently perforate [8]. In our case, apart from the perforations observed, denudation of the serosa was also noticed and was expected to heal spontaneously.

Postoperatively, the patient developed paralytic ileus and surgical site infection. Studies reviewing operative management of TIP in other resource-poor settings report surgical site infection as the most frequent postoperative complication of TIP repair [5, 26, 27]. In our case, postoperative complications were successfully treated conservatively. According to the Clavien and Dindo classification (a validated method of reporting adverse surgical events), these complications were of Grade I or least severe complications [28], but they prolonged the hospital stay of our patient.

In conclusion, the diagnosis and management of TIP in low-income countries that are endemic for typhoid fever are challenging. The successful treatment of an ominous case of multiple typhoid ileal perforations in a very elderly patient using a less conventional approach does not discount the high case fatality in resource-limited settings nor the merits of evidence-based therapeutic modalities. Highlighting the importance of early diagnosis and the utilization of existing health facilities may help dispel patient inertia and late presentation. These, in addition to individualized and optimal surgical care, may lead to a favourable outcome even amidst resource constraints.

Acknowledgments

The authors thank all those who participated in the management of the patient.

References

[1] A. I. Ugochukwu, O. C. Amu, and M. A. Nzegwu, "Ileal perforation due to typhoid fever–review of operative management and outcome in an urban centre in Nigeria," *International Journal of Surgery*, vol. 11, no. 3, pp. 218–222, 2013.

[2] K. Anupama Pujar, A. C. Ashok, H. K. Rudresh, H. C. Srikantaiah, K. S. Girish, and K. R. Suhas, "Mortality in typhoid intestinal perforation-a declining trend," *Journal of Clinical and Diagnostic Research*, vol. 7, no. 9, pp. 1946–1948, 2013.

[3] S. T. Edino, A. Z. Mohammed, A. F. Uba et al., "Typhoid enteric perforation in north western Nigeria," *Nigerian Journal of Medicine*, vol. 13, no. 4, pp. 345–349, 2004.

[4] E. Gedik, S. Girgin, I. H. Taçyildiz, and Y. Akgün, "Risk factors affecting morbidity in typhoid enteric perforation," *Langenbeck's Archives of Surgery*, vol. 393, no. 6, pp. 973–977, 2008.

[5] P. L. Chalya, J. B. Mabula, M. Koy et al., "Typhoid intestinal perforations at a University teaching hospital in Northwestern Tanzania: a surgical experience of 104 cases in a resource-limited setting," *World Journal of Emergency Surgery*, vol. 7, no. 1, p. 4, 2012.

[6] A. M. Malik, A. A. Laghari, Q. Mallah, and G. A. Qureshi, "Different surgical options and ileostomy in typhoid perforation," *World Journal of Medical Sciences*, vol. 1, no. 2, pp. 112–116, 2006.

[7] R. A. Wani, F. Q. Parray, N A. Bhat, M. A. Wani, T. H. Bhat, and F. Farzana, "Nontraumatic terminal ileal perforation," *World Journal of Emergency Surgery*, vol. 1, no. 1, p. 7, 2006.

[8] P. K. Datta, P. Lal, and S. De Bakshi, "Surgery in the tropics," in *Bailey & Love's Short Practices Surgery*, W. Norman, B. Christopher, and P. O'connel, Eds., pp. 68–70, Edward Arnold Ltd., London, UK, 25th edition, 2008.

[9] S. S. Atamanalp, B. Aydinli, G. Ozturk, D. Oren, M. Basoglu, and M. I. Yildirgan, "Typhoid intestinal perforations: twenty-six-year experience," *World Journal of Surgery*, vol. 31, no. 9, pp. 1883–1888, 2007.

[10] T. Ahmad, "Perforation operation interval as a prognostic factor in typhoid ileal perforation," *Journal of Surgery Pakistan*, vol. 14, no. 1, pp. 11–14, 2009.

[11] S. Deepak, J. A. Kumar, P. Gharde, S. D. Bala, and V. R. Sewak, "Typhoid intestinal perforation in Central India–a surgical experience of 155 cases in resource limited setting," *International Journal of Biomedical and Advance Research*, vol. 5, pp. 600–604, 2014.

[12] F. C. Eggleston, B. Santoshi, and C. M. Singh, "Typhoid perforation of the bowel. Experiences in 78 cases," *Annals of Surgery*, vol. 190, no. 1, pp. 31–35, 1979.

[13] A. Chichom-Mefire, T. A. Fon, and M. Ngowe-ngowe, "Which cause of diffuse peritonitis is the deadliest in the tropics? a retrospective analysis of 305 cases from the South-West Region of Cameroon," *World Journal of Emergency Surgery*, vol. 11, no. 1, pp. 1–11, 2016.

[14] A. Sümer, Ö. Kemik, A. C. Dülger et al., "Outcome of surgical treatment of intestinal perforation in typhoid fever," *World Journal of Gastroenterology*, vol. 16, no. 33, pp. 4164–4168, 2010.

[15] R. Caronna, A. K. Boukari, D. Zaongo et al., "Comparative analysis of primary repair vs resection and anastomosis with laparostomy in management of typhoid intestinal perforation: results of a rural hospital in northwestern Benin," *BMC Gastroenterology*, vol. 13, no. 1, pp. 1–10, 2013.

[16] G. Andualem, T. Abebe, N. Kebede, S. Gebre-Selassie, A. Mihret, and H. Alemayehu, "A comparative study of Widal test with blood culture in the diagnosis of typhoid fever in febrile patients," *BMC Research Notes*, vol. 7, no. 1, p. 653, 2014.

[17] C. M. Parry, T. T. Hien, G. Dougan, N. J. White, and J. J. Farrar, "Typhoid fever," *New England Journal of Medicine*, vol. 347, no. 22, pp. 1770–1782, 2002.

[18] W. S. Park, S. W. Kim, S. Lee, S. T. Lee, and H. S. Park, "Multiple ileal perforations due to regular diclofenac sodium injections: a case report," *BMC Research Notes*, vol. 6, no. 1, p. 129, 2013.

[19] P. Chaudhary, I. Nabi, G. Ranjan et al., "Prospective analysis of indications and early complications of emergency temporary loop ileostomies for perforation peritonitis," *Annals Gastroenterology*, vol. 28, no. 1, pp. 135–140, 2015.

[20] K. W. Ecker, G. Pistorius, M. D. Menger, and G. Feifel, "Long-term function of experimental substitutes of the ileocecal valve," *European Surgical Research*, vol. 29, no. 2, pp. 75–83, 1997.

[21] M. S. Steiner and R. A. Morton, "Nutritional and gastrointestinal complications of the use of bowel segments in the lower urinary tract," *Urologic Clinics of North America*, vol. 18, no. 4, pp. 743–754, 1991.

[22] D. P. Connolly, B. T. Ugwu, and B. A. Eke, "Single-layer closure for typhoid perforations of the small intestine: case report," *East African Medical Journal*, vol. 75, no. 7, pp. 439-440, 1998.

[23] A. K. Sharma, R. K. Sharma, S. K. Sharma, A. Sharma, and D. Soni, "Typhoid intestinal perforation: 24 perforations in one patient," *Annals of Medical and Health Sciences Research*, vol. 3, no. 5, pp. S41–S43, 2013.

[24] J. O. Adeniran, J. O. Taiwo, and L. O. Abdur-Rahman, "Salmonella intestinal perforation: (27 perforations in one patient, 14 perforations in another) are the goal posts changing?," *Journal of Indian Association of Pediatric Surgeons*, vol. 10, no. 4, pp. 248–251, 2005.

[25] E. A. Ameh, P. M. Dogo, M. M. Attah, and P. T. Nmadu, "Comparison of three operations for typhoid perforation," *British Journal of Surgery*, vol. 84, no. 4, pp. 558-559, 1997.

[26] N. Charles and E. Lucia, "Improvement in survival from typhoid ileal perforation results of 221 operative cases," *Annals of Surgery*, vol. 215, no. 3, pp. 244–249, 1991.

[27] S. T. Edino, A. A. Yakubu, A. Z. Mohammed, and I. S. Abubakar, "Prognostic factors in typhoid ileal perforation: a prospective study of 53 cases," *Journal of the National Medical Association*, vol. 99, pp. 1042–1045, 2007.

[28] D. Dindo, M. K. Muller, M. Weber, and P. A. Clavien, "Obesity in general elective surgery," *The Lancet*, vol. 361, no. 9364, pp. 2032–2035, 2003.

55

A Giant Duodenal Leiomyoma Showing Increased Uptake on 18F-Fluorodeoxyglucose Positron Emission Tomography

Keisuke Nonoyama ⓘ, Hidehiko Kitagami, Akira Yasuda, Shiro Fujihata, Minoru Yamamoto, Yasunobu Shimizu, and Moritsugu Tanaka

Department of Gastroenterological Surgery, Kariya Toyota General Hospital, Kariya, Japan

Correspondence should be addressed to Keisuke Nonoyama; nonoyama_tennis@yahoo.co.jp

Academic Editor: Giovanni Mariscalco

Background. Although 18F-fluorodeoxyglucose positron emission tomography (FDG-PET/CT) is now widely used in their differential diagnosis, it is sometimes difficult to distinguish between benign and malignant diseases. *Case Presentation.* A 44-year-old woman was found to have abnormalities on health screening. Magnetic resonance imaging for detailed examination showed an intra-abdominal tumor measuring 12 cm in the major axis near the cranial end of the uterus. Upper gastrointestinal tract endoscopy showed a tumor with an ulcer in the third part of the duodenum, involving half the circumference. Heterogeneous uptake was observed within the tumor on FDG-PET/CT. Based on these findings, the patient underwent surgery for suspected primary malignant lymphoma of the duodenum or gastrointestinal stromal tumor. Laparotomy revealed a 12 cm tumor in the third part of the duodenum. Partial duodenectomy and end-to-end duodenojejunostomy were performed. Pathological findings showed a solid tumor growing from the muscle layer of the duodenum to outside the serous membrane; based on immunostaining, it was diagnosed as a leiomyoma. *Conclusions.* Duodenal leiomyomas are originally benign; to date, there have been no reports of uptake in duodenal leiomyomas on FDG-PET/CT; therefore, our case is rare. Leiomyomas should be considered in the differential diagnosis of duodenal neoplastic diseases.

1. Background

18F-fluorodeoxyglucose positron emission tomography (FDG-PET/CT) is now widely used in the differential diagnosis of benign and malignant diseases [1]. In general, no increased uptake is observed in duodenal leiomyomas, which are benign tumors. We herein report our experience with a case of a giant duodenal leiomyoma showing increased uptake on FDG-PET/CT.

2. Case Presentation

A 44-year-old woman was diagnosed with iron deficiency anemia but showed no abnormalities on gastrointestinal tract endoscopy 5 years prior to the current presentation. A blood test for health screening showed anemia with hemoglobin 7.6 g/dL, and uterine fibroids were suspected on abdominal ultrasonography. She was diagnosed as having an intra-abdominal tumor on magnetic resonance imaging (MRI) for detailed examination and was referred to our hospital.

The abdomen was flat and soft, with an elastic mass of poor mobility which was the size of an infant's head was palpable below the umbilicus to above the pubis. There were no blood test abnormalities; CEA, CA19-9, SCC, and the interleukin 2 receptor level were within normal limits. Abdominal MRI revealed a homogeneous and well-demarcated $74 \times 98 \times 122$ mm mass near the cranial end of the uterus, with a low signal intensity on T1-weighted image, and mostly low signal intensity and partially high intensity on T2-weighted image (Figures 1(a) and 1(b)). Abdominal-enhanced computed tomography (CT) showed a well-demarcated and contrast-enhanced oval mass with a smooth margin in the pelvis. The tumor was supplied by the superior mesenteric artery, and the surrounding lymph nodes were enlarged (Figures 1(c) and 1(d)). Upper gastrointestinal tract endoscopy showed an easily bleeding tumor with an ulcer in the third part of the duodenum, involving half the circumference (Figure 2(a)).

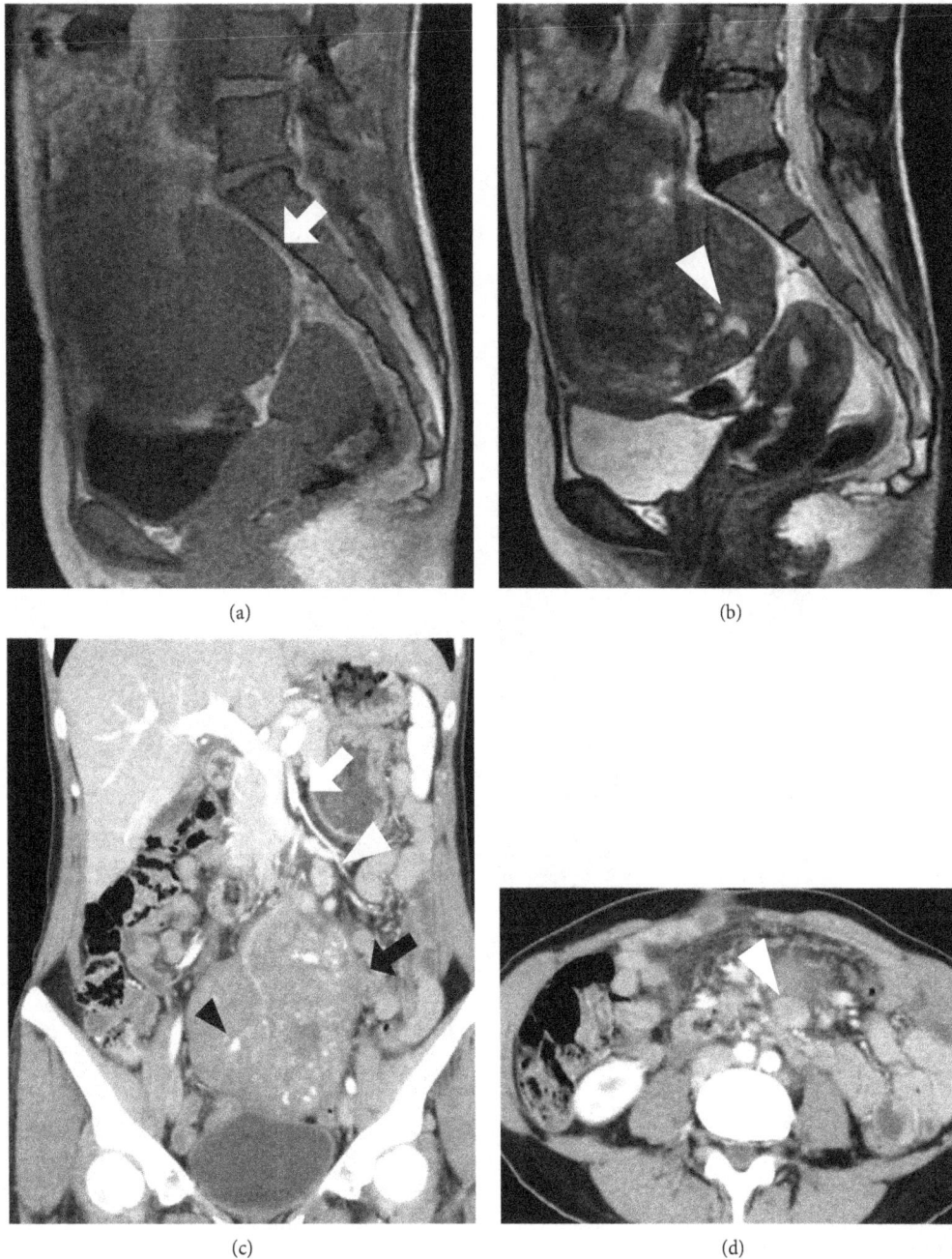

FIGURE 1: Abdominal MRI and abdominal contrast-enhanced CT. Abdominal MRI shows a homogeneous and well-demarcated 74 × 98 × 122 mm mass at the cranial part of the uterus (arrow), with a low signal intensity on T1-weighted image (a) and mostly low signal intensity and partially high intensity on T2-weighted image (b) (arrowhead). Abdominal contrast-enhanced CT shows a well-demarcated oval mass with a smooth margin and enhancement in the pelvis (black arrow). The enhanced arteries in the tumor are detected (black arrowhead). The tumor is supplied by the superior mesenteric artery (white arrow), and the surrounding lymph nodes are enlarged (white arrowhead) (c, d).

The biopsy results were inflammatory exudates and granulation tissues. FDG-PET/CT showed heterogeneous uptake inside the tumor with SUVmax 6.3 (Figures 2(b)–2(d)). A slight 18F-FDG uptake was observed in the enlarged lymph nodes with SUVmax 2.6. Along with the facts that there were no malignant cells detected by endoscopic biopsy and the CT image showing enlarged surrounding lymph nodes, the patient was suspected of nonepithelial malignancy of the duodenum such as gastrointestinal stromal tumor (GIST) and malignant lymphoma. As we could not make a definite diagnosis preoperatively, she underwent surgery for an accurate diagnosis and treatment.

Surgery was performed under general anesthesia; laparotomy was performed via midline incision from 5 cm above the umbilicus to above the pubis. There was a 12 cm tumor centered on the third part of the duodenum, extending to

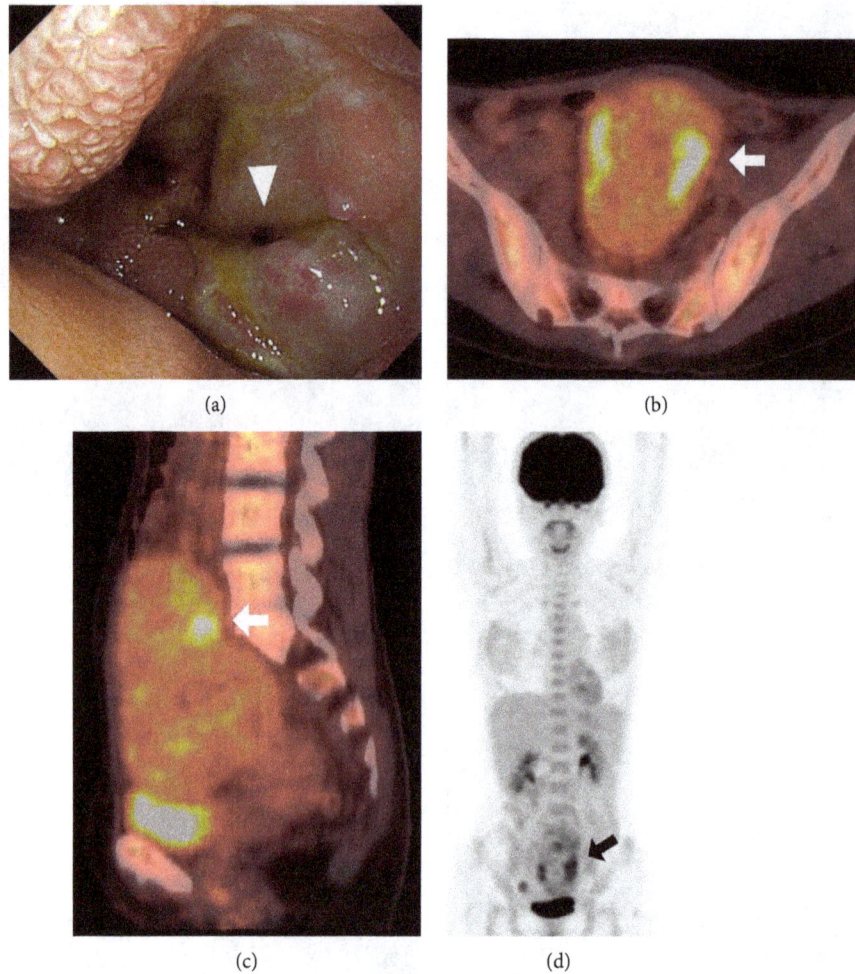

FIGURE 2: Upper gastrointestinal tract endoscopy and FDG-PET/CT. Upper gastrointestinal tract endoscopy shows a tumor with ulcer formation (arrowhead) in the third part of the duodenum, involving half the circumference (a). FDG-PET/CT axial image (b) and sagittal image (c) show heterogeneous uptake inside the tumor (white arrow) with SUVmax 6.3. FDG-PET/CT whole body image (d) also reveals heterogeneous uptake inside the tumor (black arrow).

the fourth part. The tumor extended into the pelvis and pulled the duodenum and the ligament of Treitz caudally (Figure 3(a)). There was no infiltration of the tumor into the pancreas or the small intestine. The duodenum was transected at the third part of the duodenum on the oral side. On the anal side of the tumor, the jejunum immediately after the ligament of Treitz was transected, and the tumor was resected. The enlarged lymph nodes sampling were also performed. In reconstruction, end-to-end duodenojejunostomy was performed (Figure 3(b)). She had an uneventful postoperative course and was discharged 9 days after surgery.

Pathological findings showed a solid tumor growing from the muscle layer of the duodenum through the serous membrane. The duodenal mucosa was invaginated at the site of the tumor, forming a deep ulcer (Figure 4(a)). The tumor showed uniform growth of long and spindle-shaped cells in an intricate manner, and the number of nuclear divisions was 1 or less per 50 visual fields (Figure 4(b)). There were no evidence of calcification, hemorrhage, or degeneration within the tumor. On immunostaining, α-smooth muscle actin was positive, while S-100, c-kit, and CD34 were

negative (Figures 4(c)–4(f)). The MIB-1 index was low at 3% maximum, and there were no neoplastic lesions in the enlarged lymph nodes. Based on these findings, a leiomyoma was diagnosed. Since then, no relapse has occurred for two years and six months.

3. Discussion

Primary benign tumors of the duodenum are relatively rare. Darling and Welch [2] reported the frequency of primary benign tumor of the duodenum as 0.12% (21 of 17,070 autopsy patients), Ebert et al. [3] as 0.03% (8 of 25,000 autopsy patients), and Raiford [4] as 0.02% (13 of 56,500 operated and autopsy patients). The percentage of benign tumors of the duodenum among all benign tumors of the small intestine was 30% (35 of 115 patients) in the report by Darling and Welch [2] and 15% (208 of 1399 patients) in the report by River et al. [5], with slightly lower frequency than those in the jejunum and ileum. Among benign tumors of the small intestine, the frequency of primary leiomyoma is

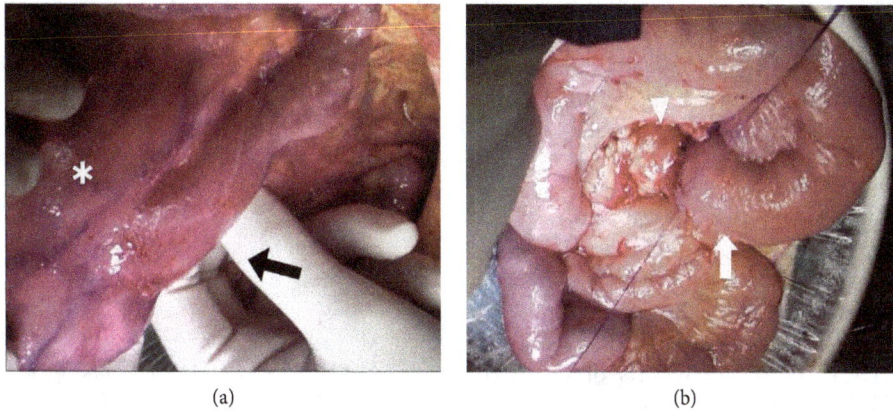

(a)   (b)

FIGURE 3: Surgical findings. Surgical findings show a 12 cm tumor mainly in the third part of the duodenum (asterisk); the duodenum and the ligament of Treitz (black arrow) are pulled in a caudal direction by the tumor (a). The horizontal part of the duodenum (arrowhead) is end-to-end anastomosed to the jejunal stump (white arrow) (b).

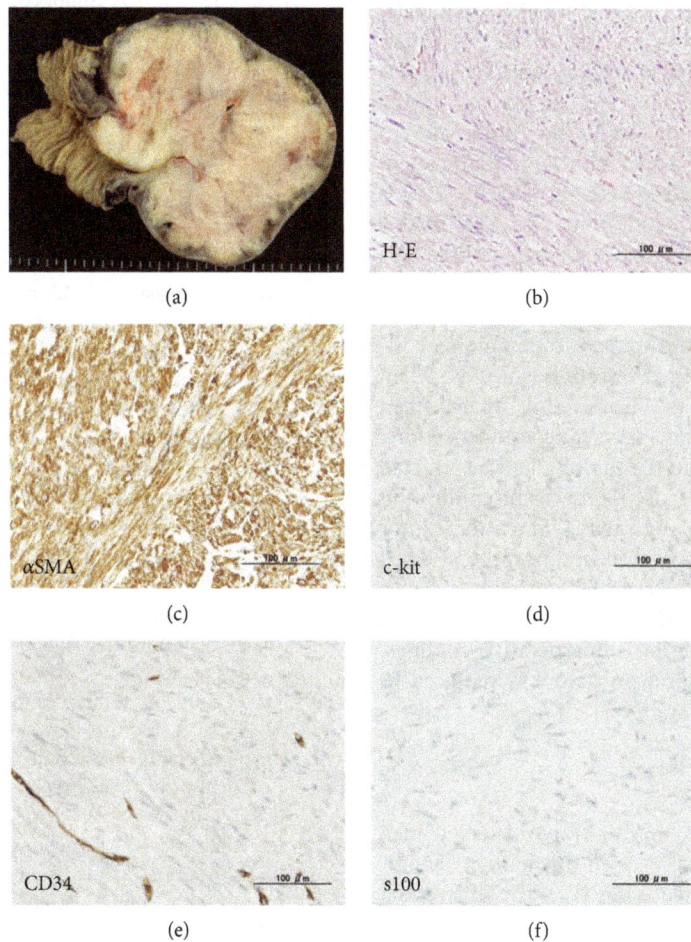

(a)   (b)
(c)   (d)
(e)   (f)

FIGURE 4: Pathological findings. Pathological testing shows a solid tumor growing from the muscle layer of the duodenum through the serous membrane (a). Hematoxylin and eosin staining show uniform growth of spindle cells in an intricate manner (b). On immunostaining, α-smooth muscle actin is positive (c), and S-100, c-kit, and CD34 are negative (d–f).

the highest after adenoma and lipoma, of which 25.3% are accounted to be duodenal primary [5, 6].

The second portion of the duodenum is the most common site affected by leiomyoma of the duodenum, accounting for more than 50% of all cases [7]. The most common clinical symptom is melena resulting from ulcer formation; abdominal pain, diarrhea, and constipation may also occur [7]. The incidence of extraductal growth is three times greater than that of intraductal growth; therefore, ductal obstruction is unlikely to occur [7]. It is presumed that this tumor was present when the patient was diagnosed with iron deficiency anemia 5 years prior to the current presentation. Possible reasons for nondiagnosis include the location of the tumor (centered in the third part of the duodenum) and absence of obstructive symptoms, probably due to extraductal growth.

Although FDG-PET/CT is widely performed for differential diagnosis of benign and malignant diseases, a gastrointestinal leiomyoma, which is a benign tumor, rarely shows uptake. A literature search of PubMed (1950–2015), using "leiomyoma" and "FDG-PET/CT" as keywords, found no report of leiomyoma of the duodenum showing increased uptake on FDG-PET/CT. There are reports of increased uptake on FDG-PET/CT in primary leiomyomas of the esophagus [8], stomach [9], and jejunum. However, it is unclear why increased uptake was observed in the gastrointestinal leiomyoma presented herein.

Increased uptake on FDG-PET/CT has been reported in leiomyomas of the uterus, and Chura et al. [10] stated that the uptake is associated with vascular growth in the tumor. Kitajima et al. [11] reported that there was a mildly positive correlation between the SUVmax of a leiomyoma of the uterus and the tumor size. In our patient, the tumor showed contrast enhancement on CT and had a large diameter of 12 cm, suggesting that increased uptake on FDG-PET/CT is associated with vascular growth and tumor size. The inflammation due to the invagination could also be one of the reasons of positive FDG uptake.

This patient was suspected of having a malignant lymphoma or GIST and underwent tumor resection alone without lymphadenectomy. Combined resection is needed when there is tumor infiltration into the surrounding organs; when the tumor involves the pancreas, pancreaticoduodenectomy may be required. In this patient, the tumor could be resected with partial duodenectomy because there was no infiltration into the pancreas or surrounding organs. Since the tumor was benign based on the pathological findings, the selected procedure was appropriate. However, when a tumor shows increased uptake on FDG-PET/CT, it is highly likely to be malignant. Therefore, considering intraoperative findings, selecting the appropriate surgical procedure is required to avoid excessive or insufficient surgery.

4. Conclusions

Increased uptake on FDG-PET/CT may be observed in a leiomyoma of the duodenum as seen in this patient. Therefore, a leiomyoma should be considered in the differential diagnosis of neoplastic diseases of the duodenum showing increased uptake on FDG-PET/CT.

Abbreviations

MRI: Magnetic resonance imaging
FDG-PET/CT: 18F-fluorodeoxyglucose positron emission
              tomography
CT: Computed tomography
SUV: Standardized uptake value
GIST: Gastrointestinal stromal tumor.

Authors' Contributions

KN, AY, SF, and MT participated in the care of the patient. KN contributed to the writing of the manuscript. KN, HK, and AY participated in the critical revision of the manuscript. All authors read and approved the final manuscript.

References

[1] M. Ide, "Cancer screening with FDG-PET," *The Quarterly Journal of Nuclear Medicine and Molecular Imaging*, vol. 50, no. 1, pp. 23–27, 2006.

[2] R. C. Darling and C. E. Welch, "Tumors of the small intestine," *The New England Journal of Medicine*, vol. 260, no. 9, pp. 397–408, 1959.

[3] R. E. Ebert, G. F. Parkhurst, O. A. Melendy, and M. P. Osborne, "Primary tumors of the duodenum," *Surgery, Gynecology & Obstetrics*, vol. 97, no. 2, pp. 135–139, 1953.

[4] T. S. Raiford, "Tumors of the small intestine," *Archives of Surgery*, vol. 25, no. 1, p. 122, 1932.

[5] L. River, J. Silverstein, and J. W. Tope, "Benign neoplasma of the small intestine. A critical comprehensive review with reports of 20 new cases," *Surgery, Gynecology & Obstetrics*, vol. 102, no. 1, pp. 1–38, 1956.

[6] J. E. Skandalakis, S. W. Gray, and D. Shepard, "Smooth muscle tumors of the small intestine," *The American Journal of Gastroenterology*, vol. 42, pp. 172–190, 1964.

[7] A. I. Mittelpunkt, N. J. Capos, and A. Bernstein, "Benign leiomyomas of the duodenum. A report of three cases and a review of the literature," *Archives of Surgery*, vol. 88, no. 2, pp. 308–313, 1964.

[8] K. Miyoshi, M. Naito, T. Ueno, S. Hato, and H. Ino, "Abnormal fluorine-18-fluorodeoxyglucose uptake in benign esophageal leiomyoma," *General Thoracic and Cardiovascular Surgery*, vol. 57, no. 11, pp. 629–632, 2009.

[9] Y. Hirose, H. Kaida, A. Kawahara, S. Kurata, M. Ishibashi, and T. Abe, "18F-FDG PET/CT and contrast enhanced CT in differential diagnosis between leiomyoma and gastrointestinal stromal tumor," *Hellenic Journal of Nuclear Medicine*, vol. 18, no. 3, pp. 257–260, 2015.

[10] J. C. Chura, A. M. Truskinovsky, P. L. Judson, L. Johnson, M. A. Geller, and L. S. Downs Jr., "Positron emission tomography and leiomyomas: clinicopathologic analysis of 3 cases of PET scan-positive leiomyomas and literature review," *Gynecologic Oncology*, vol. 104, no. 1, pp. 247–252, 2007.

[11] K. Kitajima, K. Murakami, E. Yamasaki, Y. Kaji, and K. Sugimura, "Standardized uptake values of uterine leiomyoma with 18F-FDG PET/CT: variation with age, size, degeneration, and contrast enhancement on MRI," *Annals of Nuclear Medicine*, vol. 22, no. 6, pp. 505–512, 2008.

56

Flare-Up Diverticulitis in the Terminal Ileum in Short Interval after Conservative Therapy

**Kensuke Nakatani,[1] Takaharu Kato,[1,2] Shinichiro Okada,[1]
Risa Matsumoto,[1] Kazuhiro Nishida,[1] Hiroyasu Komuro,[1] Maki Iida,[3]
Shiro Tsujimoto,[3] and Toshiyuki Suganuma[1]**

[1]*Department of Surgery, Yokosuka General Hospital Uwamachi, 2-36 Uwamachi Yokosuka City, Kanagawa 238-8567, Japan*

[2]*Department of Surgery, Saitama Medical Center, Jichi Medical University, 1-847 Amanuma-cho, Omiya-ku, Saitama 330-8503, Japan*

[3]*Department of Pathology, Yokosuka General Hospital Uwamachi, 2-36 Uwamachi, Yokosuka, Kanagawa 238-8567, Japan*

Correspondence should be addressed to Takaharu Kato; tkato@jichi.ac.jp

Academic Editor: Dimitrios Mantas

Diverticulitis in the terminal ileum is uncommon. Past reports suggested that conservative therapy may be feasible to treat terminal ileum diverticulitis without perforation; however, there is no consensus on the therapeutic strategy for small bowel diverticulitis. We present a 37-year-old man who was referred to our hospital for sudden onset of abdominal pain and nausea. He was diagnosed with diverticulitis in the terminal ileum by computed tomography (CT). Tazobactam/piperacillin hydrate (18 g/day) was administered. The antibiotic treatment was maintained for 7 days, and the symptoms disappeared after the treatment. Thirty-eight days after antibiotic therapy, he noticed severe abdominal pain again. He was diagnosed with diverticulitis in terminal ileum which was flare-up of inflammation. He was given antibiotic therapy again. Nine days after antibiotic therapy, laparoscopy assisted right hemicolectomy and resection of 20 cm of terminal ileum were performed. Histopathology report confirmed multiple ileal diverticulitis. He was discharged from our hospital 12 days after the surgery. Colonoscopy was performed two months after the surgery and it revealed no finding suggesting inflammatory bowel disease. Surgical treatment should be taken into account as a potential treatment option to manage the diverticulitis in the terminal ileum even though it is not perforated.

1. Introduction

Diverticulitis in the terminal ileum is an uncommon entity except for Meckel's diverticulum. Pathologically, the diverticulosis in small bowel is characterized by herniation of the mucosa and the submucosa through the muscular layer of the bowel wall [1, 2]. Some case reports showed patients who received surgery for perforated diverticulitis in the small intestine [3–7]. But the standardized therapy has not been established in the patient with diverticulitis which was not perforated. We present a case of diverticulitis in the terminal ileum in a middle-aged man which was flare-up of inflammation in short interval after antibiotic therapy and needed surgical treatment.

2. Case Presentation

A 37-year-old man woke up at midnight with severe abdominal pain and nausea. The patient consulted local clinic and was diagnosed with acute abdomen. He was referred to Yokosuka General Hospital Uwamachi for further examination and treatment. On physical examination, his blood pressure was 118/67 mmHg with a pulse rate of 103 beats and respiratory rate of 18 per minute and body temperature of 38.2 degrees C. He had rebound tenderness in his right lower quadrant. Laboratory analysis showed a C-reactive protein level of 2.6 mg/L, and white blood cell count was 20,700/μL. Computed tomography (CT) revealed sequential diverticula in the wall thickening terminal ileum

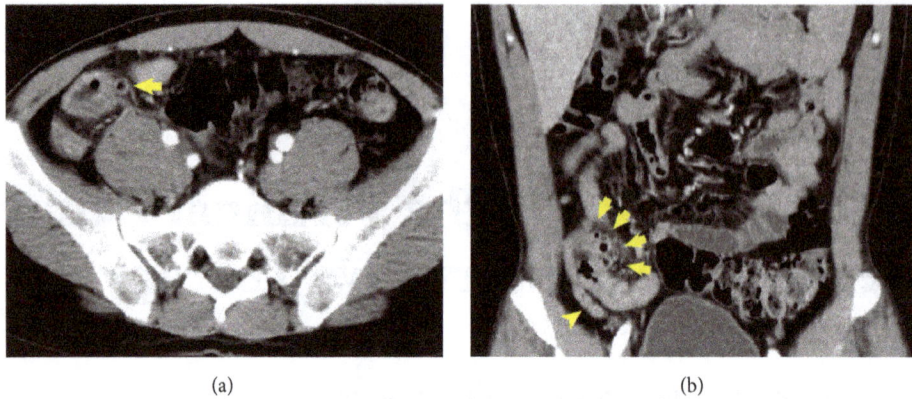

(a)

(b)

FIGURE 1: Computed tomography revealed diverticula sequentially located in the wall thickening terminal ileum (arrows); surrounding abdominal fat was developing high density suggesting inflammation. The appendix was not swollen (arrow head).

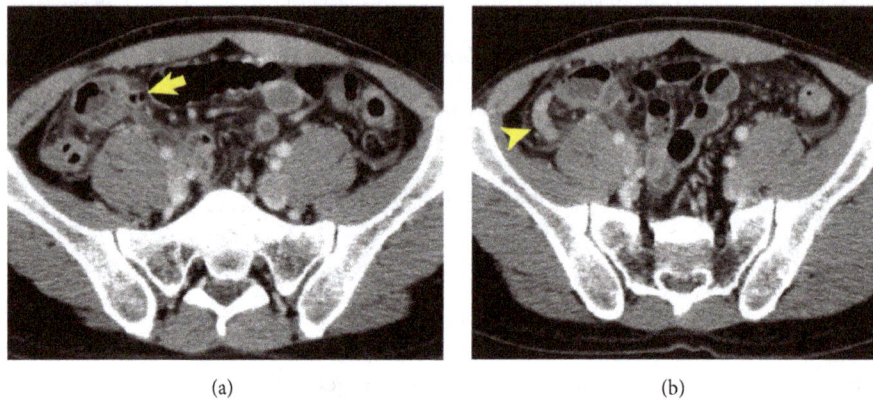

(a)

(b)

FIGURE 2: Computed tomography revealed diverticula in the terminal ileum (arrow) and swollen appendix with 10 mm in the diameter (arrow head).

with high density of surrounding fat (arrows in Figures 1(a) and 1(b)) and appendix without swelling (Figure 1(b) arrow head) and also multiple uncomplicated diverticula in the ascending colon separated from the panniculitis lesion were detected. He was diagnosed with diverticulitis in the terminal ileum. Tazobactam/piperacillin hydrate (18 g/day) was administered. Antibiotic therapy was maintained for 7 days and the symptoms disappeared. While the peak level was 12.89 mg/dL, C-reactive protein level was deceased to 0.92 mg/dL after the treatment. Following this treatment, the patient was started on potassium clavulanate and amoxicillin hydrate (1500 mg/day) and discharged from our hospital 10 days after the admission. Nineteen days after his discharge, he had been seen in the follow-up consultation without any inflammatory findings. Three weeks after his last consultation, 38 days after antibiotic therapy was finished, he noticed severe abdominal pain and nausea again and was carried to the local hospital. He was diagnosed with diverticulitis in the terminal ileum and acute appendicitis by CT examination performed in the local hospital. He was referred to our hospital for possible surgery. On physical examination, his blood pressure was 111/70 mmHg with a pulse rate of 90 beats and respiratory rate of 20 per minute and body temperature of

37.2 degrees C. He had rebound tenderness in his right lower quadrant. Laboratory analysis showed a C-reactive protein level of 1.2 mg/L, and white blood cell count was 13,600/μL. Abdominal enhanced CT performed at previous hospital which showed diverticula in the terminal ileum with high density of surrounding fat (Figure 2(a) arrows) and appendix with 10 mm swelling (Figure 2(b) arrow head). On the whole, CT findings were similar with those of primary diverticulitis. He was diagnosed with diverticulitis in the terminal ileum which was flare-up of inflammation and acute appendicitis. Tazobactam/piperacillin hydrate (18 g/day) was administered again. Since the diverticulitis was flare-up of inflammation in short interval after conservative therapy, we decided to perform surgery. Nine days after antibiotic therapy, laparoscopy assisted right hemicolectomy and resection of 20 cm of terminal ileum were performed. Meckel's diverticulum was not found in the ileum. The resected specimen revealed diverticulitis in the terminal ileum on the mesentery side (Figures 3(a) and 3(b), arrows). On microscopic evaluation, the nodular areas correspond to points of mucosal invagination into the surrounding muscular layer, creating diverticula (Figure 3(c)). There was inflammatory granuloma that consisted of foreign body giant cells (Figure 3(d) arrows)

(a)

(b)

(c)

(d)

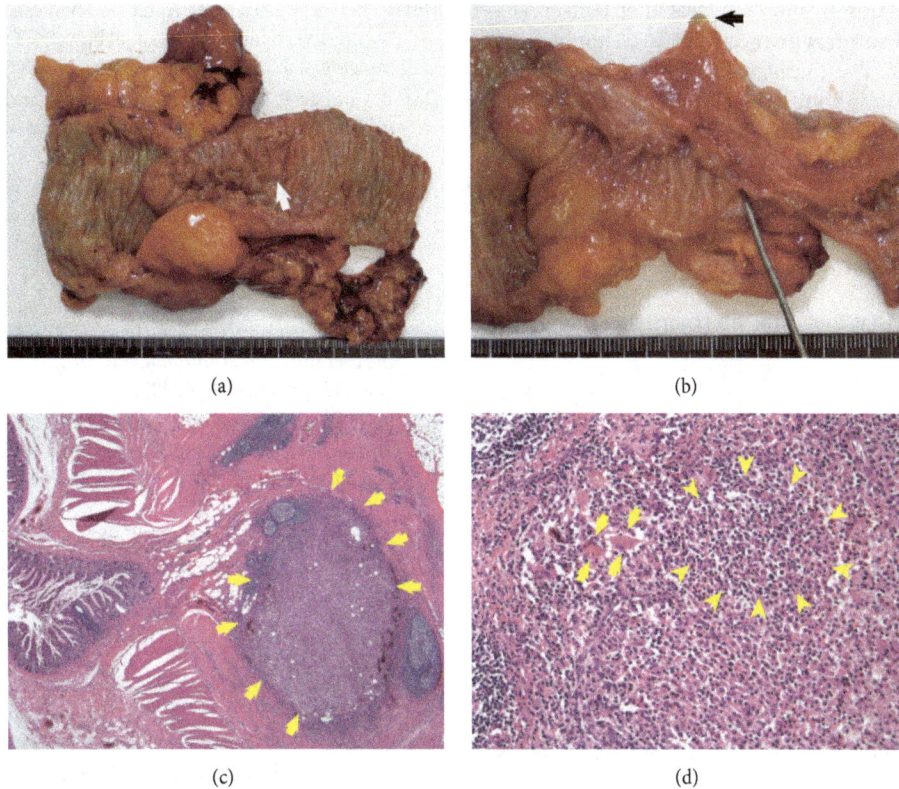

FIGURE 3: Surgically resected specimen revealed diverticula on the mesenteric side in the terminal ileum ((a) and (b)). Microscopically, the nodular areas correspond to points of mucosal invagination into the surrounding muscular layer, creating diverticula (c). There is inflammatory granuloma that consisted of foreign body giant cells (arrows in (d)) and foam cells (arrow heads in (d)) in the invaginated area.

and foam cells (Figure 3(d) arrow heads) in the invagination area. The swelling appendix did not have any inflamed mucosa, however, it showed serosal marked inflammation with hemorrhage, which was associated with ileal diverticulitis. He was discharged 12 days after the surgery without any complication. Two months after the surgery, colonoscopy was performed that showed no finding suggesting inflammatory bowel disease or other diseases.

3. Discussion

We present a case of diverticulitis in the terminal ileum which was flare-up of inflammation in 38 days after conservative therapy and needed surgical treatment. Diverticulitis in the terminal ileum is uncommon [8–10]. Diverticular disease is more common in the proximal jejunum (75%), followed by the distal jejunum (20%) and the ileum (5%) [11]. As previous reports had showed that associated colonic diverticulosis is frequently found in the patients with small bowel diverticulosis [12, 13], the present patient also developed coexistent diverticula in the ascending colon. The present patient was not elderly, but most patients were in the sixth and seventh decade of life in the previous reports [14–17]. Barton et al. [18] reported a patient with familial jejunoileal diverticulitis, but the present patient does not have familial history of diverticulitis in the small intestine. Although the etiology of

small bowel diverticula has been unknown, this condition is believed to develop from a combination of intestinal motility disorders, focal weakness of the muscle, and high segmental intraluminal pressure [6, 19]. The majority of small bowel diverticula are asymptomatic, but a wide range of less common complications has been reported, including abscess formation, chronic abdominal pain, malabsorption, anemia, volvulus, biliary tract disease, and enterolith formation [20]. Compared with duodenal diverticula, small bowel diverticula were nearly 4 times more likely to develop complications and nearly 18 times more likely to perforate and develop abscesses [20]. Several reports suggested that conservative management may be feasible to treat terminal ileum diverticulitis without perforation [21–23]; however there is no consensus on the therapeutic strategy of the symptomatic small bowel diverticulitis. In the previous reports, small bowel diverticula have a risk of perforation [4, 16, 24, 25]. Surgical intervention might be one option for diverticulitis without perforation. To prevent development of acute diverticulitis, high-fiber diet is commonly recommended to optimize their bowel movement for the patients with colon diverticulosis [26–28]. But recent studies have not supported recommendation of high-fiber diet [29, 30]. The patient does not have an unbalanced diet but has average Japanese dietary habits.

In conclusion, we present a case of diverticulitis in the terminal ileum in a healthy middle-aged man which was flare-up of inflammation in short interval after conservative therapy and needed surgical intervention. We should follow up with the patients cautiously who finished conservative therapy for diverticulitis without perforation in the terminal ileum not to overlook the flare-up diverticulitis. Surgical treatment might be considered as a potential treatment option to manage the small bowel diverticulitis.

Competing Interests

The authors declare that they have no competing interests.

References

[1] R. D. Wilcox and C. H. Shatney, "Surgical implications of jejunal diverticula," *Southern Medical Journal*, vol. 81, no. 11, pp. 1386–1391, 1988.

[2] J. S. Zager, J. E. Garbus, J. P. Shaw, M. G. Cohen, and S. M. Garber, "Jejunal diverticulosis: a rare entity with multiple presentations, a series of cases," *Digestive Surgery*, vol. 17, no. 6, pp. 643–645, 2000.

[3] S. C. Cunningham, C. J. Gannon, and L. M. Napolitano, "Small-bowel diverticulosis," *American Journal of Surgery*, vol. 190, no. 1, pp. 37–38, 2005.

[4] I. Kirbaş, E. Yildirim, A. Harman, and Ö. Başaran, "Perforated ileal diverticulitis: CT findings," *Diagnostic and Interventional Radiology*, vol. 13, no. 4, pp. 188–189, 2007.

[5] L. Graña, I. Pedraja, R. Mendez, and R. Rodríguez, "Jejuno-ileal diverticulitis with localized perforation: CT and US findings," *European Journal of Radiology*, vol. 71, no. 2, pp. 318–323, 2009.

[6] R. Kassir, A. Boueil-Bourlier, S. Baccot et al., "Jejuno-ileal diverticulitis: etiopathogenicity, diagnosis and management," *International Journal of Surgery Case Reports*, vol. 10, pp. 151–153, 2015.

[7] N. Tenreiro, H. Moreira, S. Silva et al., "Jejunoileal diverticulosis, a rare cause of ileal perforation—case report," *Annals of Medicine and Surgery*, vol. 6, pp. 56–59, 2016.

[8] K. Ietsugu, H. Nakashima, M. Kosugi, T. Misaki, K. Kakuda, and S. Terahata, "Multiple ileal diverticula causing an ileovesical fistula: report of a case," *Surgery Today*, vol. 32, no. 10, pp. 916–918, 2002.

[9] A. Matsumoto, O. Saitoh, H. Matsumoto et al., "Acquired ileal diverticulum: an unusual bleeding source," *Journal of Gastroenterology*, vol. 35, no. 2, pp. 163–167, 2000.

[10] S. G. Parulekar, "Diverticulosis of the terminal ileum and its complications," *Radiology*, vol. 103, no. 2, pp. 283–287, 1972.

[11] C.-Y. Liu, W.-H. Chang, S.-C. Lin, C.-H. Chu, T.-E. Wang, and S.-C. Shih, "Analysis of clinical manifestations of symptomatic acquired jejunoileal diverticular disease," *World Journal of Gastroenterology*, vol. 11, no. 35, pp. 5557–5560, 2005.

[12] S. B. Palder and C. B. Frey, "Jejunal diverticulosis," *Archives of Surgery*, vol. 123, no. 7, pp. 889–894, 1988.

[13] K. Makris, G. G. Tsiotos, V. Stafyla, and G. H. Sakorafas, "Small intestinal nonmeckelian diverticulosis," *Journal of Clinical Gastroenterology*, vol. 43, no. 3, pp. 201–207, 2009.

[14] E. de Bree, J. Grammatikakis, M. Christodoulakis, and D. Tsiftsis, "The clinical significance of acquired jejunoileal diverticula," *The American Journal of Gastroenterology*, vol. 93, no. 12, pp. 2523–2528, 1998.

[15] G. Gayer, R. Zissin, S. Apter, E. Shemesh, and E. Heldenberg, "Acute diverticulitis of the small bowel: CT findings," *Abdominal Imaging*, vol. 24, no. 5, pp. 452–455, 1999.

[16] B. Coulier, P. Maldague, A. Bourgeois, and B. Broze, "Diverticulitis of the small bowel: CT diagnosis," *Abdominal Imaging*, vol. 32, no. 2, pp. 228–233, 2007.

[17] W. Staszewicz, M. Christodoulou, S. Proietti, and N. Demartines, "Acute ulcerative jejunal diverticulitis: case report of an uncommon entity," *World Journal of Gastroenterology*, vol. 14, no. 40, pp. 6265–6267, 2008.

[18] J. S. Barton, A. B. Karmur, J. F. Preston, and B. C. Sheppard, "Familial jejuno-ileal diverticulitis: a case report and review of the literature," *International Journal of Surgery Case Reports*, vol. 5, no. 12, pp. 1038–1040, 2014.

[19] K. R. Kongara and E. E. Soffer, "Intestinal motility in small bowel diverticulosis: a case report and review of the literature," *Journal of Clinical Gastroenterology*, vol. 30, no. 1, pp. 84–86, 2000.

[20] R. Akhrass, M. B. Yaffe, C. Fischer, J. Ponsky, and J. M. Shuck, "Small-bowel diverticulosis: perceptions and reality," *Journal of the American College of Surgeons*, vol. 184, no. 4, pp. 383–388, 1997.

[21] H.-C. Park and B. H. Lee, "The management of terminal ileum diverticulitis," *The American Surgeon*, vol. 75, no. 12, pp. 1199–1202, 2009.

[22] M. Veen, B. J. Hornstra, C. H. M. Clemens, H. Stigter, and R. Vree, "Small bowel diverticulitis as a cause of acute abdomen," *European Journal of Gastroenterology and Hepatology*, vol. 21, no. 1, pp. 123–125, 2009.

[23] N. Fidan, E. U. Mermi, M. B. Acay, M. Murat, and E. Zobaci, "Jejunal diverticulosis presented with acute abdomen and diverticulitis complication: a case report," *Polish Journal of Radiology*, vol. 80, no. 1, pp. 532–535, 2015.

[24] S. Greenstein, B. Jones, E. K. Fishman, J. L. Cameron, and S. S. Siegelman, "Small-bowel diverticulitis: CT findings," *American Journal of Roentgenology*, vol. 147, no. 2, pp. 271–274, 1986.

[25] A. D. Kelekis and P. A. Poletti, "Jejunal diverticulitis with localized perforation diagnosed by ultrasound: a case report," *European Radiology*, vol. 12, supplement 3, pp. S78–S81, 2002.

[26] L. Köhler, S. Sauerland, and E. Neugebauer, "Diagnosis and treatment of diverticular disease: results of a consensus development conference. The Scientific Committee of the European Association for Endoscopic Surgery," *Surgical Endoscopy*, vol. 13, no. 4, pp. 430–436, 1999.

[27] N. H. Stollman and J. B. Raskin, "Diagnosis and management of diverticular disease of the colon in adults. Ad Hoc Practice Parameters Committee of the American College of Gastroenterology," *The American Journal of Gastroenterology*, vol. 94, no. 11, pp. 3110–3121, 1999.

[28] W. Kruis, C.-T. Germer, and L. Leifeld, "Diverticular disease: guidelines of the German society for gastroenterology, digestive and metabolic diseases and the German society for general and visceral surgery," *Digestion*, vol. 90, no. 3, pp. 190–207, 2014.

[29] F. L. Crowe, P. N. Appleby, N. E. Allen, and T. J. Key, "Diet and risk of diverticular disease in Oxford cohort of European Prospective Investigation into Cancer and Nutrition (EPIC): prospective study of British vegetarians and non-vegetarians," *BMJ*, vol. 343, Article ID d4131, 2011.

[30] A. F. Peery, P. R. Barrett, D. Park et al., "A high-fiber diet does not protect against asymptomatic diverticulosis," *Gastroenterology*, vol. 142, no. 2, pp. 266.e1–272.e1, 2012.

57

Successful Outcome and Biliary Drainage in an Infant with Concurrent Alpha-1-Antitrypsin Deficiency and Biliary Atresia

Andrew W. Wang,[1] Kimberly Newton,[2,3] and Karen Kling[4,5]

[1]*Department of Surgery, Naval Medical Center San Diego, San Diego, CA 92134, USA*
[2]*Division of Pediatric Gastroenterology, Hepatology, and Nutrition, Rady Children's Hospital, San Diego, CA 92123, USA*
[3]*Department of Pediatrics, School of Medicine, University of California, La Jolla, San Diego, CA 92093, USA*
[4]*Department of Surgery, School of Medicine, University of California San Diego, La Jolla, San Diego, CA 92093, USA*
[5]*Division of Pediatric Surgery, Rady Children's Hospital, San Diego, CA 92123, USA*

Correspondence should be addressed to Andrew W. Wang; wanga53@gmail.com

Academic Editor: Gabriel Sandblom

We describe the rare instance of concomitant biliary atresia and alpha-1-antitrypsin deficiency and the first documented successful portoenterostomy in this scenario. The potential for dual pathology must be recognized and underscores that prompt diagnosis of biliary atresia, despite concomitant alpha-1-antitrypsin deficiency, is essential to afford potential longstanding native liver function.

1. Introduction

For infants presenting with direct (conjugated) hyperbilirubinemia, the differential diagnosis remains vast, encompassing a wide array of medical and surgical liver diseases. As such, multiple serologic, radiologic, and histologic tests are employed simultaneously to make the correct diagnosis. Biliary atresia (BA) is diagnosed in approximately 1 in 19,000 live births [1]; it is the second most common underlying diagnosis in infants with liver disease [2] and is the most common indication for liver transplantation in the pediatric population [3]. In the case of BA, timely diagnosis and surgical intervention are critical to optimize liver function and overall outcome. When BA is suspected based on the overall clinical picture, an intraoperative cholangiogram is performed followed by corrective portoenterostomy (Kasai procedure) once the diagnosis is confirmed. There is urgency in making the diagnosis because delay in surgical treatment is associated with progression to liver failure. In contrast, alpha-1-antitrypsin deficiency (A1AT) can be seen more frequently in up to 1 in 1500 people [4], and its hepatic manifestations can present as cholestasis in the newborn period with a virtually overlapping clinical profile as that of biliary atresia. However,

its management does not involve urgent surgical reconstruction as in BA. Abnormal folding of the A1AT Z (or S) mutant protein leads to intracellular accumulation which leads to degradation mechanisms thought to trigger cellular injury and apoptosis [5], and treatment is supportive. We describe a patient who presented with both A1AT and BA in whom the diagnosis of BA was simultaneously made early enough to perform corrective portoenterostomy before progression of liver damage.

2. Case Report

An 11-day-old male infant presented for evaluation of direct (conjugated) hyperbilirubinemia. His prenatal studies were unremarkable; he was born at 38 weeks' gestation via Cesarean section due to breech presentation. The immediate postnatal course was pertinent for neonatal jaundice. A follow-up evaluation of serum bilirubin revealed a transition towards direct (conjugated) hyperbilirubinemia prompting referral to the gastroenterologist for further evaluation. The baby's parents noted his stools had become pale. His physical exam was remarkable for jaundice and hepatomegaly. Serum bilirubin was 4.7 mg/dL with a direct fraction of 3.2 mg/dL,

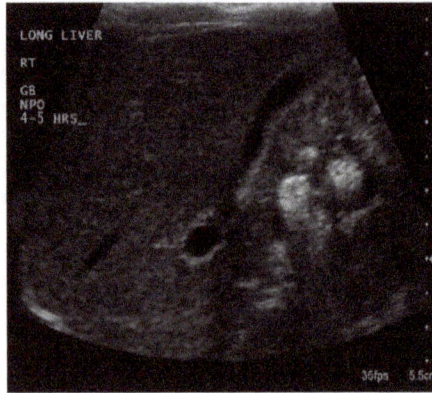

FIGURE 1: Abdominal ultrasound demonstrating a present gallbladder.

and gamma glutamyl transferase was elevated to 600 U/L. Hematologic and coagulation studies were normal. Laboratory evaluation for metabolic causes of jaundice, including alpha-1-antitrypsin deficiency, cystic fibrosis, viral hepatitis, and glycogen storage disease, was performed, and while awaiting these results, an evaluation for BA and other surgical causes of conjugated hyperbilirubinemia was concurrently initiated. An abdominal ultrasound had no evidence of choledochal cyst and demonstrated the presence of a gallbladder but was equivocal for presence of the common bile duct (Figure 1). However, presence or absence of bile ducts on US does not provide conclusive evidence of BA as ductal structures seen on US may represent obliterated remnants of the biliary tree. A hepatobiliary iminodiacetic acid (HIDA) scan was performed to assess for biliary patency, and this failed to demonstrate excretion of the radioactive tracer into the duodenum (Figure 2). Percutaneous liver biopsy could not be obtained due to technical limitations.

Given this convincing clinical picture specifically in conjunction with an abnormal HIDA scan, at 3 weeks of age, the patient underwent cholangiogram to evaluate for BA. Intraoperatively, only a hydropic gallbladder was identified consistent with nonpatency of at least part of the biliary tree. Although the subsequent cholangiogram demonstrated both the cystic and common bile ducts, the hepatic ducts were absent, suggesting that this proximal component of the biliary tree was atretic. Even with distal occlusion of the common bile duct and application of a significant amount of pressure instilling contrast in an attempt to distend and visualize a potentially small common hepatic duct, none was seen proving obstruction of the proximal biliary tree. While this is not the most typical finding associated with BA, patency of the gallbladder, cystic duct, and common bile duct with fibrosis of the hepatic ducts and porta can be seen [6]. While parts of the biliary system were patent, communication between the porta hepatitis and duodenum was absent consistent with BA; furthermore, dissection revealed the characteristic fibrosis of the hilar plate associated with BA. Thus, with a confirmed diagnosis of BA, portoenterostomy was performed without complication. Interestingly, during the Kasai reconstruction, the results of the serum alpha-1-antitrypsin analysis returned at 36 mg/dL, positive

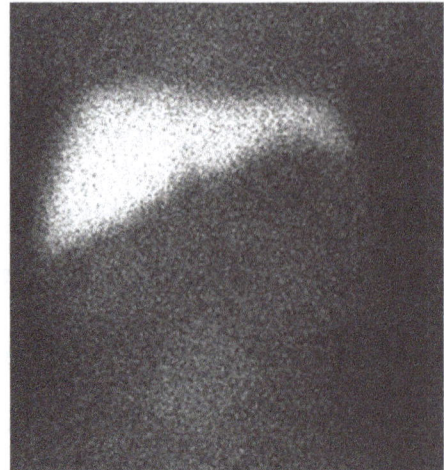

FIGURE 2: HIDA scan without excretion into the intestine.

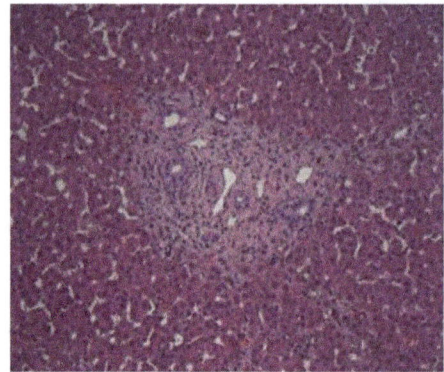

FIGURE 3: Intraoperative biopsy demonstrating bile duct proliferation.

for alpha-1-antitrypsin disease. Liver biopsy routinely obtained intraoperatively ultimately confirmed both diagnoses. Histopathology demonstrated bile duct proliferation (Figure 3), cholestasis (Figure 4), chronic inflammation, and periportal fibrosis without bridging, consistent with the diagnosis of BA; additionally, hepatocytes with PAS-positive, diastase-resistant globules (Figure 5) were seen supporting the additional diagnosis of A1AT. Subsequent genotypic evaluation showed the PiZZ mutation, the most severe form of the disease. The patient recovered well postoperatively, and successful biliary drainage was achieved with his bilirubin and transaminases normalizing.

Over the next several years, the patient has continued to do well. Between 1 and 2 years of age, he had 3 very mild episodes of cholangitis which all resolved with antibiotics. The patient has not had any additional hospitalizations for cholangitis since that time and is now 8 years old. He has normal growth, near-normal liver function tests, and normal bilirubin, with normal coagulation and hematological parameters (direct bilirubin 0.1 mg/dL, AST 35 U/L, ALT 55 U/L, GGT 40 U/L, PTT 34, PT 11.7, PLT 310, and WBC 7.9). A recent abdominal ultrasound was unremarkable with normal hepatic echogenicity, without intrahepatic ductal dilatation, with normal spleen size, and with normal portal

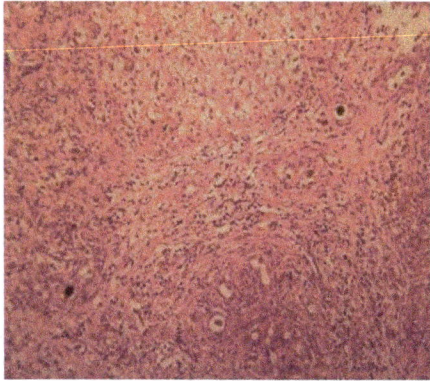

FIGURE 4: Intraoperative biopsy showing cholestasis and bile duct plugging.

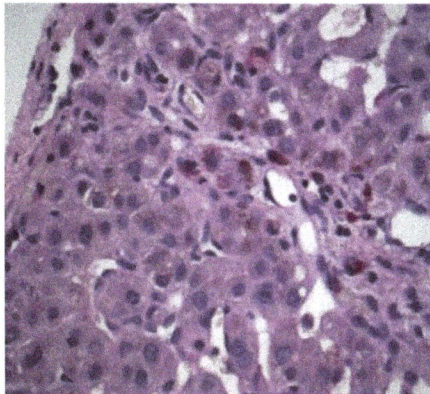

FIGURE 5: Intraoperative biopsy, hepatocytes with PAS-positive, diastase-resistant globules.

vein flow. An EGD performed in June 2016 was normal without evidence of varices. The patient is evaluated at regular intervals by pediatric hepatology and pulmonology. To date, there are no clinical signs of portal hypertension or lung disease.

3. Discussion

We present a patient with a dual diagnosis of A1AT and BA who was treated with a timely Kasai portoenterostomy with excellent outcome and 8-year survival to date with his native liver. Long-term prognosis for patients with A1AT deficiency who present with evidence of liver disease in infancy is reasonably favorable with approximately 80% manifesting no clinical evidence of chronic liver disease when followed into early adulthood [7]. In contrast, BA requires timely diagnosis and surgical treatment to achieve biliary drainage and prevent or delay progressive biliary disease. Currently, when appropriately identified and treated, biliary drainage is achieved in approximately 60% of cases leading to acceptable long term survival as part of a multimodality approach to management including the eventual need for liver transplantation [8]. Delayed diagnosis of BA can lead to progressive cirrhosis necessitating primary liver transplantation [9]. The importance of prompt investigation of

direct (conjugated) hyperbilirubinemia in infants presenting with acholic stools cannot be overemphasized.

Determining the underlying diagnosis in an infant with neonatal cholestasis can be challenging from both a clinical and a histopathological perspective. Biopsy results are not always straightforward as there can be substantial overlap among multiple hepatic diseases. Bile duct proliferation with plugging and fibrosis is characteristic of biliary atresia, but small-gauge percutaneous biopsies in infants may provide suboptimal tissue and insufficient portal tracts for adequate evaluation. At times, fibrosis and cholestasis without definitive evidence of proliferation and plugging is all that can be definitively demonstrated. Other diagnoses such as Alagille disease usually demonstrate bile duct paucity; however, this may not be apparent in very young infants. In A1AT, the characteristic PAS-positive globules can often be absent in very young infants leaving only nonspecific features of mild portal inflammation and fibrosis making definitive diagnosis elusive. Multiple diagnoses explaining neonatal cholestasis can have overlapping pathologic findings. A scenario lacking definitive diagnosis mandates cholangiogram to evaluate for biliary atresia and allow for timely surgical intervention if necessary. However, if a secure histopathologic diagnosis is established other than biliary atresia, such as A1AT, the workup usually ceases and treatment based on that diagnosis is begun. Biopsy in our case, if done preoperatively, most likely would have demonstrated PAS-positive, diastase-resistant globules and may or may not have demonstrated features of biliary atresia depending upon sample adequacy. Had the diagnosis of A1AT been made in the absence of convincing evidence of biliary obstruction, there would have likely been significant delay or complete failure to perform a cholangiogram and portoenterostomy, thereby resulting in increased liver damage and decreased or absent potential for biliary drainage. Although our usual practice is to obtain biopsy preoperatively, serendipitously, the inability to obtain biopsy, in this case, did not present us with a diagnosis of A1AT and therefore did not distract from prompt cholangiogram and portoenterostomy. Specifically, having considered other common confounding medical diagnoses (such as viral hepatitis, cystic fibrosis, TORCH infections, thyroid disease, pituitary issues, metabolic causes, cholesterol abnormalities, and bile acid diseases), given the time-sensitive nature of outcomes after portoenterostomy, we did not delay in obtaining cholangiogram. The cholangiogram did prove diagnostic of BA and made possible early portoenterostomy likely contributing to the good outcome for this patient. This underscores the importance of cholangiogram in determining the correct diagnosis and affording timely surgical reconstruction when appropriate.

Given the overlap among histopathologic findings in biliary atresia and other entities [10], this case illustrates that with sufficient clinical suspicion (as in our case of an infant with acholic stools, direct (conjugated) hyperbilirubinemia, and suggestive HIDA scan), despite other presumed diagnoses, cholangiogram, the gold standard for evaluation of biliary atresia, should still be pursued to definitively rule out BA. A HIDA scan without excretion despite a biopsy suggesting concomitant diagnoses such as A1AT or nonspecific neonatal giant cell hepatitis may still warrant cholangiogram. While operative cholangiogram does subject infants to anesthetic risks as well as a surgical scar, the operative morbidity is low. These risks must also be weighed in the context of potentially avoiding the lifelong morbidity of a missed diagnosis of BA and the missed opportunity for portoenterostomy. Additionally, in centers with the available resources and expertise, alternative techniques to operative cholangiography are becoming feasible including endoscopic retrograde cholangiopancreatography (ERCP) and percutaneous transhepatic cholecystocholangiography (PTC). These have been demonstrated to be useful and safe diagnostic alternatives to an open operative approach [10], potentially sparing some patients open operative procedures and a surgical scar. Endoscopic and percutaneous techniques may obviate operation for those in whom a patent ductal system can be demonstrated and may make cholangiography more palatable. These modalities were not available at our institution at the time of the evaluation of this infant. Ultimately, inability to complete a minimally invasive cholangiogram necessitates operative cholangiography.

More interestingly, this case report confirms that multiple etiologies can contribute to hepatic dysfunction; our patient had both A1AT and BA, and identifying the underlying diagnosis was essential in optimal management. This dual diagnosis is a very rare phenomenon; patients with BA almost universally have biopsy performed during their evaluation, yet there are only sparse case reports of synchronous A1AT and BA in the literature. Nord et al. and Tolaymat et al. previously report separate cases of patients found to have concomitant diagnoses of A1AT and BA. However, successful biliary drainage in this situation has not been reported to date and could not be achieved in either aforementioned patient; one patient underwent liver transplantation [11], and the other was being evaluated for future liver transplantation [12] by 9 months of age. Operative cholangiogram in patients known to have A1AT deficiency is not typically performed as the cholestasis associated with isolated A1AT is not mechanical. This is supported by a previous study of 11 patients with isolated A1AT deficiency evaluated with cholangiography that revealed normal extrahepatic biliary anatomy [13]. In isolated A1AT deficiency, this is a reasonable approach as the associated hepatic disease has an overall good prognosis. However, our case illustrates that there may exist concurrent diagnoses of BA and A1AT. The A1AT genotype in an infant may not yet be phenotypically expressed and may not therefore be the driving factor for the cholestatic picture; BA, as evidenced in this case, may be the predominant culprit. Thus, rarely, A1AT does not exclude BA, and securing the diagnosis of A1AT without ruling out BA may not be sufficient. This potential for synchronous diagnoses is an essential clinical situation to entertain because we demonstrate that Kasai portoenterostomy has the ability to preserve native liver in patients with this set of dual diagnoses.

4. Conclusions

We describe the very rare case of a patient who presented with both A1AT and BA and the first documented good outcome in the literature. He was successfully treated with Kasai portoenterostomy and currently survives with his native liver in situ and essentially normal liver function at age 8. This favorable outcome was achieved through early recognition of hyperbilirubinemia by the pediatrician accompanied by persistence to fully evaluate for BA. This was enhanced by the serendipity that evidence of a concurrent alpha-1-antitrypsin deficiency did not delay timely surgical cholangiography and biliary reconstruction. Our aim is not to suggest that one should abandon consideration of medical causes for hyperbilirubinemia or that all conjugated hyperbilirubinemia needs a cholangiogram, but rather to emphasize that all data must be considered and applied in the clinical context. Medical and surgical evaluations in these cases frequently proceed in a "shotgun" fashion due to the urgency of diagnosis; cholestasis should not be too quickly attributed to A1AT (a largely benign cause of cholestasis in infancy), when some elements of the workup suggest that biliary atresia (a more aggressive disease) may still be in play. This report illustrates that rarely dual diagnoses may exist. Despite what appears to be a nonsurgical diagnosis for hyperbilirubinemia, when the clinical scenario and HIDA scan do not completely rule out a diagnosis of BA, cholangiography should be pursued early enough that reconstruction can still effect a benefit. This is especially true as the recent advent of less invasive cholangiography techniques may alleviate some of the concern regarding committing an infant to open cholangiogram with a result negative for mechanical obstruction. A missed diagnosis of BA is a missed opportunity to surgically intervene and afford potential longstanding native liver function; this results in profoundly negative clinical consequences.

References

[1] R. A. Schreiber, C. C. Barker, E. A. Roberts et al., "Biliary atresia: the Canadian experience," *Journal of Pediatrics*, vol. 151, no. 6, pp. 659–665, 2007.

[2] K. M. Emerick and P. F. Whitington, "Neonatal liver disease," *Pediatric Annals*, vol. 35, no. 4, pp. 280–286, 2006.

[3] B. H. Saggi, D. G. Farmer, and R. W. Busuttil, "Liver Transplantation," in *Pediatric Surgery*, A. G. Coran, N. S. Adzick, A. A. Caldamone, T. M. Krummel, and R. C. S. Jean-Martin Laberge, Eds., pp. 643–652, Elsevier, Philadelphia, PA, USA, 7th edition, 2012.

[4] Genetics Home Reference, "Alpha-1 antitrypsin deficiency," pp. 1–8, 2017, https://ghr.nlm.nih.gov/condition/alpha-1-antitrypsin-deficiency.

[5] J. H. Teckman, "Liver disease in alpha-1 antitrypsin deficiency: current understanding and future therapy," *Journal of Chronic Obstructive Pulmonary Disease*, vol. 10, no. 1, pp. 35–43, 2013.

[6] R. P. Altman, J. R. Ully, J. Greenfeld, A. Weinberg, K. van Leeuwen, and L. Flanigan, "A multivariable risk factor analysis of the portoenterostomy (Kasai) procedure for biliary atresia twenty-five years of experience from two centers," *Annals of Surgery*, vol. 226, no. 3, pp. 348–355, 1997.

[7] T. Sveger and S. Eriksson, "The liver in adolescents with alpha 1-antitrypsin deficiency," *Hepatology*, vol. 22, no. 2, pp. 514–517, 1995.

[8] B. Lakshminarayanan and M. Davenport, "Biliary atresia: a comprehensive review," *Journal of Autoimmunity*, vol. 73, pp. 1–9, 2016.

[9] P. Wang, P. Xun, K. He, and W. Cai, "Comparison of liver transplantation outcomes in biliary atresia patients with and without prior portoenterostomy: a meta-analysis," *Digestive and Liver Disease*, vol. 48, no. 4, pp. 347–352, 2016.

[10] M. K. Jensen, V. F. Biank, D. C. Moe et al., "HIDA, percutaneous transhepatic cholecysto-cholangiography and liver biopsy in infants with persistent jaundice: can a combination of PTCC and liver biopsy reduce unnecessary laparotomy?," *Pediatric Radiology*, vol. 42, no. 1, pp. 32–39, 2012.

[11] K. S. Nord, S. Saad, V. V. Joshi, and L. C. McLoughlin, "Concurrence of alpha 1-antitrypsin deficiency and biliary atresia," *Journal of Pediatrics*, vol. 111, no. 3, pp. 416–418, 1987.

[12] N. Tolaymat, R. Figueroa-Colon, and F. A. Metros, "Alpha 1-antitrypsin deficiency (Pi SZ) and biliary atresia," *Journal of Pediatric Gastroenterology and Nutrition*, vol. 9, no. 2, pp. 256–269, 1989.

[13] G. Nebbia, M. Hadchouel, M. Odievre, and D. Alagille, "Early assessment of evolution of liver disease associated with alpha 1-antitrypsin deficiency in childhood," *Journal of Pediatrics*, vol. 102, no. 5, pp. 661–665, 1983.

58

The Close Relationship between Large Bowel and Heart: When a Colonic Perforation Mimics an Acute Myocardial Infarction

Maria Francesca Secchi,[1] **Carlo Torre,**[2] **Giovanni Dui,**[3] **Francesco Virdis,**[4] **and Mauro Podda** (iD)[5]

[1]*Department of Emergency and Acute Care Medicine, San Francesco Hospital, Nuoro, Italy*
[2]*Department of Gastrointestinal Endoscopy, San Francesco Hospital, Nuoro, Italy*
[3]*Department of Radiology, San Francesco Hospital, Nuoro, Italy*
[4]*Department of Trauma and Emergency Surgery, King's College Hospital, London, UK*
[5]*Department of General, Emergency, and Robotic Surgery, San Francesco Hospital, Nuoro, Italy*

Correspondence should be addressed to Mauro Podda; mauropodda@ymail.com

Academic Editor: Boris Kirshtein

Colonoscopic perforation is a serious and potentially life-threatening complication of colonoscopy. Its incidence varies in frequency from 0.016% to 0.21% for diagnostic procedures, but may be seen in up to 5% of therapeutic colonoscopies. In case of extraperitoneal perforation, atypical signs and symptoms may develop. The aim of this report is to raise the awareness on the likelihood of rare clinical features of colonoscopic perforation. A 72-year-old male patient with a past medical history of myocardial infarction presented to the emergency department four hours after a screening colonoscopy with polypectomy, complaining of neck pain, retrosternal oppressive chest pain, dyspnea, and rhinolalia. Right chest wall and cervical subcutaneous emphysema, pneumomediastinum, pneumoretroperitoneum, and bilateral subdiaphragmatic free air were reported on the chest and abdominal X-rays. The patient was treated conservatively, with absolute bowel rest, total parental nutrition, and broad-spectrum intravenous antibiotics. Awareness of the potentially unusual clinical manifestations of retroperitoneal perforation following colonoscopy is crucial for the correct diagnosis and prompt management of colonoscopic perforation. Conservative treatment may be appropriate in patients with a properly prepared bowel, hemodynamic stability, and no evidence of peritonitis. Surgical treatment should be considered when abdominal or chest pain worsens, and when a systemic inflammatory response arises during the conservative treatment period.

1. Introduction

Colonoscopy has become a standard tool for colorectal cancer screening worldwide. As endoscopists have gained increased experience performing the procedure, the incidence of colonoscopic complications shows a decreasing trend [1]. Overall morbidity following colonoscopy is 0.2% and 1.2% for diagnostic and therapeutic procedures, respectively [2].

In particular, colonoscopic perforation (CP) is one of the most serious and potentially life-threatening complications of colonoscopy.

CP is usually categorized into intraperitoneal, extraperitoneal, or intra- and extraperitoneal. Extraperitoneal CP is extremely rare. This occurs when the perforation site is located in the segments of the colonic wall which are attached to the extraperitoneal planes, such as the posterior walls of the ascending, descending sigmoid, rectosigmoid colon, and rectum [3].

In case of extraperitoneal perforation, atypical signs and symptoms, such as rhinolalia, pneumomediastinum, pneumoretroperitoneum, subcutaneous emphysema, dyspnea, and chest discomfort may develop [4, 5].

We present the clinical case of a patient admitted to the emergency department (ED) for cardiac-type chest pain, abdominal and thoracic subcutaneous emphysema, and rhinolalia, following operative colonoscopy and resection of a polypoid neoplasm of the cecum. The aim of this report is to raise the awareness on the likelihood of these rare clinical features of CP.

2. Case Presentation

A 72-year-old male patient presented to the emergency department (ED) complaining of neck pain, retrosternal oppressive chest pain, and progressive dyspnea, reporting also a change of the voice with rhinolalia. The patient's past medical history was significant for coronary heart disease. The patient was diagnosed with ST-elevation myocardial infarction (STEMI) in 2001, and non-ST-elevation myocardial infarction (NSTEMI) in 2006. A permanent pacemaker was positioned in 2009 for sinus node dysfunction.

In order to investigate iron deficiency anemia and a positive immunochemical fecal occult blood, the patient had undergone an outpatient screening colonoscopy four hours earlier.

The colonoscopy revealed three potential neoplastic lesions. The first one was a sessile polyp of 10 mm in diameter sited in the cecum, close to the ileocecal valve. It was removed with the diathermic loop, after infiltration of the mucosa with adrenaline.

A further two polyps were found in the ascending colon, both of about 7 mm in diameter.

As the cecal polyp exeresis was complicated by bleeding, a hemostatic clip was placed near the ileocecal valve. No obvious perforations were seen during the procedure (Figure 1), and no symptoms related to perforations, such as abdominal distension, abdominal and chest pain, or dyspnea were identified at the physical examination immediately after the procedure.

However, two hours after the completion of the procedure, the patient started complaining of abdominal, chest, and neck pain and shortness of breath.

Additional information was obtained from the endoscopist who performed the procedure. He mentioned extensive diverticular disease of the sigmoid colon and good mechanical preparation (Boston Bowel Preparation Scale: BBPS 2-3-3).

On ED arrival, the patient was apyretic. He had a blood pressure of 140/80 mmHg, a heart rate of 65 bpm, and an oxygen saturation on room air of 96%. The patient described the chest pain as a constriction, not radiated, and exacerbated by deep breaths.

The airway was intact and he was able to talk, although with rhinolalia. The abdomen was slightly distended and soft, although abdominal pain without signs of peritoneal irritation was located mainly on the right quadrants.

Subcutaneous emphysema, with a clear crepitus on palpation, was apparent on the neck, right anterior chest wall, and anterior and right lateral abdominal wall.

Due to the reported anamnesis of cardiovascular pathology, an electrocardiogram was performed. It showed a T wave inversion in the inferior and lateral leads, without any pacemaker activity (Figure 2). However, cardiac enzymes, as well as blood tests, inflammatory markers, and hemogas analysis were all unremarkable. Neck, chest, and

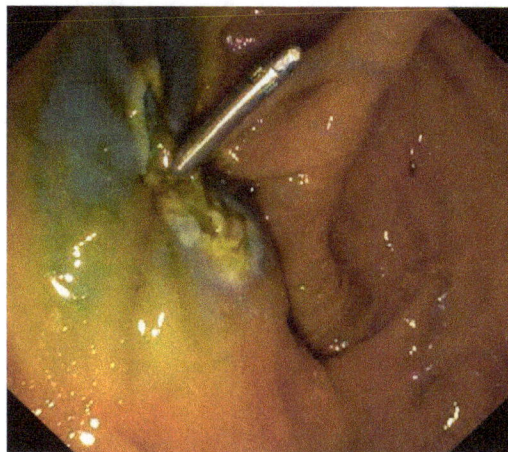

FIGURE 1: Colonoscopic finding. No definite perforation is seen. Hemostatic clipping and hot biopsy coagulation near the ileocecal valve were done.

abdominal X-rays were then requested to rule out the clinical suspicion of CP.

Right chest wall and cervical subcutaneous emphysema, pneumomediastinum, pneumoretroperitoneum, and bilateral subdiaphragmatic free air were reported on the chest and abdominal X-rays (Figure 3).

The abdominal and lower thorax contrast-enhanced computed tomography (CT) scan revealed pneumoperitoneum and pneumoretroperitoneum, mainly located at the epimesogastrium, at the right anterior and posterior pararenal and perihepatic spaces, as well as diverticulosis of the sigmoid colon (Figure 4). No questionable findings, such as an obvious intestinal perforation, peritoneal fluid, or radiological signs of peritonitis, were noted.

In view of the clinical and radiological findings, the patient's good general condition and hemodynamic stability, and the absence of peritoneal irritation and signs of inflammatory syndrome, the patient was admitted to the surgical department and treated conservatively, with absolute bowel rest, total parental nutrition, broad-spectrum intravenous antibiotics (ciprofloxacin 500 mg × 2 and metronidazole 500 mg × 3), and symptomatic care.

Vital signs on the day after the procedure included a blood pressure of 125/80 mmHg, a pulse rate of 75 bpm, a respiratory rate of 16 breaths/min, and a body temperature of 36.7°C. Follow-up chest and abdominal X-rays exhibited a resolving pneumomediastinum and pneumoretroperitoneum 48 hours after the admission. C-reactive protein was slightly raised to 0.86 mg/dl, without any other laboratory sign of inflammation. The patient's subcutaneous emphysema markedly resolved on the third postprocedure day.

Diet was started from water intake at the 5th day after the procedure, and oral antibiotics were administered instead of intravenous antibiotics. The patient recovered uneventfully and was discharged on the 12th day after admission.

The condition of the patient was observed in the outpatient clinic one week after his leaving the hospital, and was confirmed to be fully recovered without any further complications.

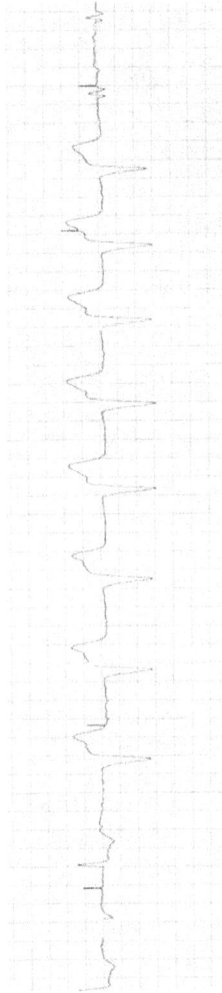

FIGURE 2: Electrocardiogram showing T wave inversion in the inferior and lateral leads.

3. Discussion

3.1. Epidemiology and Pathogenesis. The incidence of CP varies in frequency from 0.016% to 0.21% for diagnostic procedures, but may be seen in up to 5% of therapeutic colonoscopies [6, 7].

Many factors, related both to the patient (advanced age, diabetes, chronic pulmonary disease, myocardial infarction, cerebrovascular disease, congestive heart failure, renal insufficiency, peripheral vascular disease, diverticular disease, and previous abdominal surgery) and to the procedure itself (therapeutic colonoscopy with polypectomy, pneumatic dilatation, and endoscopic mucosal resection) may be related to the incidence of CP [8]. Convincing evidence shows that with polypectomies the risk of CP rises to 0.3–1%, and with hydrostatic balloon dilatation of colonic strictures, higher rates (4-5%) may be expected [9, 10].

CP may be caused by one of the following three mechanisms: (1) mechanical trauma by instrumentation, (2) barotrauma by excessive air inflation, and 3) thermal injury by electric current during colonoscopy [11].

The sigmoid colon is the most affected site of CP, followed in frequency by the rectum [12, 13].

Although the cecum and the ileocecal valve are rarely involved in perforations, the thin wall layer and the large lumen of the cecum make this colonic segment more vulnerable to injury by polypectomy, as reported in the present case [14].

Since the peritoneum, retroperitoneum, mediastinum, and thorax are anatomically connected, when perforation occurs, intraluminal compressed air may escape into either the peritoneum and the retroperitoneum. Once in the retroperitoneum, air may travel along the mesentery, large vessels, and through the diaphragmatic hiatus, and then further spread to the mediastinum and subcutaneous tissues [15]. Eventual rupture of the mediastinal pleura allows air to decompress into the pleural cavity and cause pneumothorax. Pneumothorax can also develop when the pneumoperitoneum extends to the intrapleural space through the diaphragmatic fenestrations [16].

In the present report, extraluminal air probably entered the body due to a cecal perforation following polypectomy, leading to an extremely rare combined pattern of intra- and extraperitoneal perforation.

3.2. Clinical Presentation. Key points from diagnosis to treatment of CP are summarized in Table 1.

The most common presenting symptom after CP is abdominal pain, although clinical manifestations may be variable according to the location, size, mechanism of the perforation, the extent of the soiling, and bowel preparation.

If the perforation site is in the retroperitoneum, peritoneal irritation signs may not be evident, resulting in unusual presentation, as in the current report. The review of the literature published by Cirt et al., found 24 reported cases of retroperitoneal CP with various clinical presentations. Among them, 14 cases were associated with polypectomies. Cases involving both intraperitoneal and extraperitoneal CP following colonoscopy were extremely rare, with only 11 such cases reported [10].

CP into the retroperitoneum can spread to the other areas, resulting in unusual clinical manifestations which offer important clues for early diagnosis. Voice changes, such as hoarseness and rhinolalia, have been reported as rare signs of CP, which may be caused by changes in the anatomy of the pharyngeal region due to the presence of emphysema [17, 18].

3.3. Diagnosis. To avoid any delay before the correct diagnosis, clinicians should suspect a CP if any patient recently submitted to colonoscopy develops subcutaneous emphysema, fever, and abdominal or chest pain. These clinical features should be kept in mind even if the patient presents the symptoms several days after the procedure [12, 13].

The recent review conducted by Tiwari et al. revealed that about 50% of CPs are detected immediately or within 1 hour, whereas 30% are found within 1–24 hours and 20% found after 24 hours from the procedure [16].

When CP is suspected, key diagnostics are chest and abdominal X-rays. These may demonstrate

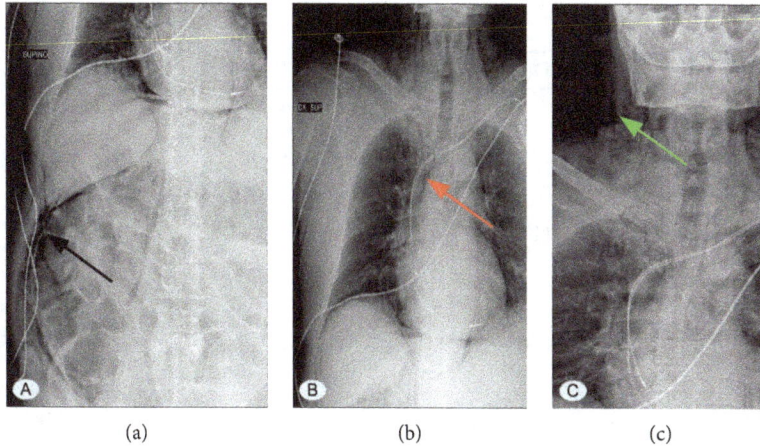

FIGURE 3: (a) Abdominal X-ray showing subcutaneous emphysema, pneumomediastinum, pneumoretroperitoneum, and right subdiaphragmatic free air (black arrow). (b) Chest X-ray showing pneumomediastinum (red arrow). (c) Neck X-ray showing right cervical subcutaneous emphysema (green arrow).

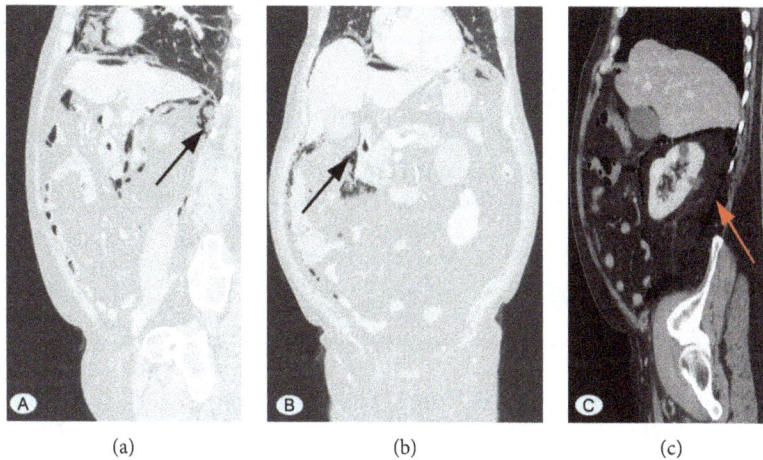

FIGURE 4: Abdominal CT scan showing pneumoperitoneum and pneumoretroperitoneum (a, b), mainly located at the epimesogastrium, at the right anterior and posterior pararenal and perihepatic spaces (c) (black arrows, red arrow).

pneumoperitoneum, pneumomediastinum, pneumoretroperitoneum, pneumothorax, and subcutaneous emphysema.

However, in cases of retroperitoneal perforation, free air might not be visible on plain X-rays. In such cases, CT scan, eventually with double contrast (intravenous and rectal) is a more effective diagnostic modality for detecting pneumoretroperitoneum [19, 20].

CT is also mandatory in those patients with CP who are eligible for conservative management because it can detect not only a small amount of free intra-abdominal gas but also the presence of free fluid and other typical features of peritonitis [21].

3.4. Treatment Strategies.
Historically, surgery with explorative laparotomy was the mainstay of treatment for the majority of patients. However, the likelihood of nonoperative treatment has increased. Conservative treatment should be reserved for patients in good general conditions, without any sign of generalized peritonitis, perforation unnoticed by the endoscopist, a good degree of bowel preparation, early detection of the CP, and no underlying disease requiring surgery [13, 21].

The conservative approach involves intravenous fluids, bowel rest, and intravenous administration of broad-spectrum antibiotics [10].

The overall success rate of a nonoperative treatment for CP ranges from 33% to 73%, and small perforations caused by therapeutic colonoscopy have been shown to have a better success rate with medical treatment [12].

Conversely, primary surgical management is recommended in patients with extensive peritoneal contamination, poor general condition, hemodynamic instability, and presence of concurrent colonic lesions which require surgery [22].

The type of surgical treatment should be tailored on a case-by-case basis. Simple closure with sutures may be appropriate in the case of small CP (<50% of bowel circumference), without significant fecal contamination and concomitant intestinal pathology requiring bowel resection [12].

Conversely, segmental bowel resection is required when the perforation is large, or when the primary closure of the

TABLE 1: Key points for early diagnosis and treatment of patients with CP.

Clinical features	Diagnostic workup	Treatment strategies

(1) Abdominal pain (diffuse or localized)
(2) Abdominal tenderness (diffuse or localized)
(3) Abdominal guarding (diffuse or localized)
(4) Ileus
(5) Chest pain
(6) Voice changes (hoarseness, rhinolalia)
(7) Subcutaneous emphysema (abdomen, chest, and neck)
(8) Fever (>38°C)
(9) Tachycardia (>100 beats/min)
(10) Tachypnea (>20 breaths/min)
(11) Oliguria (urine output <21 ml/h)
	(1) *Blood tests*
	  (i) Leukocytosis
	  (ii) Neutrophilia
	(2) *Inflammatory markers*
	  (i) High levels of C-reactive protein
	  (ii) High levels of procalcitonin
	(3) *Abdominal X-ray*
	  (i) Pneumoperitoneum
	  (ii) Pneumoretroperitoneum
	  (iii) Subcutaneous emphysema
	(4) *Chest X-ray*
	  (i) Pneumothorax
	  (ii) Pneumomediastinum
	  (iii) Subcutaneous emphysema
	(5) *Abdominal CT scan with oral and rectal contrast*
	  (i) Typical features of peritonitis
	  (ii) Free intra-abdominal gas
	  (iii) Free intra-abdominal fluid
	  (iv) Peritoneal and mesenteric thickening
		(1) *Conservative treatment (intravenous fluids, bowel rest, and intravenous administration of broad-spectrum antibiotics)*
		  (i) Patients in good general conditions
		  (ii) No signs of generalized peritonitis
		  (iii) Perforation unnoticed by the endoscopist
		  (iv) Good degree of bowel preparation
		  (v) Early detection of the CP
		  (vi) No underlying disease requiring surgery
		(2) *Surgery (simple closure with sutures)*
		  (i) Small CP < 50% of bowel circumference
		  (ii) No fecal contamination
		  (iii) No concomitant intestinal pathology requiring bowel resection
		(3) *Colonic resection (Hartmann's versus colectomy and primary anastomosis)*
		  (i) Depending on the grade of intra-abdominal contamination and the general condition of the patient
		(4) *Endoscopic clipping followed by conservative treatment*
		  (i) Early recognition of the CP
		  (ii) Small CP < 10 mm
		  (iii) No signs of peritonitis
		  (iv) Good bowel preparation

perforation could compromise the lumen, or when there is concomitant colorectal pathology (cancer, severe colonic stricture, and large sessile polyp) that requires bowel resection. The choice between bowel resection with primary anastomosis and Hartmann's procedure is related to the grade of intra-abdominal contamination, the timing of the diagnosis, and the general condition of the patient [12].

All patients under nonoperative treatment should be closely monitored. If conservative management is successful, the patient's clinical appearance should improve gradually within the first 48 hours, as reported also in our case [12]. Conversely, when pain worsens, or a systemic inflammatory response manifests with fever, tachycardia, tachypnea, and elevated inflammatory markers, complicated intra-abdominal infections (intra-abdominal abscesses or generalized fecal peritonitis) should be suspected, and thus further investigations and prompt surgical treatment should be considered [13].

Endoscopic clipping followed by conservative treatment has been recently reported and could be a valid approach in patients with small lesions and without signs of peritonitis [11]. In general, the size of the perforation suitable for endoscopic closure is less than 10 mm, but some reports showed successful endoscopic repairs of perforations larger than 10 mm [12]. A review of 75 cases of CP repaired by endoclipping, by Trecca et al. in 2008,

reported a success rate of 69%–93%. Early recognition of the CP, prompt complete endoscopic repair, and good bowel preparation are the keys to the success of endoscopic treatment for CP [23].

4. Conclusion

Awareness of the potentially unusual clinical manifestations of retroperitoneal perforation following colonoscopy is crucial for the correct diagnosis and prompt management of CP.

Treatment strategies for patients with CP should be patient-tailored, based on clinical presentation, patient's general condition, grade of colonic preparation, nature of perforation, and underlying colorectal pathologies.

Conservative treatment may be appropriate in patients with a properly prepared bowel, hemodynamic stability, and no evidence of peritonitis. However, prompt surgical treatment should be considered when abdominal or chest pain worsens, and when a systemic inflammatory response arises during the conservative treatment period.

Abbreviations

CP: Colonic perforation
ED: Emergency department
STEMI: ST-elevation myocardial infarction

NSTEMI: Non-ST-elevation myocardial infarction
CT: Computed tomography.

Authors' Contributions

Maria Francesca Secchi, Carlo Torre, and Mauro Podda contributed to the conception, design, drafting of the paper, and critical revision of the article for important intellectual content. Francesco Virdis contributed to the conception, drafting, and revision of the paper. Giovanni Dui contributed to the conception and revision of the paper. Maria Francesca Secchi and Mauro Podda did the literature review. All authors read and approved the final paper.

References

[1] V. Panteris, J. Haringsma, and E. J. Kuipers, "Colonoscopy perforation rate, mechanisms and outcome: from diagnostic to therapeutic colonoscopy," *Endoscopy*, vol. 41, no. 11, pp. 941–951, 2009.

[2] G. Dafnis, A. Ekbom, L. Pahlman, and P. Blomqvist, "Complications of diagnostic and therapeutic colonoscopy within a defined population in Sweden," *Gastrointestinal Endoscopy*, vol. 54, no. 3, pp. 302–309, 2001.

[3] H. C. Jung, H. J. Kim, S. B. Ji et al., "Pneumoretroperitoneum, pneumomediastinum, subcutaneous emphysema after a rectal endoscopic mucosal resection," *Annals of Coloproctology*, vol. 32, no. 6, pp. 234–238, 2016.

[4] R. Denadai, C. C. Medeiros, A. P. Toledo, A. F. Carvalho Jr., and C. A. S. Muraro, "Rectal perforation after colonoscopic polypectomy presented as subcutaneous emphysema, pneumomediastinum and pneumoretroperitoneum successfully treated conservatively in an elderly adult," *Journal of the American Geriatrics Society*, vol. 61, no. 8, pp. 1433–1435, 2013.

[5] M. Cappello, C. Randazzo, S. Peralta, and G. Cocorullo, "Subcutaneous emphysema, pneumomediastinum and pneumoperitoneum after diagnostic colonoscopy for ulcerative colitis: a rare but possible complication in patients with multiple risk factors," *International Journal of Colorectal Disease*, vol. 26, no. 3, pp. 393–394, 2011.

[6] A. Repici, R. Pellicano, G. Strangio, S. Danese, S. Fagoonee, and A. Malesci, "Endoscopic mucosal resection for early colorectal neoplasia: pathologic basis, procedures, and outcomes," *Diseases of the Colon and Rectum*, vol. 52, no. 8, pp. 1502–1515, 2009.

[7] H. H. Kim, J. H. Kim, S. J. Park, M. I. Park, and W. Moon, "Risk factors for incomplete resection and complications in endoscopic mucosal resection for lateral spreading tumors," *Digestive Endoscopy*, vol. 24, no. 4, pp. 259–266, 2012.

[8] M. La Torre, F. Velluti, G. Giuliani, E. Di Giulio, V. Ziparo, and F. La Torre, "Promptness of diagnosis is the main prognostic factor after colonoscopic perforation," *Colorectal Disease*, vol. 14, no. 1, pp. e23–c26, 2012.

[9] G. Arora, A. Mannalithara, G. Singh, L. B. Gerson, and G. Triadafilopoulos, "Risk of perforation from a colonoscopy in adults: a large population-based study," *Gastrointestinal Endoscopy*, vol. 69, no. 3, pp. 654–664, 2009.

[10] N. Cirt, A. S. D. Lajarte-Thirouard, D. Olivié, M. Pagenault, and J. F. Bretagne, "Subcutaneous emphysema, pneumomediastinum, pneumoperitoneum and retropneumoperitoneum following a colonoscopy with mucosectomy," *Gastroentérologie Clinique et Biologique*, vol. 30, no. 5, pp. 779–782, 2006.

[11] N. S. Park, J. H. Choi, D. H. Lee et al., "Pneumoretroperitoneum, pneumomediastinum, peumopericardium, and subcutaneous emphysema after colonoscopic examination," *Gut and Liver*, vol. 1, no. 1, pp. 079–081, 2007.

[12] V. Lohsiriwat, "Colonoscopic perforation: incidence, risk factors, management and outcome," *World Journal of Gastroenterology*, vol. 16, no. 4, pp. 425–430, 2010.

[13] D. Y. Won, I. K. Lee, Y. S. Lee et al., "The indications for nonsurgical management in patients with colorectal perforation after colonoscopy," *The American Surgeon*, vol. 78, no. 5, pp. 550–554, 2012.

[14] R. L. Foliente, A. C. Chang, A. I. Youssef, L. J. Ford, S. C. Condon, and Y. K. Chen, "Endoscopic cecal perforation: mechanisms of injury," *American Journal of Gastroenterology*, vol. 91, no. 4, pp. 705–708, 1996.

[15] C. G. Ball, A. W. Kirkpatrick, S. Mackenzie et al., "Tension pneumothorax secondary to colonic perforation during diagnostic colonoscopy: report of a case," *Surgery Today*, vol. 36, no. 5, pp. 478–480, 2006.

[16] A. Tiwari, H. Sharma, K. Qamar, T. Sodeman, and A. Nawras, "Recognition of extraperitoneal colonic perforation following colonoscopy: a review of the literature," *Case Reports in Gastroenterology*, vol. 11, no. 1, pp. 256–264, 2017.

[17] J. Kirk, E. D. Staren, J. Franklin, and T. J. Saclarides, "Voice changes: an initial manifestation of colonic perforation," *Gastrointestinal Endoscopy*, vol. 40, no. 1, p. 125, 1994.

[18] J. C. Kipple, "Bilateral tension pneumothoraces and subcutaneous emphysema following colonoscopic polypectomy: a case report and discussion of anesthesia considerations," *AANA Journal*, vol. 78, no. 6, pp. 462–467, 2010.

[19] A. Y. Teoh, C. M. Poon, J. F. Lee et al., "Outcomes and predictors of mortality and stoma formation in surgical management of colonoscopic perforations: a multicenter review," *Archives of Surgery*, vol. 144, no. 1, pp. 9–13, 2009.

[20] C. W. Iqbal, D. C. Cullinane, H. J. Schiller, M. D. Sawyer, S. P. Zietlow, and D. R. Farley, "Surgical management and outcomes of 165 colonoscopic perforations from a single institution," *Archives of Surgery*, vol. 143, no. 7, pp. 701–706, 2008.

[21] H. Y. Kang, H. W. Kang, S. G. Kim et al., "Incidence and management of colonoscopic perforations in Korea," *Digestion*, vol. 78, no. 4, pp. 218–223, 2008.

[22] C. M. Mai, C. C. Wen, S. H. Wen et al., "Iatrogenic colonic perforation by colonoscopy: a fatal complication for patients with a high anesthetic risk," *International Journal of Colorectal Disease*, vol. 25, no. 4, pp. 449–454, 2010.

[23] A. Trecca, F. Gaj, G. Gagliardi, K. Fu, and T. Fujii, "Our experience with endoscopic repair of large colonoscopic perforations and review of the literature," *Techniques in Coloproctology*, vol. 12, no. 4, pp. 315–322, 2008.

59

Necrotizing Fasciitis Resulting from an Anastomotic Leak after Colorectal Resection

Anthony Nagib,[1] **Chauniqua Kiffin,**[2] **Eddy H. Carrillo ⓘ,**[2] **Andrew A. Rosenthal ⓘ,**[2] **Rachele J. Solomon,**[3] **and Dafney L. Davare ⓘ**[2]

[1]*Nova Southeastern University, College of Osteopathic Medicine, 3301 College Avenue, Fort Lauderdale, FL 33314, USA*

[2]*Memorial Regional Hospital, Division of Acute Care Surgery and Trauma, 3501 Johnson Street, Hollywood, FL 33021, USA*

[3]*Memorial Regional Hospital, Office of Human Research, 4411 Sheridan Street, Hollywood, FL 33021, USA*

Correspondence should be addressed to Dafney L. Davare; ddavare@mhs.net

Academic Editor: Gregorio Santori

One of the most feared complications in colorectal surgery is an anastomotic leak (AL) following a colorectal resection. While various recommendations have been proposed to prevent this potentially fatal complication, anastomotic leaks still occur. We present a case of an AL resulting in a complicated and fatal outcome. This case demonstrates the importance of high clinical suspicion, early recognition, and immediate management.

1. Introduction

Colorectal anastomotic leaks (AL) are a common, yet serious complication of colorectal resections, with occurrence rates of 2–21% and mortality rates of 3–33% [1–6]. AL may have various clinical presentations throughout a patient's postoperative course. Due to its nonspecific presentation, few clinical criteria exist to define the development of an AL [2, 3, 7, 8]. Thus, a high index of suspicion and clinical judgment are paramount to the early recognition and prevention of fatal outcomes. We present a case of an AL with a unique presentation that occurred 8 years after a colorectal resection.

2. Case Presentation

A 76-year-old female presented to the emergency department with complaints of the left thigh and hip pain and swelling for five days. She reported having a history of chronic left leg sciatic pain that contributed to a fall two days prior to the onset of these symptoms. Her past medical history was significant for colon cancer requiring a low anterior resection, which is eight years ago. The patient was noted to be confused and tachycardic. She was afebrile but had

leukocytosis of 14,000. On physical examination, she was noted to have a significant crepitus to the left thigh and knee. Radiographs of the left leg confirmed subcutaneous emphysema consistent with necrotizing fasciitis (Figure 1). Prior to surgical consultation, the patient also received a pelvic computed tomography (CT) scan to evaluate for hip fractures. This further confirmed the necrotizing fasciitis (Figures 2(a) and 2(b)) but also identified a collection in the presacral space (Figure 3) that communicated to the left leg through the left sciatic notch, which is consistent with an AL. The patient was immediately taken to the operating room for debridement of the thigh and diverting colostomy.

An exploratory laparotomy with diverting colostomy was created to control ongoing contamination of the leg. Intra-abdominally, there were no abnormal findings, which is consistent with the extraperitoneal nature of the disease process. The decision, at this point, was to access the extraperitoneal collection through interventional radiology so as to minimize intra-abdominal contamination. After the colostomy was completed, the left thigh and hip were incised revealing a significant amount of feculent and purulent drainage. Necrotic, nonviable tissue was debrided down towards the knee, and the wound was left open and dressed. The patient was septic

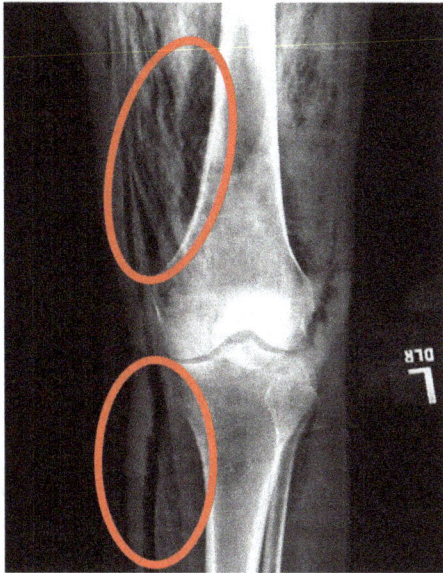

FIGURE 1: AP radiograph of the left lower extremity demonstrating subcutaneous emphysema (red ovals).

during the procedure and remained septic postoperatively. After an initial discussion with the patient's family, the plan was to perform percutaneous drainage of the presacral abscess postoperatively and obtain an orthopedic consultation as the hip joint was actively infected from the AL.

Recommendations by orthopedic and trauma consultants were that the patient would initially need an above the knee amputation due to the significant soft tissue loss and function from the extensive debridement. Furthermore, their concern was that this patient may ultimately need disarticulation of the left hip with potential hemipelvectomy if severe and recurrent osteomyelitis developed.

The patient's family ultimately decided to withdraw care, and the patient died in the hospital on day three.

3. Discussion

Colorectal anastomotic leaks have an incidence that varies from 2–30% [3, 4, 9]. The development of this complication leads to increased lengths of hospital stay, significant morbidity, and mortality rates of 6–32% [2, 4, 9]. There are several studies that have identified risk factors that contribute to the breakdown of a colorectal anastomosis. These include operative duration, male sex, diabetes, tobacco use, obesity, and immunosuppression [3, 9]. In addition, the type of anastomosis created can be a risk factor for its break down. For example, low anterior resections have been seen to have higher rates of anastomotic breakdown when compared to more proximal anastomoses [1, 6]. Some studies found that an anastomosis within 7 cm of the anal verge was an independent risk factor for AL [1, 8].

Presentation of ALs can vary in time of development and in symptomology. Anastomotic leaks can present as early as within the first postoperative week or as late as several years after the operation, as seen in our case. Early leaks, those presenting within 5 days of surgery, will present with nonspecific

findings of pain, fever, tachycardia, and leukocytosis. It is imperative to suspect and identify this complication as early as possible. The utilization of CT scan or water-soluble contrast enema can assist in determining the presence of an anastomotic breakdown and can guide the surgeon in appropriate management [2, 7]. Leaks that occur after 5 days can also present with nonspecific findings, with a wide range of signs and symptoms. Examples include low-grade fever, prolonged ileus, urinary symptoms, and diet intolerance. Utilization of the aforementioned diagnostic studies can guide management.

Timing of ALs can affect the presentation as well as the location of the anastomotic breakdown. Extraperitoneal leaks are less likely to present with a severe septic picture, when compared to intraperitoneal leaks. An extraperitoneal leak could have an insidious onset and therefore be discovered after harm has already occurred, as seen in our case [2]. On the other hand, an intraperitoneal leak usually presents earlier with a clinical picture of peritonitis and sepsis due to peritoneal contamination.

In this case, the location of the anastomotic breakdown leads to extraperitoneal drainage into the sciatic canal with subsequent contamination of the left lower extremity and necrotizing fasciitis. This is a very rare occurrence with limited research and case studies discussing this type of presentation. On exam, the patient painted a clinical picture of necrotizing fasciitis, which was thought to be related to a recent trauma. However, her history of chronic left-sided sciatica may have been an indication of a very small persistent leak that over time contributed to her overall presentation.

The management of ALs should begin before surgery. If possible, preoperative optimization should be considered; this includes smoking cessation, weight loss, and improving nutritional status. Intraoperatively, the meticulous surgical technique must be utilized to ensure that the anastomosis is free of tension and remains well-vascularized. Consideration of a proximal stoma should be entertained in complex surgical cases to protect the anastomosis. Evaluation of the anastomosis can also include the use of air-leak testing, which is a common intraoperative practice. This involves manual obstruction proximal to the anastomosis while the peritoneal cavity is filled with saline. The introduction of the proctoscope and colorectal insufflation of air should create bubbling in the presence of an anastomotic breakdown. Multiple studies have shown that air-leak testing decreases the rate of leaks due to early detection. In one study, 77% of anastomoses that tested positive on air-leak testing had a confirmed leak postoperatively [7].

Postoperative management of an AL can either be nonsurgical or surgical. Nonoperative management is utilized when the leak is a localized abscess. These events can be treated with percutaneous drainage and antibiotics. In the presence of sepsis and peritoneal contamination, abdominal reexploration is warranted with the creation of a proximal diverting stoma. The choice of operative management is done on a case-by-case basis with clinical judgment being the ultimate determining factor. Of note, simple suture repairs of an AL are often unsuccessful and have been shown to cause further disruption of the anastomotic breakdown [2].

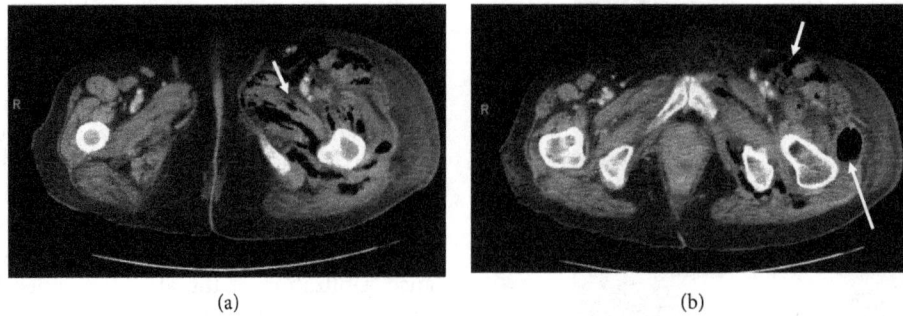

(a)   (b)

FIGURE 2: Axial CT images with IV contrast of the lower pelvis (a and b) demonstrating extensive subcutaneous emphysema consistent with necrotizing fasciitis around the left femur (short arrows). Note the air filled abscess cavity (b) filled along the posterior aspect of the left hip (long arrow).

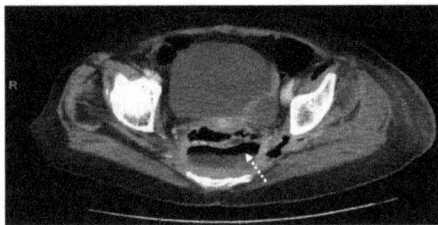

FIGURE 3: Axial CT images with IV contrast of the pelvis showing the extraperitoneal abscess (dotted arrow) derived from a previous colorectal anastomosis.

With the incidence of colorectal ALs as high as 30% in some studies, its recognition and management are of utmost importance [3, 4, 9]. Unfortunately, there is a paucity of literature providing clinicians with precise definitions and algorithms for recognizing and managing this potentially lethal complication. Computed tomography can be very helpful in both diagnosing and planning management of an AL. In this case, the utilization of CT imaging was very helpful in identifying the cause of this patient's presentation. However, under different circumstances, the patient may have undergone an emergent debridement without such imaging. The identification of stool drainage from the leg and the history of colorectal surgery should be a red flag for the anastomotic breakdown, prompting intervention.

4. Conclusion

This case highlights that ALs can occur at any time following colorectal surgery. In addition, this case demonstrates a unique presentation of an AL. In our patient, the presentation was 8 years after her original surgery. Furthermore, it is difficult to ascertain the cause for the delayed breakdown. The patient's age, nutritional status, and site of resection and anastomosis are potential contributing factors to this complication. It is important to consider an AL as a potential differential diagnosis in any patient with a history of colorectal surgery presenting with abdominal pain, fever, and leukocytosis.

ALs are a significant complication with severe consequences. In our case, it resulted in mortality due to delay in both presentation and diagnosis. Early identification and high clinical suspicion are critical to mitigating morbidity

and mortality. Furthermore, the clinician must keep this potentially lethal complication in mind, even in the patient with a remote history of colorectal surgery. In all, the most reliable way of preventing morbidity and mortality from AL is by having a high index of suspicion to ensure early detection, workup, and intervention.

References

[1] N. Damen, K. Spilsbury, M. Levitt et al., "Anastomotic leaks in colorectal surgery," *ANZ Journal of Surgery*, vol. 84, no. 10, pp. 763–768, 2014.

[2] R. G. Landmann, "Surgical management of anastomotic leak following colorectal surgery," *Seminars in Colon and Rectal Surgery*, vol. 25, no. 2, pp. 58–66, 2014.

[3] V. C. Nikolian, N. S. Kamdar, S. E. Regenbogen et al., "Anastomotic leak after colorectal resection: a population-based study of risk factors and hospital variation," *Surgery*, vol. 161, no. 6, pp. 1619–1627, 2017.

[4] C. C. M. Marres, A. W. H. van de Ven, L. G. J. Leijssen, P. C. M. Verbeek, W. A. Bemelman, and C. J. Buskens, "Colorectal anastomotic leak: delay in reintervention after false-negative computed tomography scan is a reason for concern," *Techniques in Coloproctology*, vol. 21, no. 9, pp. 709–714, 2017.

[5] C. Alexandra and A. Mironiuc, "Anastomotic leaks after colorectal surgery: a prognostic score," *Acta Medica Marisiensis*, vol. 60, no. 1, pp. 3–6, 2014.

[6] A. A. Khan, J. M. D. Wheeler, C. Cunningham, B. George, M. Kettlewell, and N. J. M. C. Mortensen, "The management and outcome of anastomotic leaks in colorectal surgery," *Colorectal Disease*, vol. 10, no. 6, pp. 587–592, 2008.

[7] M. C. Audett and I. M. Paquette, "Intraoperative and postoperative diagnosis of anastomotic leak following colorectal resection," *Seminars in Colon and Rectal Surgery*, vol. 25, no. 2, pp. 54–57, 2014.

[8] C. Platell, N. Barwood, G. Dorfmann, and G. Makin, "The incidence of anastomotic leaks in patients undergoing colorectal surgery," *Colorectal Disease*, vol. 9, no. 1, pp. 71–79, 2007.

[9] T. P. Kingham and H. L. Pachter, "Colonic anastomotic leak: risk factors, diagnosis, and treatment," *Journal of the American College of Surgeons*, vol. 208, no. 2, pp. 269–278, 2009.

60

Gallbladder Mucus Plug Mimicking Ascaris Worm: An Ambiguous cause of Biliary Colic

Salah Termos, Mohammad Alali, Majd Alkabbani, Abdullah AlDuwaisan, Ahmad Alsaleh, Khalifa Alyatama, and Hussein Hayati

Hepatobiliary and Transplant Unit, Department of Surgery, Al-Amiri Hospital, Kuwait City, Kuwait

Correspondence should be addressed to Salah Termos; salahtermos@gmail.com

Academic Editor: Gregorio Santori

Biliary colic is a visceral pain caused by attempts of the gallbladder or bile duct to overcome the obstruction in the cystic duct or ampulla of Vater. Obstruction can be due to different etiologies such as stone, mass, worm, and rarely by mucus plug. We report the case of a 31-year-old gentleman who presented with recurrent biliary colic and weight loss. Work-up showed linear calcifications in the gallbladder extending to the common bile duct suggesting hepatobiliary ascariasis. Further investigations including stool analysis, upper endoscopy, endoscopic ultrasonography (EUS), and endoscopic retrograde cholangiopancreatography (ERCP) did not support our provisional diagnosis. Laparoscopic cholecystectomy was performed. Histopathological finding was grossly ambiguous; a rope-like mucus plug resembling ascaris worm was noted. The patient's condition improved instantly after the procedure. To our knowledge, we are reporting the first case in the English literature describing this unique entity of symptomatic gallbladder disease to increase awareness and improve its management.

1. Introduction

Biliary colic is usually caused by the gallbladder contraction in response to hormonal or neural stimulation, forcing a stone or possibly sludge and rarely a worm or a mucus plug against the gallbladder outlet or cystic duct opening, leading to increased intravesicular pressure [1]. We describe an unusual cause of obstruction due to a mucus plug resembling a worm that was diagnosed and managed as biliary ascaris.

2. Case Presentation

In our manuscript, we report the case of a 31-year-old Syrian gentleman, who was previously healthy, presenting to the emergency room with repeated bouts of biliary colic. His pain was frequent, lasting for about two hours, and alleviated with pain killers and antispasmodics. The symptoms were exacerbated by heavy meals. He also reported a significant weight loss of 10 kilograms in two months. His vital signs and laboratory tests were all within the normal ranges. Ultrasound abdomen showed a contracted gallbladder with

intraluminal calcification. Initial work-up began with an enhanced computed tomography (CT) scan, which revealed linear dense calcifications within the gallbladder extending into the cystic duct to the junction of the common bile duct (Figure 1). Further investigations were conducted. Stool analysis did not detect any egg or parasite. Upper endoscopy and ERCP showed the absence of worms in the duodenum or inside the biliary tree, respectively. The patient did not note any family history of biliary cancers. Tumor markers were within the normal ranges, and MRCP showed a 3-line sign and was unremarkable for any other abnormalities (Figure 2). EUS elicited a hyperechoic calcified linear structure measuring 4×0.5 cm. We proceeded for laparoscopic cholecystectomy. Intraoperatively, the liver looked normal and the gallbladder appeared contracted with no sign of inflammation or malignancy. It was easily removed, and frozen section of the cystic duct was negative for any pathology.

Gallbladder gross examination was suggestive of a parasitic worm with some sludge (Figure 3). However, the definitive histopathological study revealed a chronic cholecystitis with

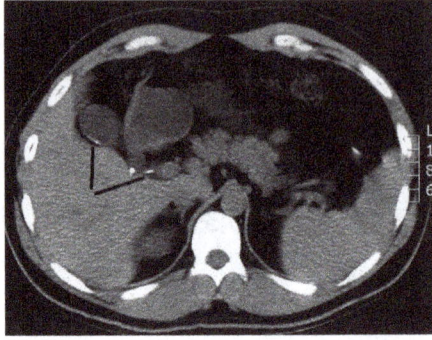

FIGURE 1: CT abdomen: linear calcification extending from the gallbladder through the cystic duct (dashes).

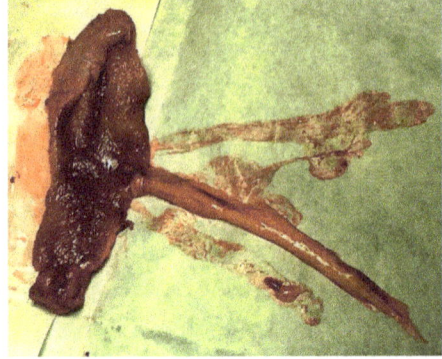

FIGURE 3: Gross specimen of the gallbladder with a mucus plug mimicking a worm.

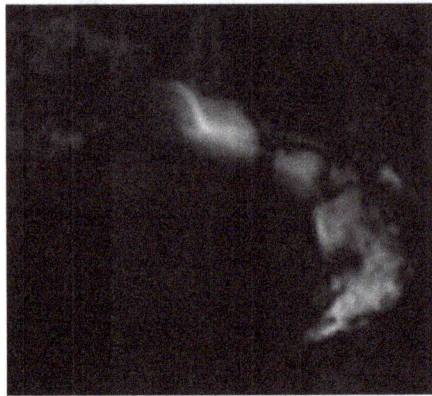

FIGURE 2: Magnetic resonance cholangiopancreatography (MRCP) demonstrating the 3-line sign typical for ascaris worm (arrow).

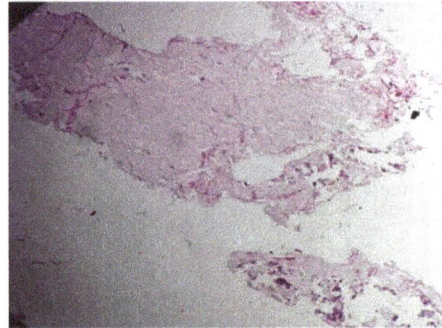

FIGURE 4: Microscopic examination of the tubular structure confirming a thick mucus content and absence of parasitic infestation.

thick mucus content and no evidence of a parasitic infection, worm, larva, or ova (Figure 4). The mucus plug in the gallbladder was seen wrapped in a tubular fashion mimicking ascaris. The patient had an uneventful postoperative hospital stay. He is currently asymptomatic on follow-up one year after his surgery and regained his weight.

3. Discussion

Biliary colic can present with different manifestations and due to many causes. Our patient is a young gentleman who suffered from typical colicky right upper quadrant pain, moderate in severity over a period of six months. It was associated with weight loss, which was likely due to fear of triggering the pain, and in part due to anxiety from the extensive work-up and the unusual etiology of his condition. Our differential diagnosis leant towards a parasitic disease based on results of his imaging studies. His stool analysis, however, was negative for any egg or helminth, and upper endoscopy did not show any sign of parasites or abnormalities.

Helminthic infestation occurs most commonly with *Ascaris lumbricoides*, *Clonorchis sinensis*, *Opisthorchis felineus*, and *Fasciola hepatica* [2]. Ascaris is a roundworm and is one of the most prevalent helminthic hepatobiliary parasites in humans worldwide. Fortunately, it only infrequently produces symptomatic disease. *Ascaris lumbricoides* normally reside in the jejunum but are actively motile and can invade the papilla

and thus migrate into the biliary system causing biliary obstruction with a variety of hepatobiliary complications. Biliary colic (56%), acute cholangitis (24%), acute cholecystitis (13%), acute pancreatitis (6%), and rarely hepatic abscess have all been reported as complications of this parasite [3].

Radiographic imaging of biliary ascariasis is usually pathognomonic. On ultrasound, we may find long, linear, parallel echogenic structures without acoustic shadowing or the presence of "four-line sign." Nonshadowing echogenic strips with a central anechoic tube representing the parasite's digestive tract, indicative of the worm and its intestines, may also be seen [4]. On CT scan, a nonenhancing coiled tubular structure of soft tissue density with specks of curvilinear disk-like lesion or linear calcification may be seen. In other situations, such ovoid lesions may represent a neoplasm in the absence of clinical suspicion of ascaris.

MR cholangiogram may show intraductal worms as a linear low-intensity filling defect in the bile ducts. The "three-line sign" appears to be a characteristic sign of biliary ascariasis on 3D magnetic resonance cholangiopancreatography (MRCP) [5]. ERCP is highly sensitive in detecting parasites in the biliary and pancreatic ducts. Worms can be seen in the duodenum and very often across the ampulla of Vater during endoscopy [6]. Cholangiographic findings of the ascaris worm during ERCP include long, smooth, linear filling defects with tapering ends as well as parallel, smooth filling defects, curves, and loops crossing the hepatic ducts transversely and dilation of the bile ducts (usually the common bile duct).

Our case is ambiguous due to the paucity of these radiological signs in such a common medical illness. It is well known that ill-defined lesions may simulate the presence of a neoplasm in the absence of clinical suspicion of ascaris. We investigated the patient thoroughly for malignancy using laboratory and radiological testing, in addition to intraoperative frozen section analysis which was also negative for malignancy. Our preoperative and postoperative diagnosis favored gallbladder ascariasis as the patient was from Syria, as the condition is endemic in this region [7]. However, the microscopic examination surprisingly excluded our provisional diagnosis.

According to the literature, similar conditions may occur if the cystic duct is atretic or stenotic due to inspissated mucus or mucosal hyperplasia. This usually leads to a contracted gallbladder with some sludge. Our patient denied any past antecedent of jaundice or family history of cystic fibrosis or any metabolic disease [8]. The mechanism of mucus secretion remains unclear, and the secretory granules in the chief cell of the gallbladder epithelium were microscopically observed to secrete mucus by a mechanism similar to that of merocrine secretion [9]. Mucus glycoprotein overproduction has been investigated as an important factor during the formation of gallbladder stones. Experimental results note that the increase in the cholesterol content of bile can stimulate gallbladder mucus hypersecretion [10].

The presence of thick mucus sludge in the gallbladder can be encountered in conditions associated with endocrine disorders, such as hypothyroidism, and in mucoceles. A mucocele refers to an overdistended gallbladder filled with mucoid fluid. It results from outlet obstruction of the gallbladder in the neck of the gallbladder or in the cystic duct [11]. Roundworms can cause this due to bile duct obstruction; however, our case presented with a clinical picture of acute on the top of chronic cholecystitis with no evidence of parasitic infection or mucocele. A mucus plug etiology in a case such as ours is unusual. It is known that mucus formation can be a result of lithogenic bile, and it is associated with biliary sludge. In a literature review, we did not find any similar condition that had been described in the past. Presence of contracted gallbladder and absence of plentiful Rokitansky–Aschoff sinuses preclude the diagnosis of mucocele [12].

4. Conclusion

Biliary colic is a common clinical manifestation that occurs due to various causes. Linear ground-glass opacification inside the gallbladder usually indicates hepatobiliary ascariasis. Absence of objective findings may suggest different pathologies. A rope-like mucus plug in our case was a unique entity, presented with symptomatic biliary colic with a picture resembling a parasitic worm.

Acknowledgments

Special thanks are due to Dr. Ayman Adi, Department of Histopathology, Al-Amiri Hospital, for his great efforts in sorting out the diagnosis.

References

[1] A. K. Diehl, N. J. Sugarek, and K. H. Todd, "Clinical evaluation for gallstone disease: usefulness of symptoms and signs in diagnosis," *American Journal of Medicine*, vol. 89, no. 1, pp. 29–33, 1990.

[2] A. E. Yellin and A. J. Donovan, "Biliary lithiasis and helminthiasis," *American Journal of Surgery*, vol. 142, no. 1, pp. 128–136, 1981.

[3] M. S. Khuroo, S. A. Zargar, and R. Mahajan, "Hepatobiliary and pancreatic ascariasis in India," *Lancet*, vol. 335, no. 8704, pp. 1503–1506, 1990.

[4] M. S. Khuroo, S. A. Zargar, R. Mahajan, R. L. Bhat, and G. Javid, "Sonographic appearances in biliary ascariasis," *Gastroenterology*, vol. 93, no. 2, pp. 267–272, 1987.

[5] Z. X. Ding, J. H. Yuan, V. Chong, D. J. Zhao, F. H. Chen, and Y. M. Li, "3 T MR cholangiopancreatography appearances of biliary ascariasis," *Clinical Radiology*, vol. 66, no. 3, pp. 275–277, 2011.

[6] B. Mijandrusić-Sincić, D. Štimac, B. Kezele, D. Miletić, N. Brnčić, and G. Poropat, "Acute pancreatitis caused by *Ascaris lumbricoides*: a case report," *Gastrointestinal Endoscopy*, vol. 67, no. 3, pp. 541-542, 2008.

[7] F. Sandouk, S. Haffar, M. M. Zada, D. Y. Graham, and B. S. Anand, "Pancreatic-biliary ascariasis: experience of 300 cases," *American Journal of Gastroenterology*, vol. 92, no. 12, pp. 2264–2267, 1997.

[8] E. Gilbert-Barness, L. A. Barness, and P. M. Farrell, *Metabolic Disease, Foundation of Clinical Management, Genetics and Pathology*, p. 527, IOS Press BV, Amsterdam, Netherlands, 2nd edition, 2017.

[9] S. P. Lee, "The mechanism of mucus secretion by the gallbladder epithelium," *British Journal of Experimental Pathology*, vol. 61, no. 2, pp. 117–119, 1980.

[10] S. P. Lee, J. T. LaMont, and M. C. Carey, "Role of gallbladder mucus hypersecretion in the evolution of cholesterol gallstones," *Journal of Clinical Investigation*, vol. 67, no. 6, pp. 1712–1723, 1981.

[11] S. Agrawal and S. Jonnalagadda, "Gallstones, from gallbladder to gut. Management options for diverse complications," *Postgraduate Medicine*, vol. 108, no. 3, pp. 143–153, 2000.

[12] I. Damjanov and J. Linder, "Diseases of the digestive system: gallbladder and extrahepatic ducts," in *Anderson's Pathology*, vol. 2, Mosby-Year Book, St. Louis, MO, USA, 10th edition, 1996.

Permissions

All chapters in this book were first published in CRS, by Hindawi Publishing Corporation; hereby published with permission under the Creative Commons Attribution License or equivalent. Every chapter published in this book has been scrutinized by our experts. Their significance has been extensively debated. The topics covered herein carry significant findings which will fuel the growth of the discipline. They may even be implemented as practical applications or may be referred to as a beginning point for another development.

The contributors of this book come from diverse backgrounds, making this book a truly international effort. This book will bring forth new frontiers with its revolutionizing research information and detailed analysis of the nascent developments around the world.

We would like to thank all the contributing authors for lending their expertise to make the book truly unique. They have played a crucial role in the development of this book. Without their invaluable contributions this book wouldn't have been possible. They have made vital efforts to compile up to date information on the varied aspects of this subject to make this book a valuable addition to the collection of many professionals and students.

This book was conceptualized with the vision of imparting up-to-date information and advanced data in this field. To ensure the same, a matchless editorial board was set up. Every individual on the board went through rigorous rounds of assessment to prove their worth. After which they invested a large part of their time researching and compiling the most relevant data for our readers.

The editorial board has been involved in producing this book since its inception. They have spent rigorous hours researching and exploring the diverse topics which have resulted in the successful publishing of this book. They have passed on their knowledge of decades through this book. To expedite this challenging task, the publisher supported the team at every step. A small team of assistant editors was also appointed to further simplify the editing procedure and attain best results for the readers.

Apart from the editorial board, the designing team has also invested a significant amount of their time in understanding the subject and creating the most relevant covers. They scrutinized every image to scout for the most suitable representation of the subject and create an appropriate cover for the book.

The publishing team has been an ardent support to the editorial, designing and production team. Their endless efforts to recruit the best for this project, has resulted in the accomplishment of this book. They are a veteran in the field of academics and their pool of knowledge is as vast as their experience in printing. Their expertise and guidance has proved useful at every step. Their uncompromising quality standards have made this book an exceptional effort. Their encouragement from time to time has been an inspiration for everyone.

The publisher and the editorial board hope that this book will prove to be a valuable piece of knowledge for researchers, students, practitioners and scholars across the globe.

List of Contributors

Laura F. Tait
Howard University College of Medicine, Washington, DC 20059, USA

Gezzer Ortega, Daniel D. Tran and Terrence M. Fullum
Division of Bariatric and Minimally Invasive Surgery, Howard University Hospital, Washington, DC 20060, USA

Daniela Berritto, Francesca Iacobellis, Francesca Iasiello, Nunzia Luisa Pizza and Roberto Grassi
Depatment of Radiology, Second University of Naples, P.za Miraglia 2, 80138 Napoli, Italy

Raffaello Crincoli
Depatment of Radiology, Ospedale Landofi ASL, Solofra Indirizzo, Via Melito, 83029 Solofra, Italy

Francesco Lassandro
Depatment of Radiology, Azienda ospedaliera "V. MONALDI," Via Leonardo Bianchi, 80131 Napoli, Italy

Lanfranco Musto
Depatment of Radiology, Ospedale Criscuoli. Via Quadrivio, Sant'Angelo dei Lombardi, 83054 Avellino, Italy

Beth-Ann Shanker and Oliver S. Eng
Department of Surgery, Rutgers-RobertWood Johnson Medical School, New Brunswick, NJ 08903, USA

Vyacheslav Gendel and John Nosher
Division of Interventional Radiology, Department of Radiology, Rutgers-RobertWood Johnson Medical School, New Brunswick, NJ 08903, USA

Darren R. Carpizo
Division of Surgical Oncology, Department of Surgery, Rutgers Cancer Institute of New Jersey, Rutgers-RobertWood Johnson Medical School, New Brunswick, NJ 08903, USA

Ibrahim Uygun, Selcuk Otcu, Bahattin Aydogdu, Mehmet Hanifi Okur and Mehmet Serif Arslan
Department of Pediatric Surgery, Medical Faculty of Dicle University, 21280 Diyarbakir, Turkey

Lior Menasherian-Yaccobe, Nathan T. Jaqua and Patrick Kenny
Department of Internal Medicine, Tripler Army Medical Center, 1 JarrettWhite Road, Honolulu, HI 96859, USA

Patrick Kenny
Gastroenterology Service, Tripler Army Medical Center, USA

Omar Bellorin, Alexander Ramirez-Valderrama and Armando Castro
Department of General Surgery, New York Hospital Medical Center of Queens/Weill Cornell Medical College, 5645 Main Street, Flushing, NY 11355, USA

Anna Kundel
Department of Endocrine Surgery, New York University Langone Medical Center, 550 First Avenue, New York, NY 10016, USA

Yoko Yamamoto and Ken Kodama
Department of Thoracic Surgery, Yao Municipal Hospital, Yao City, Osaka 581-0069, Japan

Shigekazu Yokoyama
Department of Gastroenterological Surgery, Yao Municipal Hospital, Yao City, Osaka 581-0069, Japan

Masashi Takeda
Department of Pathology, Yao Municipal Hospital, Yao City, Osaka 581-0069, Japan

Shintaro Michishita
Department of Breast and Endocrine Surgery, Osaka University, Osaka 565-0871, Japan

Vinay Rai, Akin Beckley and Charles F. Bellows
Department of Surgery, University of New Mexico, Albuquerque, NM 87131, USA

Anna Fabre
Department of Radiology, University of New Mexico, Albuquerque, NM 87131, USA

Mesut Sipahi, Kasim Caglayan, Ergin Arslan and Faruk Onder Aytekin
Department of General Surgery, School of Medicine, Bozok University, 66100 Yozgat, Turkey

Mustafa Fatih Erkoc
Department of Radiology, School of Medicine, Bozok University, 66100 Yozgat, Turkey

Tahsin Colak, Tolga Olmez, Ozgur Turkmenoglu and Ahmet Dag
Department of General Surgery, Medical Faculty, Mersin University, 33079 Mersin, Turkey

Yavuz Savas Koca and Mustafa Tevfik Bülbül
Department of General Surgery, School of Medicine, Suleyman Demirel University, 32200 Isparta, Turkey

Bünyamin AydJn and Mehmet Numan Tamer
Division of Endocrinology and Metabolism, Department of Internal Medicine, School of Medicine, Suleyman Demirel University, 32200 Isparta, Turkey

Tugba Koca
Department of Pediatric Gastroenterology, Hepatology and Nutrition, School of Medicine, Suleyman Demirel University, 32200 Isparta, Turkey

Evgeni Brotfain, Leonid Koyfman, Amit Frenkel, Jochanan G. Peiser, Abraham Borer, Benjamin F. Gruenbaum, Alexander Zlotnik and Moti Klein
Department of Anesthesiology and Critical Care, Soroka Medical Center, Ben-Gurion University of the Negev, 84105 Beer Sheva, Israel

Kodai Tomioka and Masahiko Murakami
Department of Gastroenterological and General Surgery, Showa University Hospital, 1-5-8 Hatanodai, Shinagawa, Tokyo 142-8666, Japan

Kodai Tomioka, Hitoshi Ojima, Makoto Sohda, Akiko Tanabe, Yasuyuki Fukai, Akihiko Sano and Takahiro Fukuda
Department of Gastroenterological Surgery, Gunma Prefectural Cancer Center, 617-1 Takabayashi-Nishi, Ota, Gunma 373-8550, Japan

Ali H. Zakaria and Salam Daradkeh
Istishari Hospital, The University of Jordan, P.O. Box 13261, Amman 11942, Jordan

Alfin Okullo and Ghiyath Alsnih
Department of Surgery, Blacktown-MtDruittHospital, Blacktown Road, Blacktown, Sydney, NSW2148, Australia

Titus Kwok
Department of Surgery, Concord Repatriation and General Hospital, Hospital Road, Concord, Sydney, NSW2139, Australia

Yoshinori Handa, Mikihiro Kano and Naoki Hirabayashi
Department of Surgery, Hiroshima City Asa Hospital, 2-1-1 Kabeminami, Asakita-ku, Hiroshima 731-0293, Japan

Mayumi Kaneko
Department of Pathology, Hiroshima City Asa Hospital, 2-1-1 Kabeminami, Asakita-ku, Hiroshima 731-0293, Japan

Metin Ertem, Emel Ozveri, Hakan Gok and Volkan Ozben
General Surgery Clinic, Kozyatagi Acibadem Hospital, 34742 Istanbul, Turkey

Metin Ertem
Department of General Surgery, Cerrahpasa Medical Faculty, Istanbul University, Cerrahpasa, Fatih, 34098 Istanbul, Turkey

Sheraz Yaqub, Øystein Mathisen, Bjørn Edwin and Knut Jørgen Labori
Department of Hepato-Pancreato-Biliary Surgery, Oslo University Hospital, Sognsvannsveien 20, 0317 Oslo, Norway

Tom Mala
Department of Gastrointestinal Surgery, Oslo University Hospital, Sognsvannsveien 20, 0317 Oslo, Norway

Bjarte Fosby
Department of Transplantation Surgery, Oslo University Hospital, Sognsvannsveien 20, 0317 Oslo, Norway

Dag Tallak Kjærsdalen Berntzen and Andreas Abildgaard
Department of Radiology, Oslo University Hospital, Sognsvannsveien 20, 0317 Oslo, Norway

Caroline C. Jadlowiec, Beata E. Lobel, Namita Akolkar, Michael D. Bourque and David W. McFadden
University of Connecticut General Surgery Residency Program, Farmington, CT 06030, USA

Michael D. Bourque
Connecticut Children's Medical Center, Department of Pediatric Surgery, Hartford, CT 06106, USA

Thomas J. Devers
University of Connecticut Health Center, Division of Gastroenterology, Farmington, CT 06030, USA

David W. McFadden
Department of Surgery, University of Connecticut Health Center, Farmington, CT 06030, USA

Heshmatollah Salahi
Transplant Research Center, Shiraz University of Medical Sciences, Shiraz, Iran

Mehdi Tahamtan
Colorectal Research Center, Shiraz University of Medical Sciences, Shiraz, Iran

Bijan Ziaian
Department ofThoracic Surgery, Shiraz University of Medical Sciences, Shiraz, Iran

Mansoor Masjedi
Department of Anesthesiology, Shiraz University of Medical Sciences, Shiraz, Iran

Zahra Saadati and Nazanin Hoseini
Shiraz University of Medical Sciences, Shiraz, Iran

Elahe Torabi
Department of Internal Medicine, Shiraz University of Medical Sciences, Shiraz, Iran

Nadim Al Hajjar, Calin Popa and Florin Graur
Department of Surgery, Regional Institute of Gastroenterology and Hepatology "Prof. Dr. Octavian Fodor", Croitorilor Street, No. 19-21, 400162 Cluj-Napoca, Romania

Nadim Al Hajjar
3rd Surgical Clinic, Iuliu Hatieganu University of Medicine and Pharmacy, Croitorilor Street, No. 19-21, 400162Cluj-Napoca, Romania

Calin Popa and Tareg Al-Momani
Training and Research Center "Prof. Dr. Sergiu Duca", Petre Ispirescu Street, No. 1, 400090 Cluj-Napoca, Romania

Tareg Al-Momani
Department of Oncological Surgery, The Oncology Institute "Prof. Dr. Ion Chiricuța" Republicii Street, No. 34-36, 400015 Cluj-Napoca, Romania

Simona Margarit
Department of Intensive Care Unit, Regional Institute of Gastroenterology and Hepatology "Prof. Dr. Octavian Fodor", Croitorilor Street, No. 19-21, 400162 Cluj-Napoca, Romania
1st Anesthesiology and Critical Care Clinic, Iuliu Hatieganu University of Medicine and Pharmacy, Croitorilor Street, No. 19-21, 400162 Cluj-Napoca, Romania

Marcel Tantau
Department of Gastroenterology, Regional Institute of Gastroenterology and Hepatology "Prof.Dr.Octavian Fodor", Croitorilor Street, No. 19-21, 400162 Cluj-Napoca, Romania
3rd Medical Clinic, Iuliu Hatieganu University of Medicine and Pharmacy, Croitorilor Street, No. 19-21, 400162Cluj-Napoca, Romania

Federico Sista, Valentina Abruzzese, Mario Schietroma and Gianfranco Amicucci
Dipartimento di Scienze Cliniche Applicate e Biotecnologie, Università degli Studi di L'Aquila, 67100 Coppito, Italy

Hideki Katagiri, Shozo Kunizaki, Mayu Shimaguchi, Yasuo Yoshinaga, Yukihiro Kanda and Ken Mizokami
Department of Surgery, Tokyo Bay Urayasu Ichikawa Medical Center (Noguchi Hideyo Memorial International Hospital), 3-4-34 Todaijima, Urayasu, Chiba 279-0001, Japan

Alan T. Lefor
Department of Surgery, Jichi Medical University, 1-3311 Yakushiji, Shimotsuke, Tochigi 329-0498, Japan

Osama Shaheen, Samer Sara, Mhd Firas Safadi and Bayan Alsaid
Department of Surgery, Almouwasat University Hospital, Damascus, Syria

Bayan Alsaid
Laboratory of Anatomy, Faculty of Medicine, University of Damascus, Damascus, Syria

Charalampos G. Markakis, Eleftherios D. Spartalis, Emmanouil Liarmakopoulos and Periklis Tomos
Second Department of Propedeutic Surgery, University of Athens, Medical School, "Laiko" General Hospital, AgiouThoma 17, 11527 Athens, Greece

Evangelia G. Kavoura
First Department of Pathology, University of Athens, Medical School, 11527 Athens, Greece

David G. Darcy, Ali H. Charafeddine, Jenny Choi and Diego Camacho
Department of Surgery, Montefiore Medical Center, New York, NY 10467, USA

Michael Donaire, James Mariadason, Daniel Stephens, Sitaram Pillarisetty and Marc K. Wallack
Department of Surgery, Metropolitan Hospital, New York Medical College, USA

Clara Kimie Miyahira, Jéssyca Fernanda de Lima Farto, Annelise de Figueiredo Calili and Nathalia Rabello da Silva Sousa
São José do Rio Preto Medical School, São José do Rio Preto, SP, Brazil

Miguel Bonfitto
Hospital de Base de São José do Rio Preto, São José do Rio Preto, SP, Brazil

Ana Paula de Figueiredo Calili
Marília Medical School, Marília, SP, Brazil

Haijing Zhang and Todd V. Brennan
Department of Surgery, Duke University Medical Center, Durham, NC 27710, USA

Stephanie L. Jun
Department of Radiology, University of California San Francisco, San Francisco, CA 94122, USA

M. Uittenbogaart, M. N. Sosef and J. van Bastelaar
Department of Surgery, Atrium Medical Centre, Henri Dunantstraat 5, 6419 PC Heerlen, The Netherlands

C. Spitali, K. De Vogelaere and G. Delvaux
UZ Brussel, Brussels 1090, Belgium

Zijah Rifatbegovic, Zlatan Mehmedovic, Jasmin Hasanovic and Amra Mestric
Department of General Abdominal Surgery, Clinic for Surgery, University Clinical Center Tuzla, Tuzla, Bosnia and Herzegovina

Majda Mehmedovic
Department of Gastroenterology and Hepatology, Clinic for Internal Diseases, University Clinical Center Tuzla, Tuzla, Bosnia and Herzegovina

Constantinos Nastos, Dimitrios Giannoulopoulos, Dionysios Dellaportas, Ioannis Papaconstantinou, Theodosios Theodosopoulos and Georgios Polymeneas
Second Department of Surgery, National and Kapodistrian University of Athens, School of Medicine, Aretaieion University Hospital, Athens, Greece

Ioannis Georgopoulos
First Department of Pediatric Surgery, National and Kapodistrian University of Athens, School of Medicine, Agia So$a University Hospital, Athens, Greece

Christos Salakos
Department of Pediatric Surgery, National and Kapodistrian University of Athens, School of Medicine, Attikon University Hospital, Athens, Greece

Abdalla Mohamed, Jamshed Zuberi and Tanuja Damani
Department of Medicine, St. Joseph's University Medical Center, Paterson, NJ, USA

Youssef Botros and Walid Baddoura
Division of Gastroenterology and Hepatology, St. Joseph's University Medical Center, Paterson, NJ, USA

Paul Hanna and Sang Lee
Department of Surgery, St. Joseph's University Medical Center, Paterson, NJ, USA

Joseph Gutowski
Rutgers Robert Wood Johnson Medical School, Piscataway Township, NJ 08854, USA

Rachel NeMoyer
Rutgers Robert Wood Johnson Medical School, New Brunswick, NJ 08901, USA

Glenn S. Parker
Jersey Shore University Medical Center, Neptune City, NJ 07753, USA

Jad A. Degheili, Mohammed H. Abdallah, Ahmad Moukalled and Ali H. Hallal
Division of General Surgery, Department of Surgery, American University of Beirut Medical Center, Riad El-Solh, Beirut 1107 2020, Lebanon

Ali A. Haydar
Division of Interventional Radiology, Department of Diagnostic Radiology, American University of Beirut Medical Center, Riad El-Solh, Beirut 1107 2020, Lebanon

Chalerm Eurboonyanun, Somchai Ruangwannasak and Anan Sripanaskul
Department of Surgery, Faculty of Medicine, Khon Kaen University, Khon Kaen 40002, Thailand

Kulyada Somsap
Department of Radiology, Faculty of Medicine, Khon Kaen University, Khon Kaen 40002, Thailand

Mauro Podda, Jenny Atzeni, Antonio Messina Campanella, Alessandra Saba and Adolfo Pisanu
Department of Surgical Science, General, Emergency and Laparoscopic Surgery, University of Cagliari, Blocco G, 09042 Monserrato, Italy

Khuram Khan, Saqib Saeed, Haytham Maria, Mohammed Sbeih, Alexius Ramcharan and Brian Donaldson
Department of Surgery, Harlem Hospital Center, Columbia University, New York, NY, USA

Farhana Iqbal
Department of Medicine, Richmond University Medical Center, Staten Island, New York, NY, USA

Hideki Katagiri, Kana Tahara, Kentaro Yoshikawa, Tadao Kubota and Ken Mizokami
Department of Surgery, Tokyo Bay Urayasu Ichikawa Medical Center, 3-4-32 Todaijima, Urayasu, Chiba 279-0001, Japan

Alan Kawarai Lefor
Department of Surgery, Jichi Medical University, 1-3311 Yakushiji, Shimotsuke, Tochigi Prefecture 329-0498, Japan

Krish Kulendran, Kay Tai Choy, Cian Keogh and Dinesh Ratnapala
Cairns Hospital, Cairns, QLD, Australia
Ipswich Hospital, Ipswich, QLD, Australia

Tiziana Casiraghi
Azienda Socio-Sanitaria di Vimercate, Presidio di Carate, Via Mos`e Bianchi 9, 20841 Carate Brianza, Italy

Alessandro Masetto
Azienda Socio-Sanitaria di Vimercate, Presidio di Vimercate, Via Santi Cosma e Damiano 10, 20871 Vimercate, Italy

Massimo Beltramo, Mauro Girlando and Camillo Di Bella
Azienda Ospedaliera di Desio e Vimercate, Presidio di Carate, Via Mosè Bianchi 9, 20841 Carate Brianza, Italy

Holly Mulinder, Allison Ammann, Yana Puckett and Sharmila Dissanaike
Department of General Surgery, School of Medicine, Texas Tech University, Lubbock, TX 79409, USA

Christos Plataras, Efstratios Christianakis, Dimitrios Bourikas and Khalil Eirekat
Pediatric Surgery Department, Penteli Children's Hospital, Ippokratous 8, Penteli 15236, Greece

Florentia Fostira
Department of Genetics, Demokritos Research Center, Neapoleos 10, Agia Paraskevi 153 10, Greece

George Bourikis
General Surgery Department, Tzanio General Hospital, Leoforos Afentouli ke Zanni, Piraeus 185 36, Greece

Maria Chorti
Histopathology Department, Sismanoglio General Hospital, Sismanogliou 37, Marousi 151 26, Greece

Nikolaos Fotopoulos
General Surgery Department, Sismanoglio General Hospital, Sismanogliou 37, Marousi 15126, Greece

Konstantinos Damalas
General Surgery Department, Agios Savvas Regional Cancer Hospital, Leof. Alexandras 171, Athens 11522, Greece

Asem Ghanim, Joseph Martinez, Melanie S. Morris and John R. Porterfield
Department of Surgery, University of Alabama at Birmingham, Birmingham, AL, USA

Benjamin Smood
School of Medicine, University of Alabama at Birmingham, Birmingham, AL, USA

Francesca D'Auria and Vincenzo Consalvo
General Surgery, Università degli Studi di Salerno, Via Giovanni Paolo II, 132, 84084 Fisciano, Italy

Vincenzo Consalvo
Clinique Clementville, rue de Clementville, Montpellier, France

Antonio Canero, Maria Russo, Carmela Rescigno and Domenico Lombardi
Azienda Ospedaliera Universitaria San Giovanni di Dio e Ruggi d'Aragona, Via San Leonardo, 1, Salerno, Italy

Dionysios Dellaportas, James A. Gossage and Andrew R. Davies
Department of Oesophagogastric Surgery, St Thomas' Hospital, King's College London, London, UK

Gael Kuhn, Jean Bruno Lekeufack, Michael Chilcott and Zacharia Mbaidjol
Hôpital Fribourgeois Riaz, Rue de l'Hôpital 9, Case Postale 70, Riaz, 1632 Fribourg, Switzerland

Jayan George, Michael Peirson, Samuel Birks and Paul Skinner
Department of General Surgery, Northern General Hospital, Herries Road, Sheffield S5 7AU, UK

Apiradee Pichaichanlert and Vor Luvira
Department of Surgery, Faculty of Medicine, Khon Kaen University, Khon Kaen, Thailand

Nakhon Tipsunthonsak
Surgery Unit, Khon Kaen Hospital, Khon Kaen, Thailand

Surasak Puvabanditsin, Marissa Botwinick, Charlotte Wang Chen, Aditya Joshi and Rajeev Mehta
Department of Pediatrics, Rutgers Robert Wood Johnson Medical School, One Robert Wood Johnson Place, New Brunswick, NJ 08903, USA

Houssam Khodor Abtar, Mostapha Mneimneh, MazenM. Hammoud and Ahmed Zaaroura
Makassed General Hospital, Department of Surgery, Beirut, Lebanon

Yasmina S. Papas
Saint George Hospital University Medical Center, Department of Surgery, Beirut, Lebanon

Jun-ichiro Harada, Takeshi Matsutani, Nobutoshi Hagiwara, Yoichi Kawano, Akihisa Matsuda, Nobuhiko Taniai, Tsutomu Nomura and Eiji Uchida
Department of Gastrointestinal and Hepato-Biliary-Pancreatic Surgery, Nippon Medical School, 1-1-5 Sendagi, Bunkyo-ku, Tokyo 113-8603, Japan

Benjamin Momo Kadia
Foumbot District Hospital, Foumbot, Cameroon

Benjamin Momo Kadia and Martin Hongieh Abanda
Grace Community Health and Development Association, Kumba, Cameroon

Desmond Aroke, Tsi Njim and Christian Akem Dimala
Health and Human Development (2HD) Research Network, Douala, Cameroon

Desmond Aroke
Mbengwi District Hospital, Mbengwi, Cameroon

Martin Hongieh Abanda
Non-Communicable Disease Unit, Clinical Research Education, Networking and Consultancy (CRENC), Douala, Cameroon

Martin Hongieh Abanda
Bafang District Hospital, Bafang, Cameroon

Tsi Njim
Centre for Tropical Medicine and Global Health, Nu0eld Department of Medicine, University of Oxford, Oxford, UK

Christian Akem Dimala
Faculty of Epidemiology and Population Health, London School of Hygiene and Tropical Medicine, London, UK
Department of Orthopaedics, Southend University Hospital, Essex, UK

Keisuke Nonoyama, Hidehiko Kitagami, Akira Yasuda, Shiro Fujihata, Minoru Yamamoto, Yasunobu Shimizu and Moritsugu Tanaka
Department of Gastroenterological Surgery, Kariya Toyota General Hospital, Kariya, Japan

Kensuke Nakatani, Takaharu Kato, Shinichiro Okada, Risa Matsumoto, Kazuhiro Nishida, Hiroyasu Komuro and Toshiyuki Suganuma
Department of Surgery, Yokosuka General Hospital Uwamachi, 2-36 Uwamachi Yokosuka City, Kanagawa 238-8567, Japan

Takaharu Kato
Department of Surgery, SaitamaMedical Center, JichiMedical University, 1-847 Amanuma-cho, Omiya-ku, Saitama 330-8503, Japan

Maki Iida and Shiro Tsujimoto
Department of Pathology, Yokosuka General Hospital Uwamachi, 2-36 Uwamachi, Yokosuka, Kanagawa 238-8567, Japan

Andrew W. Wang
Department of Surgery, Naval Medical Center San Diego, San Diego, CA 92134, USA

Kimberly Newton
Division of Pediatric Gastroenterology, Hepatology, and Nutrition, Rady Children's Hospital, San Diego, CA 92123, USA
Department of Pediatrics, School of Medicine, University of California, La Jolla, San Diego, CA 92093, USA

Karen Kling
Department of Surgery, School of Medicine, University of California San Diego, La Jolla, San Diego, CA 92093, USA
Division of Pediatric Surgery, Rady Children's Hospital, San Diego, CA 92123, USA

Maria Francesca Secchi and Mauro Podda
Department of Emergency and Acute Care Medicine, San Francesco Hospital, Nuoro, Italy

Carlo Torre
Department of Gastrointestinal Endoscopy, San Francesco Hospital, Nuoro, Italy

Giovanni Dui
Department of Radiology, San Francesco Hospital, Nuoro, Italy

Francesco Virdis
Department of Trauma and Emergency Surgery, King's College Hospital, London, UK

Mauro Podda
Department of General, Emergency, and Robotic Surgery, San Francesco Hospital, Nuoro, Italy

Anthony Nagib
Nova Southeastern University, College of Osteopathic Medicine, 3301 College Avenue, Fort Lauderdale, FL 33314, USA

Chauniqua Kiffin, Eddy H. Carrillo, Andrew A. Rosenthal and Dafney L. Davare
Memorial Regional Hospital, Division of Acute Care Surgery and Trauma, 3501 Johnson Street, Hollywood, FL 33021, USA

Rachele J. Solomon
Memorial Regional Hospital, Office of Human Research, 4411 Sheridan Street, Hollywood, FL 33021, USA

Salah Termos, Mohammad Alali, Majd Alkabbani, Abdullah AlDuwaisan, Ahmad Alsaleh, Khalifa Alyatama and Hussein Hayati
Hepatobiliary and Transplant Unit, Department of Surgery, Al-Amiri Hospital, Kuwait City, Kuwait

Index

www.ingramcontent.com/pod-product-compliance
Lightning Source LLC
Chambersburg PA
CBHW080507200326

41458CB00012B/4118